Quality of life for people with disabilities

Models, research and practice

Edited by

Roy I Brown

Professor, School of Special Education and Disability Studies,
Flinders University of South Australia, Australia

Professor Emeritus, Rehabilitation Studies Programme,
Department of Educational Psychology, University of Calgary, Canada

Second Edition

Stanley Thornes (Publishers) Ltd

First published as *Quality of Life for Handicapped People*
First edition published by Chapman & Hall in 1988
(ISBN 0 412 70900 7)

Second edition under new title published in 1997 by:
Stanley Thornes (Publishers) Ltd
Ellenborough House
Wellington Street
CHELTENHAM
GL50 1YW
United Kingdom

97 98 99 00 01 / 10 9 8 7 6 5 4 3 2 1

A catalogue record for this book is available from the British
Library

ISBN 0–7487–3294–2

Typeset by Columns Design Limited of Reading
Printed and bound in Great Britain by TJ International,
Padstow, Cornwall

Contents

Acknowledgements

I was delighted when the publishers approached me regarding a new edition of *Quality of Life for Handicapped People*, first published in 1988. In the event, because of major developments that have taken place in quality of life, the new edition needed more than an update. A wide range of information was available and new chapters were required, along with substantial updating of existing material.

The present authors have produced an interesting array of chapters. I would like to thank them for their commitment to this work and also for taking into account the recommendations that were raised during the editorial stage. I am also appreciative of the helpful comments passed on to us by the external reviewer. I believe these recommendations have helped to make the book more accessible. I have had an opportunity to discuss the issues of quality of life with many of the authors throughout the development of the book and have appreciated their supportive and encouraging comments.

I would like to thank Mary Brown for reading several drafts and, particularly, for her commentary on Chapter 1. In carrying out the review process, a number of postgraduate students have read the material and to them, I wish to pass on thanks for they identified a number of errors. Vicky Duffield helped with the author index and Sharon Cock typed the extensive changes that have been made to Chapter 1. I am particularly grateful to Jenny Loveder for carrying out the detailed word processing for the final copy, to Amanda Kitson for typing the indices and I also acknowledge Flinders University of South Australia for financial support for this part of the development.

I would like to thank Sally Champion for her advice, patience and support during the development of this work and finally, thanks are due to Stanley Thornes for completing the publication of the book.

R.I.B.
1996

Contributors

Hilary Brown, Professor, School of Health and Social Welfare, Open University, Walton Hall, Milton Keynes, Bucks MK6 7AA, UK

Roy I Brown, Professor and Dean, School of Special Education and Disability Studies, Flinders University of South Australia, Box 2100 GPO, Adelaide, South Australia 5001, Australia

Robert A Cummins, Reader in Psychology, Faculty of Health and Behavioural Science, Deakin University, Burwood Campus, 221 Burwood Highway, Melbourne, Victoria 3125, Australia

Michelle Donelly, Lecturer, School of Occupational Therapy, Cumberland College of Health Sciences, University of Sydney, Sydney, New South Wales, Australia 2006

David Felce, Professor of Research in Learning Disabilities, Welsh Centre for Learning Disabilities, Applied Research Unit, Meridian Court, North Road, Cardiff CF4 3BL, Wales, UK

Roy V Ferguson, School of Child and Youth Care, University of Victoria, PO Box 1700, Victoria, BC V8W 2Y2, Canada

David Goode, Professor of Sociology, Co-ordinator, Program in Developmental Disabilities, PSA Department, College of Staten Island, Staten Island, New York 10301, USA

James Hogg, Professor and Director, White Top Research Unit, Department of Social Work, University of Dundee, Frankland Building, Dundee DD1 4HN, Scotland

Loretto Lamb, Projects Director, Profound and Multiple Impairment Service, White Top Research Unit, University of Dundee, Scotland

Patrick McGinley, Director of Psychological Services, Brothers of Charity, Woodlands Centre, Renmore, Galway, Ireland

David Mitchell, Professor and Director of International Programmes, School of Education, University of Waikato, Private Bag 3105, Hamilton, New Zealand

Aldred H Neufeldt, Associate Professor, Rehabilitation Studies, Department of Educational Psychology, University of Calgary, 413 Education Tower, 2500 University Drive NW, Calgary, Alberta, Canada T2N 1N4

Trevor R Parmenter, Professor, Centre for Developmental Disability Studies, Faculty of Medicine, the University of Sydney, PO Box 6, Ryde, New South Wales 2109, Australia

Jonathan Perry, Welsh Centre for Learning Disabilities Applied Research Unit, Meridian Court, North Road, Cardiff CF4 3BL, UK

Dimity Peter, Lecturer, School of Special Education and Disability Studies, Flinders University of South Australia, Box 2100 GPO, Adelaide, South Australia 5001, Australia

Robert L Schalock, Professor and Chair, Department of Psychology, Hastings College, Hastings, Nebraska 68962–0269, USA

Vianne Timmons, Associate Professor and Dean, Faculty of Education, University of Prince Edward Island, C1A 4P3, Canada

Beth P Velde, Associate Professor, Department of Occupational Therapy, College Misericordia, Dallas, Pennsylvania, USA

Bernie Warren, Professor, School of Dramatic Art, University of Windsor, 401 Sunset, Windsor, Ontario N9B 3P4, Canada

John Winslade, Senior Lecturer in Education, Department of Education Studies, University of Waikato, Private Bag 3105, Hamilton, New Zealand

Foreword

Around the middle of this century we were employed in a Dickensian institution for 'mental defectives', compulsorily detained under the archaic 1913 Mental Deficiency Act. The population we served ranged from the more severely retarded to large numbers of disadvantaged, mildly retarded or merely educationally backward adolescents and young adults whose lives had been marred by wartime disruption, neglect or cruelty within chaotic families. Now legally certified, they had come to the end of the road.

Roy Brown joined our team in the late 1950s. He shared our aim to better the lives of our population by means of habilitation units in which training for normal employment was undertaken, along with individual programmes of education and emotional support. We had many successes as well as occasional failures, but it seemed that the successful inculcation of social and other skills had considerable implications both for research and practice. It is strange to recall that at that period such a view was regarded as revolutionary.

At the same time that research into the social and psychological aspects of mental retardation began to make headway, parents' groups sprang up voicing deep concern at the lack of facilities for their children, especially in the very adverse conditions within institutions. Britain saw the start of a human rights movement, championed initially by the National Council for Civil Liberties. In the following decade, in Denmark and Norway, the concept of 'normalization' was born as a counter to the neglect of the quality of life for those designated mentally deficient/mentally retarded/mentally subnormal/learning disabled. So research findings, parental pressure groups and human rights issues coalesced to produce powerful social reform focusing on individual problems.

Roy Brown's interests remained in this field and he has been active in several continents. Nobody has done more in advancing the issues of habilitation and, indirectly or directly, he has contributed to the quality of life of thousands. It is appropriate, therefore, that he should have invited a broadly based group of authors to explore this topic. Although apparently disagreeing on some matters, including the details of definition, they have in common a deep humanity and interesting and unique contributions to the literature.

Quality of life studies rest at the interface between art and science and we believe that this is where they will remain. Qualitative methods, descriptive rather than inferential, seem very appropriate in investigating processes bearing on the changing patterns of an individual life path. In this domain, a detailed case history may be more revealing than a table of statistical results.

Many of the chapters adopt a holistic, non-analytic approach, entirely appropriate to the subject at hand, and a rich resource of information is presented on topics as diverse as: issues of quality of life for children with handicaps; the aged; human spirituality; creative activities; and sexual rights and wrongs. There are also outstanding chapters on assessment, emphasizing the possibility of scientific rigour.

There is a tension between the notion that personal contentment represents quality of life on the one hand and a more objective view that there are certain basic essentials, including an element of choice, on the other. Even here we may become conceptually entangled when considering the lot of those whose intellects may be unable to comprehend more than the simplest possible alternatives. But the topic is important and the reader will find much to think about in these pages.

This book reflects the profound shift over the last few decades from paternalistic notions that we, the professionals, can decide what is best for the individual or, worse, that a standard pattern is necessarily best to the view that a person-centred partnership is the only way forward. We believe that this volume will prove to be essential reading for those who are in sympathy with this notion, as well as for those who remain critical of what they regard as the excesses of the normalization movement.

Ann and Alan Clarke
Professors Emeriti
University of Hull, UK
December 1996

Quality of life: the development of an idea 1

Roy I Brown

INTRODUCTION

The first edition of *Quality of Life of Handicapped Persons* (Brown, 1988) represented one of the first attempts to bring together a wide range of knowledge in the field of disability set within the context of the developing models of quality of life. Since the publication of that book, the field of quality of life has changed dramatically which has led to new as well as substantially revised chapters in this edition. Quality of life has grown through infancy to adolescence and now represents a challenge to other ways of conceptualizing and thinking about persons with disabilities. Understandably, this has provoked controversy and there now exist a number of arguments criticizing the value of quality of life models. Yet I would argue that since 1988 the development of quality of life research has enabled us to look at the field of disability and people with disabilities themselves in a qualitatively new fashion. Quality of life is now seen by a wide range of authors as a holistic phenomenon. It is also seen as a lifespan concept and not the least of its attributes (and the criticisms about it) is the complexity of interacting forces which go to make up any individual's quality of life.

Since 1988 the concepts involving quality of life have been redefined and the definitions developed, though there is far from total consensus. Yet it is this fluidity of viewpoint that, in one sense, makes the field so attractive, for development of research and programmes in the field of quality of life shows that the related models are capable of change in a most creative and progressive fashion. The language of quality of life has grown, not only within the scientific and disability fields but also within the political and social policy domains. It is within the political and social policy areas that the language of quality of life is often used, but the underlying concepts are often eschewed. Many community programmes for persons who are disadvantaged or disabled are said to represent quality of life, yet it is difficult to see the principles of this concept truly applied. Now more than ever, social and psychological researchers need to underscore the importance of personal perception in an understanding of the individual's quality of life. It is recognized that objective parameters are important, yet it is the blending of a wide range of views, opinions and knowledge which enables us to develop constructs around quality of life.

One advantage of quality of life models is that they represent the linkage of many concepts and ideas within an ever-flowing and changing environment. This interaction leads in turn to personal changes in perception. Wolfensberger (1994) argues that quality of life models are dangerous because they can be misused by political and services systems. If authorities view quality of life of specific individuals as limited or negative, we may come to believe an individual's life is not worth preserving. But such potential negativism is inherent in many social, behavioural or biological models. Most knowledge can be employed to ill effect. It is the role of scientists to explore and uncover knowledge which can be used to develop models. This can in turn lead to greater understanding and improved intervention at a practical level. That ideas may be used for negative outcomes is an issue that requires constant vigilance, understanding and answers. This is inevitable within any applied science.

But there are also questions of a scientific nature. For example, quality of life may be an awareness-raising concept but can it be employed scientifically? There are issues which also need careful examination at a semantic level. Not least of these is the issue of subjectivity or objectivity of data. Although the various chapters cover the division of objectivity and subjectivity employed in quality of life studies, I would like to argue that such a division is confusing and arbitrary. Increasingly, we recognize that we live in a world of personal perceptions and, as Andrews (1974) has pointed out, people respond to their perceptions rather than to more objective data. In other words, the lifeblood of development and behaviour of change relates fundamentally to our perception of a variety of attributes. Insofar as such personal views can be presented orally or registered non-verbally, they represent an externalization of personal and internal processes in forms that are measurable and replicable. Such data frequently show correlations with other measures of environment and behaviour. Personal perceptions appear similar in quality to our perception of colour or temperature. They represent a system of data which we can value, not as expressions of belief or objective understanding, but as objective measures of perceived phenomena. It is the denial of the 'reality' of these stated perceptions which has caused scientists to ignore such phenomena, arguing they are not measurable. To ignore these data is to restrict scientific investigation.

There are those who argue that quality of life cannot become a scientific concept. It is suggested here that we cannot understand behaviour within its social context unless we are willing to accept such a concept. It may be that Goode (1994) is correct in stating it will not be recognized as a hard science, but I am suggesting we have overestimated the 'softness' of the data. At times, such personal perceptions differ from those of others or from external data arising from other sources. This does not make them more correct or incorrect. It simply means that they represent another useful data source, a data source to which people react and adapt. Perceptual data simply represent additional information arising from human emotion and partial awareness. Because such data can be subjected to the usual criteria of science, namely observability, reliability and validity, they should be treated with the same respect as traditional objective data. Such data contain error – our requirement is to determine the nature of this error. Personal perceptions are essential to our understanding of value systems and individual responses to events and interventions. As we shall see in the following chapters, there are various approaches to using such perceptions. Such data are often not well handled by traditional research methodology, nor do the data sit well with many current intervention or counselling procedures. The development of quality of life models does not mean that previous knowledge must be thrown out, nor that what has been developed within current quality of life models should be religiously supported.

Data and discussion are provided to support a quality of life model rather than a social movement or mission. Quality of life models are built upon previous knowledge and information and are necessarily more diverse than their predecessors, although they incorporate a considerable amount of evidence and viewpoint from preceding models. However, it is argued that the formulation of quality of life, and the evidence which backs this formulation, must be studied rigorously and perceptual data may have greater value than traditional objective information. For example, elsewhere I have argued (Brown, Bayer & Brown, 1992) that feelings of safety or lack of safety may be more critical to the development of self-image and behaviour than objective measures of safety or lack of safety. Feelings of health may be salient within a medical context of ill health which may have great effect on the client. Our society, in its treatment of people with disabilities, needs to recognize the formal means of ensuring safety, health and well-being, but it should do so in the context and awareness of perceptions of safety, health and well-being declared by the people whom society wishes to serve.

Quality of life models accept the notion of human variability both between and within subjects. This variability is seen as a critical and valuable attribute. For example, Brown, Bayer & Brown argue that the changeability of clients, which has been used by some service personnel to suggest that client statements are too fickle to be employed, represents a variability which is essential to any intervention process based on quality of life.

There are a number of other dilemmas within the area of quality of life. A central issue is the nature and role of personal choice. If it is argued that personal choice should be recognized and that variation in choices, attitudes and interventions lead to individualized service options, then there must be further debate about how the choices of others influence particular requests for individualized goals. This has not yet been recognized and should be the subject of much further research. Moreover, the issue of choice and personal expression, which appears so critical to the development of self-image, is a challenge when individuals have little knowledge of the potential choices available. Yet, to some degree this is true of all people. Choice is in part a developmental issue and needs to take place in the context of structure, with some control and support, interlaced with some element of risk and exploration. It is essential that the carers of those with disabilities do not curtail the processes of choice and exploration when exercising care. To do so is to handicap but to remove all structure also exposes the individual to handicap. Nice balance is required and this demands skill and flexibility.

Models of quality of life have changed dramatically since the late 1980s, partly in terms of the methodology employed within the scientific framework. It is important in this context not to confuse research with experimentation. Experiment represents a particular approach to research and science. Other scientific methodologies, it is argued, are more appropriate at different levels and types of analysis. Discourse analysis, phenomenological approaches and extensive use of ethnographic methods, including the use of narrative and personal stories, are now extensively employed.

The clients and other consumers have themselves become involved in the development of new methods and models. This is now accepted and encouraged. In a sense, this is paradoxical. People like myself were brought up in an era where objective data, as formally defined, were seen as the major expression of measurement for understanding behaviour. Within this approach the client's or the subject's anonymity was preserved. Indeed, it has become one of the ethical tenets of science that confidentiality and anonymity are critical. Yet the very development of narrative and discourse within scientific methodology means that the roles of researcher and consumer are complementary and therefore form a partnership. The researched becomes the researcher. It therefore becomes appropriate to ask whether, instead of anonymity, the consumer's name should (if he or she wishes) be clearly visible in order that personal contributions can be acknowledged. Who is the discoverer? It is also suggested that such methodology represents a way in which scientists can 'break into' such fields as quality of life and use the findings to develop experimental methodologies. Thus within quality of life there is a growing understanding that preliminary research will be descriptive and employ phenomenological and allied methodologies before proceeding to experimental strategies with the use of formal control.

The chapters also indicate the artificiality of the division between science and arts. The holistic and integrated quality of affective human behaviour is examined. The examples are of disability, but disability set within an artistic appreciation of humanness. It is in the quality of life approach that sharing has the potential to offer equality of opportunity.

All of these views raise some questions of direction. Over the decades services have moved from congregate administration and care to individual intervention. This in turn has led to the present consideration of individual and personal quality of life, where personal perceptions in the context of choice become relevant. This is often disregarded in relation to children and adolescents and elderly persons with disabilities. Obviously choice relates to opportunity and environment but it also relates to how individuals image choice and what they mean when they say they have need. The study of disability thus moves not just from group to individual services, but from external to internal levels of control. Internal control means the individual becomes responsible for decision making. However, we know little of such processes. Quality of life therefore poses some further and critical questions about individual consciousness. To what extent are individuals aware of choices, how do they image themselves within such a learning environment and how can our knowledge assist in such developments? These must become the challenges for any quality of life model.

The preparation of this book presented some problems of definition. Authors from different countries use different terminology concerning populations. Although one could spend some time looking at the equivalence of terms and in the text mental retardation and intellectual disability may eventually be regarded as synonymous, the whole thrust of quality of life is towards individualization and, therefore, the commentary throughout, though sometimes taking examples from specific disabilities, is in my view generic to the field of disabilities. Levels may differ, but the general principles of quality of life apply to everyone with disability. Indeed, so comprehensive is the model of quality of life that it is arguably applicable to us all, regardless of condition.

ORGANIZATION OF THE CHAPTERS

It is important to recognize that authors in this book are attempting to provide models of quality of life which depend primarily on sociological and psychological constructs of group and individual behaviour. Each author has been provided with a platform to explore the development of quality of life models within specific contexts. This has led to some overlap in ideas, but I believe it is relevant to retain such overlap because it shows the degree to which different authors in various parts of the world are drawn to similar conclusions.

Following the introduction are two chapters, one written by Beth Velde, the other by Dimity Peter, concerning individuals who have disabilities and their personal perceptions of their lives. Both are about individuals, one with a physical disability, the other with an intellectual disability. These chapters have been placed early in the book for several reasons. They describe through their personal accounts the effects disabilities can have on experience. They demonstrate the wide-ranging effects of disability across life domains, which often hamper experience and community involvement and sometimes enhance perception and understanding. In turn, each exemplifies and therefore illustrates issues which are taken up later in the theoretical models and with practice of quality of life. However, they also serve to remind us that disability is personal and understanding it requires a comprehension of each individual and some appreciation of the internal personal processes that help individuals understand themselves within the context of their experience. This aspect of disability is not always understood and is frequently forgotten when policies and services are developed and delivered. In placing these stories near the beginning of the book, I am hoping that they will give personal substance to what follows. Disability is a personal matter and although we need policies, systems and practices to enable professionals and general services to develop, there is cause for concern as economic rationalism and scientific theory polarize our thinking towards systems of affluence and desired perfection, rather than towards enlightened involvement arising from individual experiences across our society.

Links to the first edition are clearly apparent. For example, the notion of four areas of well-being was briefly put forward by Roger Blunden in the first edition. Felce now uses this model as a foundation to Chapter 3, which underscores the common views of a number of researchers and practitioners in this field. David Goode's chapter takes the model further and shows the possibilities of applying quality of life to individuals with profound and multiple handicaps. The complexity of the model provides insight into ways we can observe, evaluate and communicate with persons who are profoundly handicapped, insights that are critical for the development of both human science and service delivery. This consumer–professional interaction is seen as an essential part of developing new services based on a quality of life model.

Trevor Parmenter and Michelle Donelly build on the Parmenter chapter in the 1988 edition and include specific issues and concerns of people with

a wide range of disabilities, but particularly those with physical disabilities. The expansion of such concepts, chapter by chapter, provides an
exciting challenge for they provide ways of thinking about disability
enlightened and directed by observing and recording the perceptions of
people with disabilities.

But further challenges remain. At one level they may be thought to
represent polarized needs, one underlying the importance of scientific
measures and their validity, without which no model can be effectively
sustained, the other the need to accept the experiences of each individual
with their own needs and provide the required support. The basis of this
latter view is both humanitarian and service oriented. The importance of
the model-building chapters is that they bring both scientific and humanitarian aspects together. These two interests can be followed in subsequent chapters. The first, by Robert Cummins, provides a detailed
account of the development and analysis of assessment in the field of
quality of life. This chapter, deeply embedded in scientific rigour, provides a pathway for a more detailed evaluation of personal perceptions
and a means of utilizing data relating to quality of life, by taking into
account what several authors refer to as objective and subjective
measures.

Effective measurement must be seen as a major requirement of any
system which claims to be scientific. The model must demonstrate how it
is relevant to a wide range of issues as well as the individual concerns of
persons with disabilities. Quality of life, if it is to fulfil its potential, has to
bridge the gap from traditional science, with its accent on measurement,
including reliability and validity, along with a rigorous accounting of
error, to the newer paradigms of science which accent individual variability and personal expression. Indeed, Cummins' chapter is an attempt
to demonstrate that rigour can be achieved without doing an injustice to
the perceptual or subjective experience of individuals. Thus the initial
chapters, with their individual accounts of personal experiences of disability, lead through model building to a more measured approach to the
field. Indeed, it can be argued that quality of life structures reflect the
development of science from observation through model building with
pragmatic definition to measurement in social behavioural terms. The
methods employed in these chapters show a range of diversity including
single case studies involving ethnographic methodology to the development of instrumentation for quantifying objective and consumer-based
observations. Survey, cross-sectional and longitudinal studies involving
experimental or quasi-experimental approaches are drawn upon, as well
as more recent methodologies such as discourse analysis and phenomenology, which help to develop the overall framework.

Following Cummins' chapter there are several chapters which consider
the application of quality of life to different age groups. The chapters are

very different, yet they all attempt to apply ideas from quality of life and related fields to groups with very particular needs. The first is the chapter by David Mitchell and John Winslade which highlights systems theory. However, the same themes, depicted in early chapters, surface again as the issue of quality of life for young children and families are explored. The interacting dynamics of personal worlds within family structure are identified and the way the family affects and is affected by its cultural world is examined. In this chapter, probably more clearly than in others, the nature of political and social dynamics and their reverberating impacts lead the reader to consider the necessary involvement of various integrated approaches to an understanding of disability with its personal and cultural constraints. The notion that assessment involves evaluation of systems within the quality of life framework is brought to the fore. It is clear that management of clinical and service practices requires a clear understanding of personal and family needs within a quality of life construct. That services and systems may be decompartmentalized and prevent the application of new models is illustrated in the following chapter by Vianne Timmons and Roy Brown. Not only do they demonstrate the importance and relevance of applying a quality of life model to children, they also analyse why this application is critical to understanding how, for example, quality of life experiences relate to inclusive education within a community and family framework.

The holistic nature of the quality of life model is clearly illustrated in these two chapters and both provide examples of how different societal systems interact and affect every aspect of the individual's life. Quality of life models raise intervention issues – where, how and when should intervention take place? These chapters argue that the client must have a major and clearly documented say in this selection but, equally important, the chapters illustrate that intervention at any one point leads to change in the rest of the social system in which the individual operates. It must be stressed that when the personal choices of the individual are considered relevant we will need to answer issues of conflicting choices between the individual and society. For example, in attempting to rehabilitate through the employment of persons with disabilities our best approach may lie more effectively in other domains than the economic or political dimensions identified by society. That is, the individual's choices may indicate that initial intervention may be in areas other than employment and thus not immediately satisfy the requirements of a bureaucracy. Success in the area of choice is likely to lead to solutions in other areas of performance (Brown, Bayer & Brown, 1992).

The chapter by James Hogg and Loretto Lamb exemplifies the application of quality of life to a further group of people who have tended to be marginalized, namely the elderly who are also disabled. Here the authors examine service and personal needs of individuals through a research model. The chapter illustrates, once again, the complexity of situations viewed from a quality of life perspective. It examines the views of service providers and receivers. The need for a holistic model of disability is recognized and the chapter reflects some of the issues raised in earlier chapters, particularly that of David Goode. Increasingly, it appears that different aspects and types of disability and service can be conceptualized from the quality of life perspective.

Much of the discussion in these chapters has reflected the relevance of values and rights and the importance of choice within all life domains. Rights and choices must not be interpreted here in any simplistic way. Not only must it be recognized that social acceptance and freedom to make choices carry responsibilities, but that choices occur within both social and cultural contexts. The importance appears to lie in these personal choices being recognized and accepted and in the individual having opportunities to have a say and increased control of their life. Some personal choices have to be made recognizing the choices and rights of others, but this consideration cannot be used as a method of denying access to the choices of the consumer. Unfortunately some managers and professionals have argued that consumers are incompetent in making choices. The balances are delicate and at times formidable. This is very clearly illustrated in the chapter on sexual rights and wrongs by Hilary Brown. This chapter requires that we come to understand more fully and clearly the issues surrounding rights and what constitutes best practice. Planning and application must be understood by professionals and policymakers at both general and specific levels and the quality of life model requires that we consider both levels. Appropriate social policy requires that we recognize the practical importance of protecting individuals through the promulgation of rights, but at the same time it is necessary not to overprotect and through this deny opportunities for psychological and social growth. This is a dilemma which will be hotly debated (see Swain & Thirlaway, 1996).

To this point, the book has been concerned with disability set within a quality of life framework. However, the more the underlying principles are examined, the more apparent it is that the authors are demonstrating, in general terms, ways in which attainment and fulfilment may be optimized for all individuals as they live within increasingly complex societies. These complexities, along with modern technological resources, precipitate ethical issues which have not previously preoccupied society in such a profound manner. The model of quality of life and its expansion may be more apparent, and therefore perceived as critically necessary, within the field of disability, but the issues raised apply to society as a whole. Similar challenges face children and adults with and without disabilities and when crisis occurs, the quality of life issues become fundamental to both comprehending and handling human relationships effectively.

The next three chapters take up these wider themes. While still addressing quality of life within the field of disabilities, each in turn looks at the issues in the context of physical environment, creative activity through the arts and the need for religious and spiritual experience. By necessity the three chapters take broad perspectives. Roy Ferguson's chapter, which links clearly with the findings reported by Trevor Parmenter, demonstrates how the physical environment can be adapted and modified to expand the range of community and home access for people with disabilities. In doing so, choices for the individual are increased. The person with disability can now begin to meet more equally with those not so handicapped by environment. We begin to see how previous chapters become even more pertinent as they relate to life-span concerns and access of the individual to a wider range of activities in school, home, employment and community. In widening access to the community, infringement of rights becomes an even more critical issue. Increased access means greater social interaction, which raises new challenges which in turn result in society gaining greater insight into its own barriers and limitations. In the end, ongoing modification to the environment is likely to increase accessibility for all citizens, enhancing opportunities for contact, exploration and communication. As a result of this, issues of relationships, sexuality, family and social interactions, institutional living and community awareness will have to be re-examined through what can be termed the prism of quality of life. Bernie Warren examines these issues through the arts. He argues that the arts can increase social understanding and reduce handicap. He devotes some space to the interesting argument that dimensions to Eastern thought and practice, in drama and other artistic expression, bring new insight and skills consistent with the quality of life model. Aldred Neufeldt and Patrick McGinley consider the place of religion and spirituality in this wider framework. Although they wonder whether spirituality is a separate dimension from quality of life, they discuss how aspects of self and one's value of self, along with one's relationships to others, are deeply linked to ethical, spiritual and religious values. In this sense they explore the role of religion as a personal and societal construct in individuals' lives. They not only draw on the personal resources which spirituality and religion may engender, but consider the changes which are required of organized religion if a quality of life model is to be adopted.

In the penultimate chapter, Roy Brown has attempted to bring together some of the implications of a quality of life model for professional practice. The argument is made that if a quality of life model is to be put into effect, a fundamental change in how we teach and practise must necessarily occur. To adapt a model is simply not good enough. Changes in practice have to be taught, new insights are provided and policymakers and managers are required to change how they operate. In the final chapter,

Robert Schalock takes a broad look at the potential of quality of life as a tool for people with disabilities in the 21st century. In many ways, the chapter reiterates some of the early papers, but underscores the importance of clear conceptualization about quality of life along with the recognition that we can, as a society, embrace new opportunities and understanding of disability which focus on consumers' perceptions and needs.

The theme of this edition, therefore, is that a broad-ranging model of quality of life has been gradually taking shape amongst scientists, practitioners and consumers. It holds much optimism for the future and the attendance at quality of life seminars, workshops and conferences by many people with disabilities, their families, practitioners, managers and scientists testifies to the interest in this development. As indicated, there are critics and, rightly, there are fundamental questions to be answered. The answers probably lie in the extent to which the systems peopled by policymakers and managers will permit a reorganization of values and priorities, which can promote individuals taking responsibility for their own choices within a context of support and consultation. The challenges are clear. It is one thing to provide society with grand technical inventions, it is another to employ them as a way to minimize handicap and enhance exploration and personal control as each individual wishes, within the context of a civilized society.

REFERENCES

Andrews, F.M. (1974) Social indicators of perceived life quality. *Social Indicators Research*, **1**, 279–99.
Brown, R.I. (1988) *Quality of Life for Handicapped People*, Croom Helm, London.
Brown, R.I., Bayer, M.B. and Brown, P.M. (1992) *Empowerment and Developmental Handicaps: Choices and Quality of Life*, Chapman & Hall, London.
Goode, D. (1994) The national quality of life for persons with disabilities project: a quality of life agenda for the United States, in *Quality of Life for Persons with Disabilities: International Perspectives and Issues*, (ed. D. Goode), Brookline Books, Cambridge, MA.
Swain, J. and Thirlaway, C. (1996) 'Just when you think you've got it all sorted.' Parental dilemmas in relation to the developing sexuality of young, profoundly disabled people. *British Journal of Learning Disabilities*, **24**(2), 58–64.
Wolfensberger, W. (1994) Let's hang up 'quality of life' as a hopeless term, in *Quality of Life for Persons with Disabilities: International Perspectives and Issues*, (ed. D. Goode), Brookline, Cambridge, MA.

Quality of life through personally meaningful activity

2

Beth P Velde

INTRODUCTION

Activity which is *purposeful* and *meaningful* to the individual appears to contribute positively to an individual's perception of their own quality of life (Asker, 1990; Hoover, 1992; Kibele, 1989; Sinnott-Oswald, Gliner & Spencer, 1991; Wehman, 1993). Activities attain personal meaning through voluntary engagement of the individual's mind and body in the pursuit of an end goal which is relevant to personal needs, interest, capacities and fulfilment of one's life roles (Fidler, 1994).

EXPLAINING OUR EXPERIENCE

According to Csikszentmihalyi (1990), individuals have two options for achievement of quality of life. They may try to match external conditions to personal goals or change the way external conditions are experienced. Seligman (1991) suggests a similar approach when he describes how individuals are able to choose the way they think about and interpret the external environment – a process he calls *learned optimism*. Manz (1992) distinguishes between *opportunity thinking* and *obstacle thinking*. When someone is engaged in opportunity thinking, they see a challenge as an opportunity. In this case, the individual focuses on ways to meet the challenge. However, if the challenge is seen as an obstacle, the person focuses upon reasons to give up or run away from the problem. This is directly related to an individual's perception of their quality of life. If quality of life includes an external component and an interpretation of external conditions, then quality of life must be related to our thinking about the quality of our experience.

While these statements hold true for any person, they are especially relevant for a person with a disability. Massimini (in Csikszentmihalyi, 1990) studied a group of individuals with paraplegia. He found that while the accident causing the paralysis was tragic, the individuals often perceived the results as positive. This could be attributed to the way the research participants viewed the accident and its consequences – as a challenge which presented them with clear goals. Those interviewed interpreted their external conditions as constructive and growth inducing.

Weinberg (1984) found similar results when she interviewed 30 adults with physical disabilities. When presented with the question, 'If there were a surgery available that was guaranteed to completely cure your disability (with no risk) would you be willing to undergo the surgery?', only 50% chose the surgery. When asked why they would refuse the surgery, most replied that becoming able-bodied would change the essence of who they were. They maintained that they had satisfying lives and were happy with the identity they had built for themselves.

How does an individual use daily life experiences to frame a lifestyle which they label as satisfying? Using excerpts from an interview conducted with a 34-year-old man who has quadriplegia, this chapter will explore the relationship of meaningful activity to quality of life using a phenomenological perspective.

PAUL

Paul (an assumed name) lives in his own apartment in a large city in western Canada. Personal care aides assist in his home twice a day. He uses a manual wheelchair for mobility and for transportation, a public transit system for people with disabilities. In describing himself he says, 'I still try to think as a normal human being … well, but with the limitation of being in the chair. So I … you know, my ideas is still the same as any able-bodied person. The only problem is, is that time now is considerably jeopardized.'

Prior to his accident his work included piloting aircraft and carpentry. After his accident he worked in flight services using radar and radio. He has the equivalent of a high school diploma. He currently describes himself as retired.

Paul was recommended for the interview by several friends and acquaintances who view him as having a high quality of life. Paul's spinal cord injury was the result of a hang-gliding accident when he was 25. The injury resulted in a complete break at the C5–6 vertebrae. About the accident and hang-gliding, he says, '… that's how I got hurt but I have no malice against it …'.

DESCRIBING QUALITY OF LIFE

Quality of life has been described in a variety of ways. Hultsman (1985) attributes quality of life to three aspects: perceived freedom, intrinsic motivation and the degree of positive attribution accorded to life experiences. Brown, Bayer & MacFarlane (1989) suggest that quality of life is best explained using a combined model of objective and subjective measures. Subjective measures include unmet goals and control. Unmet goals are the discrepancy between a person's achieved and unmet needs and desires. The expression of any discrepancy is idiosyncratic and comes from the individual. The second subjective measure is the extent to which an individual controls aspects of their life. Control is identified as the amount of personal power over one's life as perceived by the individual. As the amount of control increases, the person may perceive a higher quality of life. The primary objective measures are indicators of a discrepancy between one's personal attainment of income, housing, health, mastery and the norms for one's culture. There are important subjective concepts within this objective measure as well. The individual must be the one who determines the reference group to which these objective measures are compared and they need to identify the relative importance of each component in their lifestyle.

While the objective measures may be assessed by others, it is essential to consult the individual regarding the subjective measures. 'Quality of life is an interaction between the individual and the environment. It can be described in terms of personal control that can be exerted by the individual over the environment. It must be assessed by consulting the individual directly' (Brown, Bayer & MacFarlane, 1989, p57). This orientation recognizes the importance of person–environment interactions within a cultural and ecological perspective and supports the contribution of personally relevant activities to quality of life.

McKenna (1993) suggests that quality of life can be expressed both through universal themes and as an idiosyncratic interpretation using discrete activities:

> ... I feel that quality of life has some commonalities and can be generalized, but only to a certain extent. Having autonomy and freedom; enjoying self-integrity and self-esteem; being free of illness, pain or physical restriction are features which would undoubtedly be prized by most people and would almost universally be identified as components of life's goodness. However, aside from these common denominators, there are those features which are valued to a special degree by the individual alone. To play golf, to travel, to hold a grandchild, to feel a oneness with the environment are very personal experiences identified by some participants in my research as being the key to their happiness and quality of life.
>
> (p34)

Paul describes his life as satisfying and meaningful because of his perception of activities which are a part of his lifestyle. He considers himself to be busy and engaged in productive activities. When asked what change was the most relevant to the way he views his life since his accident, he responded, '... I find if I don't feel like doing something and I'm doing it, it's not worth doing because I usually just make a mockery of what I'm doing. When I feel like doing it, I'm wholeheartedly into it and it becomes a work of art, you know'. It appears from this quote that those activities which he chooses to do, and to continue, contribute to aspects of control and goal achievement.

ACTIVITY AND QUALITY OF LIFE

According to Fidler (1996), quality of life is the most important theme in human existence. She states, '... wellness and a sense of well-being can be understood ... as a way of life that is more satisfying than not to self and to those significant others with whom one shares living' (p2). Wellness and well-being are a result of participation in 'personally and socially relevant activities that focus on and maximize individual strengths and capacities' (p2). The desire to engage in those activities is intrinsically motivated and participation is sustained because 'there is congruence between the characteristics of an activity and the biopsychosocial characteristics of the person' (p2).

Activity which is meaningful to the individual implies that the individual has had some experience with the activity. Meaning is established by 'the perceptual sense it makes to the individual as well as to the cognitive associations elicited in the individual' (Nelson, 1988, p635). Through the actual *doing* of an activity, the individual understands or makes sense out of the experience and remembers the experience by integrating their cognitive, affective and psychomotor responses to the activity. Activities may also be purposeful to the individual when the activity will assist in meeting stated or unstated goals. The individual interprets the activity based on the meaning which has been developed through past experience and its relationship to its potential for meeting a more future-oriented goal.

Paul describes how the activities in his life are tied together through their common meaning and purpose – his desire for personal growth:

> ... so a lot of people think because I'm not working for a living but I still have time, that I'm bored ... whenever they say to me, 'Aren't you bored?' it always seems to be such a, you know, like 'Who the hell do you think I am?', you know. Like, I'm more busy now than if I'm actually working. There's so many things that I want to know, there's so many things that I still want to do, you know. And I was working to try and make those things possible, you know. That's what my main objective in life is, it's not to slave for somebody else, but it's to learn, to experiment, to grow, to grow, basically inside, you know.

In Paul's case, the meaning of his life is related to personal growth. Activity which is meaningful to him provides him with a way of actualizing his life's meaning.

Many authors discuss activities in two essential categories: work and leisure (Barnes, 1990; Brown, Bayer & Brown, 1988; Clark & Hirst, 1989; Glyptis, 1989). However, with the changes in lifestyle created by employment patterns, technology and the economy (Naisbett, 1989; Popcorn, 1991), viewing activities from this dichotomous relationship may be less useful than in the past. Instead, activity can be described through its relationship to the experiences a person has every day. Fidler (1996) proposes four areas grouped according to why a person may choose to engage in the activity and why it is meaningful to them. These are: self-care and maintenance, societal contribution, interpersonal engagement and intrinsic gratification. While she suggests that any given activity may reside predominantly in one area, the areas are not mutually exclusive.

SELF-CARE AND MAINTENANCE

Activities which involve meeting one's personal needs in a manner which is self-dependent fall within the domain of self-care and maintenance. What seems to be important is that the individual is able to recognize and articulate their personal needs so they are met independently or someone is able to assist when given direction by the individual needing assistance. These needs may represent personal care such as toileting, bathing, dressing, eating and grooming (Christiansen, 1992).

Paul recognizes the importance of personal care to his overall quality of life. He shares the following:

> I always had the philosophy that the healthier you are, the more you will perceive, the more you will do, the more you will be able to do. I used to trade sleep for time, you know, for conscious time. I still sleep little actually. I'm one of those lucky people who can manage to function on just four hours, but I find any less than four hours, I can feel myself entrapped very heavily, like gravity, you know. ... [S]ometimes actually I find that I wish that I didn't have to even sleep. It's not really a pleasurable thing for me. I find that I'm wasting time, you know, and unfortunately, like anybody else, I can't live without it, you know. But it's gotten me into trouble because I'm working on a project and the feeling of working on the project is so sweet, you know, you go, 'Oh ...' You know, you say to yourself, 'At 10 o'clock I'll stop and make supper,' and you know 10 comes and you are, 'Oh, I'll do it at 10:30 and I'll do it at 11:00.' And at 2 o'clock in the morning you still haven't gotten around to eating and you think, 'Oh, it's too late to

eat.' And then the next day you're in trouble because, you know, you haven't eaten and, you know, you go off to do something and halfway through the day you're falling on your face. ... I figure because I'm paralysed I don't need as much (to eat) as an able-bodied person, but I find I still have to get that one meal because otherwise I start hacking, my skin starts breaking down, you know. Like, for example, if I develop an ulcer on my rear or anywhere like that, I can't sit up in the chair so it means having to lie down on the bed, and once I do that, I am screwed because I can't ... because I find once I'm lying down I'm even more restricted than when I'm sitting up.

Self-care may also involve functional activities of daily living. These include behaviours required to live independently in the community such as use of the telephone, food preparation, housekeeping, laundry, shopping, money management, use of transportation and medication management (Lawton, 1971). Paul describes how he views one of these aspects, money management, in his life. 'It doesn't make much sense trying to do more than I'm capable of. My finances is also very limited and that ... that seems to be, you know ... to me that was always what money was for, to buy time. I never really wanted to be rich to the point where, you know, money was all I thought about. As far as I'm concerned it was to buy time, and if I could buy time, that's what I'd do, you know.'

SOCIETAL CONTRIBUTION

Activities which contribute to the need fulfilment and welfare of others fall within the domain of societal contribution. This may come from paid work, volunteer experiences or providing a service to others. Paul expresses how refinishing and selling or giving away stereo speakers and cabinets contributes to his quality of life.

... [W]henever I can I pick up cheap speakers and usually gut them and try to refinish them in a cabinet, you know. ... You know, I've had some compliments on my work like, you know, people walk in, they hear the speaker and they say, 'Wow'. ... And when that happens it gives me a really nice feeling, you know, inside, you know, like ... I'm not saying that my ego ... well it does I guess, my ego gets boosted but it's not really that. Even if they walk in and see a model sitting there and they go, 'Wow, is that ever neat,' you know, and you know, and for a few minutes they let me blab about it. I get a feeling that I'm doing something worthwhile.

Paul also experiences frustration when put into a position where someone else is helping him and the individual does not honour the commitment. In Paul's view using personal care aides in the morning and evening can sometimes be frustrating. While the aides are in the position of working and offering service to him, he finds it 'frustrating … especially when other people waste my time, you know. Like, if I have to depend on them to do something and they seem to diddle-daddle or they, you know, they don't show up or they, you know, I get frustrated because time's precious.' While Paul is self-dependent regarding his personal care because he can direct the manner in which others help him, he loses control of his time when the aides are late.

INTERPERSONAL ENGAGEMENT

Activities which are pursued to develop and sustain relationships with others, and involve reciprocity with others, fall in the domain of interpersonal engagement. Unlike the area of societal contribution, the relationships developed here involve give and take between participants. This includes family. Paul explains, 'I'm suddenly starting to understand my father a lot more now because I'm suddenly at his age where when I was with him he made a lot of decisions that I didn't understand, you know, and now it's all becoming apparent to me why, you know'.

Reciprocal relationships also involve peers, friends and acquaintances. Paul values interactions with others and considers himself a social person.

> … every time I go to the mall I find I do that. Well, everywhere I go really. I come … just before you saw me there … I don't like to be in a crowd, eh. I was going to have a coffee and I ended up sitting over on the edge there and started watching for a while, just watching the mall buzz around and the people. … I find myself thinking about people. I've always been really social. Sometimes I get talking to people. It is kind of fun. A little hobby. Watching, listening, talking and thinking.

INTRINSIC GRATIFICATION

Activities which an individual pursues because of the pleasure and enjoyment they offer fall within the domain of intrinsic gratification. Undoubtedly, for Paul, this is a significant domain in his life. Paul describes the sense of gratification in the following excerpt where he is describing his hobby of aero-modelling.

I feel like I'm creating something and I think that's when the mind is actually very open, very loose, very ... yeah, I go into another state of thinking then. Sometimes I come out of it, when I do come out of it, I ... it's like you break into a trance and when you come out of the trance although you might not be working as hard as, say lifting weights, you are physically tired from just thinking in those depths. And, you know, I find a form of euphoria after. ... [T]hat's why I said on a lot of my projects I stop when the drive goes away, I leave, you know, I leave it there, you know. I know it will come back but sometimes it might be a design problem and I get stuck. So I go off and try and work on something else, you know. Yeah, I'd have to say that it is because if you use that, what I just said, as a mark to work on it, then, you know, you're not really forcing yourself when you don't want to and therefore you produce ... I think what you can produce under those circumstances goes far beyond what you can in a forced situation because the romance is there, you know, your heart is into it, your mind is into it, your total being is into what you're doing, you know ... because if when you're forcing yourself and you're not there, it's a shamble.

Paul also believes that through doing activities which are intrinsically gratifying, the individual is able to explore their own multidimensionality.

I often ask people what their hobbies are, you know, and a lot of them ... well, I guess because I've always grown up with a hobby or being able to do things like that. Hobbies lead your time. I'm often quite shocked when I hear them say, 'Well, I don't have a hobby'. And I think, 'Oh, God, what a boring life they must lead' or 'How can they function without, you know, that inner side being opened up'.

QUALITY OF LIFE AND BALANCE

When considering quality of life from an activities perspective, it is important to consider how the concept of balance is applied to an individual's activity pattern. Many authors consider balance to be reflected in quantifiable terms as an equal amount of time and effort devoted to activities of work and leisure (AOTA, 1994; Christiansen & Baum, 1991;

Hopkins & Smith, 1993). This balance may be measured at one point in time and over a lifetime. Within the area of leisure, authors also discuss the need for balance in the type of activities (such as sports, culture, entertainment) and level of participation (such as active, passive) (Austin & Crawford, 1991; Howe-Murphy & Charboneau, 1987; Peterson & Gunn, 1984). When the concept of activities is broadened to represent the four areas identified earlier which are not mutually exclusive, the quantitative concept of balance does not fit since equality is not an issue.

An alternative is the concept of harmony where the amount of time spent in each area does not have to be equal. Instead, each area must be related to the other areas, but the focus is upon the individual's perception of 'a pleasing arrangement or combination of parts' (Morehead & Morehead, 1981, p249). According to Paul, this harmony arises from his ability to relate the activities in his life to the meaning of his life. Much of what he chooses to do relates to his learning and personal growth. When asked if he reads and what activity domain it might fall within, he replied:

> I used to. Yeah, I haven't done that for a long time. What I mean is that I haven't really read a novel, a basic short story. I say I will but I never seem to get around to it, you know. I find now that I'm reading more with what my hobbies are concerned with or whatever I'm working on. I find if I'm working I'm reading more anything that will relate. Books on physics, books on …

This theme has been carried across his life stages. When viewing his life to date he says:

> And I have nothing against growing older, it's actually kind of fascinating a lot more. I think you learn a lot better when you're older, you know, you're more open minded. I realize now that as a kid, although I tried to keep an open mind, I wasn't because … maybe it was my age or what I was capable of, you know. One tends to be more ideal when you're younger, you know.

His sense of harmony also appears to come through both the *doing* of activity and the act of *reflecting* upon the experience. Paul describes one of the activities he identified as *societal contribution*.

I worked for an aircraft company for a while. That was a ... often you dream of things, you know. 'If I become a pilot, you know, all my problems will be solved.' I got into it and I found out that it's so regulated that the real love of it was almost destroyed. ... I eventually got out of it and became a carpenter and kept it as a hobby so that I could enjoy the pleasure, build my own plane so I could fly whenever I wanted to and enjoy what I wanted to do with it. I find the business really robbed it, really robbed the essence of flying for me.

Based on the interview with Paul, it appears that three primary themes underlie the concept of harmony as it relates to his life. These are *continuity*, *control* and *intensity*. These themes identify how harmony is created and maintained across a lifetime.

CONTINUITY

The first theme which represents the link between activities and the individual's perception of harmony is continuity. In Paul's case, continuity is reflected by maintaining engagement in activities with similar qualities. For example, one activity which dominated his life prior to his accident was hang-gliding. He explains, '... that's how I got hurt but I have no malice against it because I thought that was probably the purest form of it, you know, as far as we'll have to depend on some kind of mechanical device to get us into that ocean. I think hang-gliding is probably the best. It's light, it gives you an expression of really flying by yourself'. Paul still enjoys gliding: 'Yeah, I've been flying the last three years down in Black Diamond with this lady actually ... We fly tandem as I don't have the use of my legs so I can't work the rudder and you know, we've been talking about other devices'. The qualities may include similar equipment, similarity of environments or similar psychological requirements such as control and autonomy. In other activity domains he describes a similar continuity of experience, a continuation of an activity over several life stages.

CONTROL

A second theme relates to being in control. Paul continues to place value on his ability to maintain control of his experience and his time. One area where he expressed the most dissatisfaction is when he requires assistance and the helper does not come on time. This creates frustration because he views this as wasting his time. 'Unfortunately, I can't cut the wood myself and things so I usually have somebody come over and do it and sometimes I get left … this happens in the modelling as well … I get left, stuck because I can't move until they do, you know. What I ask them to do, it holds up the whole project, so in my frustration I'll go and do something else to try and save time.' He expresses the same level of frustration whether the domain is self-care, intrinsic gratification, interpersonal engagement or societal contribution.

Haggard & Williams (1992) suggest leisure as one area where control by the participant is an inherent part of the definition. When leisure is defined as freedom of choice, then an individual chooses what aspect of the self to focus upon at a given time. Leisure may be a time to bring the perceived self into congruence with the ideal self. 'We maintain our personal identities by affirming these specific identity images; it is through testing, adoption, and expression or affirmation, of these specific identity images that we gain self-understanding and self-expression' (p8).

Part of control may be the intrinsic motivation regarding participation, the *drive* to the experience. Harper (1986) believed that in leisure we were heeding a call which was a call to self. He explained that not only do we heed the call, we answer the call. Harper further explained, '… what we find ourselves freely consenting to is the urgent inner need to or demand to understand ourselves; and such self-understanding is furthered by ways of experiences in which we are in accord (or in greater accord) with our basic metaphysical needs' (p124). This may explain why activities which are predominantly *intrinsically gratifying* play such an important role for Paul in explaining his quality of life.

INTENSITY

The third theme revolves around the intensity of the engagement in the activity. In many ways the following excerpt reflects the intense focus Paul has in many of the activities he experiences.

> If I had the television on and I'm working on a model. It's like … oh, something … this is interesting, it just crossed my mind. I often see people, especially during athletics, wear musical devices, you know … and I remember when I was skiing, and it started back in the '70's, it started. You know, the mini-stereos started coming out and everybody, 'Oh, you got to try it. It just makes you ski so much better'. I found I got into trouble because I couldn't concentrate on the skiing and the music at the same time. They just didn't … even though it was rock and roll and a lot of times you're … I found I either had to blank one out. I'd either come down the hill, ski really well and not remember what I'd even listened or even notice what

I'd listened to or I'd pay attention to the music and end up in trouble on the hill. You know, I couldn't ... I found I couldn't cope with them both at the same time. It was almost impossible to do although I love music. I'm very much into it, but I guess a lot of times when I ... you know, when I'm in the workshop, music might be grand but I find it's a waste of time because it's ... you know, sometimes a tape had stopped hours ago and I don't even realize it. It's gone, it's gone by, you know.

PAUL'S QUALITY OF LIFE

Why was Paul recommended by his peers and by professionals who work with him to be part of the study? Perhaps it was because he had achieved, through his activity repertoire, Csikszentmihalyi's (1990) tasks of differentiation and integration. Through the activities of his life he has been able to carve a self-identity which is unique and valued. As a result of his experiences he is able to be part of a larger entity. His contributions to others, his increased self-knowledge and his learning enable him to be part of a world of ideas which develop him into a more complex self. This process or organization of self is directly related to the two subjective measures of quality of life – control and achievement of goals.

CONCLUSIONS

Brown, Bayer & MacFarlane (1989) suggested that quality of life is affected by: the discrepancy between a person's achieved and unmet needs and desires; the extent to which an individual increasingly controls aspects of their life; and the discrepancy between one's personal attainment and the norms of one's culture regarding objective measures. The intent of this chapter was to focus on the subjective measures and their relationship to meaningful and purposeful activity. Using an interview with a person who has quadriplegia, the role of activities in his life was presented from his perspective. According to Paul and others who know him, he has a high quality of life. This appears to occur because he is engaged in activities in four areas: self-care and maintenance, intrinsic gratification, societal contribution and interpersonal engagement. For Paul, the areas are seen as harmonious and contribute to his perception of a high quality of life because they relate to the meaning of his life. This life meaning of personal growth is tied to quality of life through the achievement of many of his needs by experiencing activities in the four areas. He has a relatively high level of control over his time and experience, although he does relate frustration when he requires assistance to do parts of an activity and the helpers are late or do not come.

Because subjective measures of quality of life require qualitative methodologies to gather data, the generalizability of one person's reporting of a high quality of life through four activity areas is limited. However, the value of the approach must not be devalued. Based upon this study, the following recommendations are presented.

RECOMMENDATIONS

1. The study of the contribution of activity to quality of life should be broadened to include more than a view of work and leisure. Many no longer view these two categories as mutually exclusive. In addition, these two categories fail to recognize the importance of activities related to self-care and maintenance.
2. Subjective measures require a different approach to understanding phenomena related to quality of life. Further use of ethnography and phenomenology is essential to understanding quality of life for all individuals.
3. The contribution of activity to quality of life may be similar for persons regardless of whether they have a disability or not. Further studies with a wide variety of persons is required to understand this relationship.
4. Activity is intrinsically related to context. Understanding quality of life from the perspective of meaningful and purposeful activity requires further elaboration of contextual components such as culture, ethnic origin, history, politics and environment.
5. The role and value of activity is related to gender, life stage and age. Further studies with women and men representing a variety of life stages and ages is imperative.
6. Harmony – a subjective interpretation of activity – is an important concept in understanding the role of activity in quality of life. Balance – usually conceptualized as a quantitative measure – is less meaningful in understanding the contribution of each activity area to the individual's reporting of quality of life status. Further research should be initiated to validate the themes which describe the concept of harmony and lifestyle.
7. What of activities that a person longs to try and has not had the opportunity to experience? Do these enter into the evaluation of quality or harmony? Including questions which address these activities would broaden our understanding of desired versus achieved activities.
8. Would a person with a disability and unable to work (or limited in the amount of work they could do) have more time to devote to personal growth than a person who is working long hours in a job that does not

contribute to growth and therefore to quality of life? An investigation into the role of activities and personal growth would expand our understanding of this relationship.

REFERENCES

AOTA (1994) *Uniform Terminology*, 3rd edn, AOTA, Bethesda, MD.

Asker, D. (1990) *The Interdependence of Leisure Activity and Cultural Values*, ERIC Document Reproduction Service No. ED 320889.

Austin, D. and Crawford, M. (1991) *Therapeutic Recreation: An Introduction*, Prentice-Hall, Englewood Cliffs, NJ.

Barnes, C. (1990) *'Cabbage Syndrome': The Social Construction of Dependence*, Falmer Press, New York.

Brown, R.I., Bayer, M.B. and Brown, P.M. (1988) Quality of life: a challenge for rehabilitation agencies. *Australia and New Zealand Journal of Developmental Disabilities*, **14** (3 & 4), 189–99.

Brown, R.I., Bayer, M.B. and MacFarlane, C. (1989) *Rehabilitation Programmes: Performance and Quality of Life of Adults with Developmental Handicaps*, Lugus , Toronto.

Christiansen, C. (1992) A social framework for understanding self-care intervention, in *Ways of Living: Self-Care Strategies for Special Needs, 1–26*, (ed. C. Christiansen), AOTA, Baltimore, MD.

Christiansen, C. and Baum, C. (eds) (1991) *Occupational Therapy: Overcoming Human Performance Deficits*, Slack Inc., Thorofare, NJ.

Clark, A. and Hirst, M. (1989) Disability in adulthood: ten-year follow-up of young people with disabilities. *Disability, Handicap & Society*, **4**(3), 271–83.

Csikszentmihalyi, M. (1990) *Flow: The Psychology of Optimal Experience*, Harper Perenniel, New York.

Fidler, G. (1994) Foreword, in *Ways of Living: Self-Care Strategies for Special Needs*, (ed. C. Christiansen), AOTA, Baltimore, MD.

Fidler, G. (1996) Lifestyle performance: from profile to conceptual model. *American Journal of Occupational Therapy*, **50**, 139–47.

Glyptis, S. (1989) Leisure and unemployment, in *Understanding Leisure and Recreation: Mapping the Past, Charting the Future*, (eds E. Jackson and T. Burton), Venture Publishing, State College, PA.

Haggard, L.M. and Williams, D.R. (1992) Identity, affirmation through leisure activities: leisure symbols of the self. *Journal of Leisure Research*, **24**(1), 1–18.

Harper, W. (1986) Freedom in the experience of leisure. *Leisure Sciences*, **8**(2), 115–29.

Hoover, J. (1992) Development of a leisure satisfaction scale for use with adolescents and adults with mental retardation: initial findings. *Education and Training in Mental Retardation*, **27**(2), 153–60.

Hopkins, H.L. and Smith, H.D. (eds) (1993) *Willard and Spackman's Occupational Therapy*, 8th edn, J.B. Lippincott, Philadelphia, PA.

Howe-Murphy, C. and Charboneau, B. (1987) *Therapeutic Recreation Intervention: An Ecological Perspective*, Prentice-Hall, Englewood Cliffs, NJ.

Hultsman, J. (1985) *The Relationship of the Study of Leisure to the Perception of Quality of Life*, University of Oregon, Eugene, OR.

Kibele, A. (1989) Occupational therapy's role in improving the quality of life for persons with cerebral palsy. *American Journal of Occupational Therapy*, **43**(6), 371–7.

Lawton, M.P. (1971) The functional assessment of elderly people. *Journal of the American Geriatrics Society*, **19**, 465–81.

Manz, C.C. (1992) *Mastering Self-Leadership*, Prentice-Hall, Englewood Cliffs, NJ.

McKenna, K. (1993) Quality of life: a question of functional outcomes or the fulfilment of life plans. *Australian Occupational Therapy Journal*, **40**, 33–5.

Morehead, A. and Morehead, P. (1981) *The New American Webster Handy College Dictionary*, Signet Books, New York.

Naisbett, J. (1989) *Megatrends 2000: Ten New Directions for the 1990s*, William Morrow, New York.

Nelson, D. (1988) Occupation: form and performance. *American Journal of Occupational Therapy*, **42**(10), 633–41.

Peterson, C. and Gunn, S. (1984) *Therapeutic Recreation Programme Design: Principles and Procedures* , 3rd edn, Prentice-Hall, Englewood Cliffs, NJ.

Popcorn, F. (1991) *The Popcorn Report*, Doubleday, New York.

Seligman, M. (1991) *Learned Optimism*, Alfred A. Knopf, New York.

Sinnott-Oswald, M., Gliner, J.A. and Spencer, K.C. (1991) Supported and sheltered employment: quality of life issues among workers with disabilities. *Education and Training in Mental Retardation*, **26**(4), 388–97.

Wehman, P. (1993) *The ADA Mandate for Social Change*, ERIC Document Reproduction Services No. ED 354660.

Weinberg, N. (1984) Physically disabled people assess the quality of their lives. *Rehabilitation Literature*, **45**(1/2), 12–15.

A focus on the individual, theory and reality: making the connection through the lives of individuals

3

Dimity Peter

INTRODUCTION

I am interested in promoting ideas, discussions, research and actions that will improve the lives of individuals with a disability, but what I have to say applies equally to people with and without disabilities. I believe there are some shared values within our society about what constitutes the 'good life' or quality of life for ourselves or our loved ones, with or without a disability. One does not need to be a human service worker or researcher to know if 'good' things are happening for ourselves, our sons, daughters, parents, spouse or friends within societal institutions such as schools, hospitals, recreation programmes or employment.

Taylor (1994) argues that 'quality of life' is a useful 'sensitizing concept' in that it focuses research on the broader life-defining issues by attempting to comprehend the perspective of the person with a disability. He argues that this is important because historically research has predominantly focused on outcomes or programmes and the perspective of the person being studied has often been ignored. Taylor argues further that attempts to limit, define or measure quality of life diminish the usefulness and relevance of the concept. This creates a dilemma; how can one discuss a topic that one is unwilling to define? However, the point is well taken and the question that remains is, does trying to define and research quality of life drive away its essence, the very thing one is trying to ascertain?

Many authors in this book and others have attempted to define quality of life. I am choosing to use this term as a sensitizing concept and the description of quality of life in this chapter is not intended as a definitive statement. Throughout this chapter, quality of life refers to those aspects of one's life or lifestyle that contribute to, or the absence of those things that diminish, one's well-being. Inherent in this would be opportunities to fulfil one's needs, opportunities to grow and learn and opportunities to become a participant or contributor within the larger society.

This perception of what constitutes quality of life may well reflect some of the writer's biases and should be taken into account when reading the data presented later in the chapter. The intention in this chapter is to notionally describe quality of life for an individual rather than define it or measure it.

ISSUES OF QUALITY OF LIFE

SOME COMPONENTS

I believe there are four important components in a discussion about quality of life:

1. knowledge of or 'knowing' an individual;
2. an understanding of their circumstances;
3. some insight into how they experience their circumstances;
4. a reflection of such experiences against the current mores or values of the culture.

In the current climate of human service provision it is often difficult to 'know' the individuals being supported. In particular, high caseloads, increasing bureaucratic requirements and staff turnover work against the acquisition and retention of such information. Who is the person being served or supported? What are their most pressing and important needs? How have these experiences shaped or moulded their identity? What are this person's interests and capacities? Answers to these questions are needed to begin a discourse about a person's 'quality of life.'

It is often difficult to perceive services other than through the 'eyes' of the service system. Sometimes a person's life is characterized by segregation, social isolation, lack of opportunities to learn and contribute, lack of choice and so forth. Alternatively a person's life is often considerably enriched by the involvement of their family, by a relationship with a particular person or by participation in a particular activity. It is important to be able to identify those characteristics that enrich or diminish a person's life and lifestyle.

It is also important, if not critical, to understand the way an individual perceives their life circumstances. However, it is problematic to see quality of life exclusively as a subjective experience, akin to a measure of contentment. Many people with disabilities have a very narrow range of life experiences and lack the knowledge of how things could be different. Quality of life assumes a referent. How can one think about quality of life without having something (or someone) with which to compare it?

What is one's frame of reference if one has limited experience of the world? It is hard to be discriminating about matters of quality in a world about which one knows very little. For example, people with disabilities who live in large restrictive residential settings who experience many abuses and degradations (as perceived by the larger society) may say that they have a 'good life' from a lack of understanding of how it could be different. Alternatively, such people may say they have a 'good life' for a variety of other reasons including fear, a desire to please or not understanding the question and so forth (Stensman, 1985; Wolfensberger, 1994).

Finally, the notion of quality of life is culturally specific so it is important to take into account this relativity. If it is culturally normative to have an education, employment, your own home and so on, then it is important to ascertain if an individual with a disability is extended the same opportunities, security and well-being afforded to the rest of society.

If the thrust of the notion of quality of life is to improve the lives of individuals, then research paradigms are needed that can take this into account. Most of us have aspects of our lives we find deeply satisfying. These positive aspects often coexist with other facets of our lives that are problematic. This chapter discusses the relevance and benefits of qualitative research in revealing the satisfying and the problematic as they pertain to individuals. It goes on to explore both the satisfying and problematic from the perspective of Barry,* a man who is blind and has been labelled as mentally retarded.

THE RELEVANCE AND BENEFITS OF QUALITATIVE RESEARCH TO QUALITY OF LIFE

Although this chapter will focus specifically on the benefits of qualitative research in illuminating issues relating to quality of life, it is important to note that in order to deepen our understanding of the concept of the quality of people's lives it is useful to use the broadest range of research paradigms. There are benefits to both quantitative and qualitative research paradigms and methodologies. Qualitative and quantitative methods answer different research questions and suit the different personal styles and values of the researcher (Glesne & Peshkin, 1992). Clearly, there exists a plethora of research questions which should generate the full spectrum of research methodologies, each enriching and enhancing our understanding of the issues.

Qualitative research is defined by Taylor & Bogdan (1984) as 'research that produces descriptive data: people's own written or spoken words and

* All names of people, places and services have been changed.

observable behaviour' (p5). Although qualitative research is essentially descriptive in nature, it frequently encompasses interpretation as well. Some of the following aspects of qualitative methodology suggest how well suited such an approach is to examining the complex issues around quality of life.

Qualitative research is able to shed some light on the complexities and ambiguities of what a quality lifestyle might be for a person (or persons) with a disability

Qualitative research assumes that there are multiple perspectives with which to view the world and there is no 'single truth' that needs to be revealed (Bogdan & Biklen, 1982). Eisner (1981) noted that qualitative research is 'less concerned with the discovery of truth than with the creation of meaning ... truth implies singularity and monopoly. Meaning implies relativism and diversity. Truth is more closely wedded to consistency and logic, meaning to diverse interpretation and coherence' (p9). Because the notion of quality of life is multifaceted, touching many aspects of people's lives, such a methodology is able to explore these many dimensions in a coherent way.

Therefore qualitative research can focus on how the various participants view the issue of 'quality of life'. The perspective of the person with a disability should be paramount (Schalock, 1994), but the perspective of parents and human service workers can also be captured by such a methodology. A comparison or contrast of views is likely to deepen our understanding of the issues at hand.

It is clear from the current literature that the notion of quality of life is indeed complex and encompasses complex relationships between society, human services and the person with a disability, as well as a multitude of life characteristics that could be subjectively evaluated (see for example, Brown, Bayer & McFarlane, 1989). Qualitative research is well suited to teasing out the significance of some of these relationships and the complexities of some of the more subjective issues related to individual personal characteristics.

The qualitative approach is well suited to unravelling the fundamental elements of quality of life. Is quality of life about relationships or the sorts of choices we have? Or is it about having sufficient resources to gain access to 'the good life'? Is quality of life about realizing our gifts and capacities? Or can quality of life be equated with good service quality? Within the qualitative paradigm it is possible to identify the significance and the relationship between these (and other) threads for individuals. The paradigm is well suited to clarifying the role and impact these complex and interwoven threads have in the fabric of people's lives.

Qualitative research often attempts to understand people from their own perspective

Within the paradigm of qualitative research, the researcher attempts to obtain the participant's own account of their experiences. A theme consistently arising from quality of life research is that definitions of quality of life should incorporate the subjective experiences of the individual with a disability (Goode & Hogg, 1994). As far back as 1967, the noted sociologist Becker argued that qualitative research has a growing tradition of taking the side of the oppressed, rather than the 'official' or 'systems' view. Taylor (1994) argued that the notion of quality of life had brought a renewed interest in unravelling the opinions and feelings that individuals with disabilities have.

One of the important aspects of qualitative research is that it opens the possibility that the informants can 'lead' the direction of the research. It is possible that the informants can shed light on issues not previously raised by professionals or researchers. The agenda of what is important, from the perspective of the person with a disability, can potentially be exposed by the qualitative research methodology. Alternatively, such a paradigm can also potentially be used to control the view of the world that people with disabilities have. Furthermore, it can potentially reinforce negative views/stereotypes that exist about people with disabilities. Arguably, neither of these options is likely to improve the lives of people with disabilities.

Qualitative research takes a holistic view of an informant's life

Quality of life cannot just be understood by isolating particular variables. It is important that one also has a holistic view of the informant's life. Goode (1988) noted that qualitative research 'maintain(s) that the everyday existence of human beings has an integrity or totality which cannot be dissected into variables and measures without being unfaithful to, and essentially altering our understanding of the social structures of everyday reality' (p7). Qualitative research is therefore particularly suited to maintaining a holistic view of the informant which is integral to many of the notions of quality of life.

Qualitative research contextualizes the findings within a social or cultural framework

Qualitative research is most often conducted in natural settings, in the places where people live, work and enjoy themselves (Taylor & Bogdan, 1984). These are the settings in which one is trying to gauge quality of life. The context of behaviour is a crucial factor in understanding its meaning. Because behaviour and one's perceptions are so inextricably linked to social context, it is impossible to decipher the meaning of events and feelings unless the context is understood. Because quality of life is inextricably linked to one's environment, qualitative research is able to capture the context and the informant's perspective as well as the nature of the relationship between them.

Qualitative research has strong internal validity

Taylor & Bogdan (1984) noted that qualitative research lent itself to strong internal validity as it was 'designed to ensure a close fit between the data and what people actually say and do ... the qualitative research obtains first hand knowledge of social life unfiltered through concepts, operational definitions and rating scales' (p7). This internal validity is enhanced when researchers quote extensively from the data to demonstrate their findings.

SOME ISSUES OR LIMITATIONS OF QUALITATIVE RESEARCH

Reliability and other forms of validity

Emerson (1983), in his discussion of the credibility of qualitative research findings, noted that the traditional techniques for ensuring reliability and validity do not fit qualitative analysis and data. Therefore a variety of different procedures have been developed to increase the likelihood of credible findings. Emerson suggested that 'rich data' collected over a long period of time, using a variety of procedures, are likely to increase the credibility of the findings as the likelihood of observer bias and responder duplicity diminish under these conditions.

Other authors have tried to develop analogues to the concepts of reliability and validity to apply to qualitative data (Emerson, 1983). Typically, reliability refers to the replicability of the data. Given that different researchers may be investigating different perspectives or different phenomena in the same setting, one would not anticipate two or more researchers producing the same findings (although one would hope that they would not be contradictory). Bogdan & Biklen (1982) suggested, 'Qualitative researchers tend to view reliability as a fit between what they record as data and what actually occurs in the setting under study' (p44).

The issue of generalizability

Choosing just one informant (or a small number of informants) presents the methodological dilemma of generalizability. Such studies have traded the possibility of obtaining a thinner description of a number of people for a far richer and more complete understanding of one person's life. However, what we learn from one person with a disability will not be irrelevant to other people with disabilities. Although one needs to be circumspect about the circumstances in which one can generalize, Eisner (1981) noted in his discussion about generalization from a single case that 'Generalization is possible because of the belief that the general resides in the particular and because what one learns for a particular one applies to other situations' (p7). Donmeyer (1990) and Scholfield (1990) have suggested the concept of generalizability needs to be reconceptualized and perhaps broadened to encompass the issues raised by qualitative methodology.

There is a growing tradition in sociology and anthropology of 'life stories' where one person's life provides an insight to larger social phenomena (Plummer, 1983). For example, Shaw (1930, 1931) explored the life stories of various Chicago delinquents; such studies illuminated socialization processes, social conditions and social institutions. Heyl's (1979) documentation of Ann, a prostitute, spoke to the larger issue of how women were socialized into prostitution. Similarly, Klockars' (1975) chronicles of the life of a thief shed light on the social organization of small-time theft in the USA. Lewis (1959, 1961, 1964, 1969) undertook a number of portrayals of poor families in Mexico and Puerto Rico which powerfully illustrated the propagation of poverty. Bogdan (1974) documented the life history of a transsexual. The book sheds light on both the mental health system in which she was embroiled and the nature of feminine/masculine behaviour.

Researcher bias

Becker (1967) noted that 'There is no position from which sociological research can be done that is not biased in one or another way' (p22). In sociological terms, value-free research is unattainable. The fantasy of value-free research has been adequately debunked by many other authors (Gouldner, 1970; Rist, 1977; Scriven, 1972). However, good qualitative research is empirical and strives for an honest representation and accurate descriptions of the subjective. One argument is that the impact of the researcher's opinions, prejudices and other biases can be minimized.

Most qualitative researchers are concerned with the effect their biases might have on the data they produce as it may reduce the potency and breadth of their findings. Some qualitative researchers include their own reflections on possible prejudices in their field notes or data collection. Others ask colleagues to examine their data in order to detect any aberrations. Nevertheless, these steps are only limiting, not extinguishing researcher bias.

A declaration of the researcher's biases assists the reader to interpret the findings. Such declarations do not invalidate the information, but rather enrich and contextualize the findings. For example, it would be absurd to dismiss the first-person accounts of those with a disability within the service system as biased and invalid as the very subjectivity of the material is its essence. Such accounts have served to deepen and enrich our understanding (Kennedy, 1993; Martinez, 1990; Ward, 1990).

Although qualitative research is usually not driven by overt hypothesis testing, it is still assumption driven. Researchers do not enter into research without a view of the world or some notion of what is likely to be 'discovered'. Glesne & Peshkin (1992) argue that the influences of values, attitudes and interests are in fact the strengths and insights from which the researcher can construct a narrative or make sense of what has been observed. Both arguments agree that, when presenting findings, it is helpful if researchers state their likely biases and values. In conjunction with relevant quotes from the data, the readers can decide for themselves the subjectivity of the interpretation.

Phillips (1990) argues that objectivity could be redefined as a philosophical stance where one presents rational evidence that is open to critical evaluation or refutation and hence eliminates or at least minimizes bias. Phillips argues that this stance is the hallmark of 'objectivity' and it is important to strive for within both qualitative and quantitative paradigms.

THE CONTRIBUTION OF CASE STUDIES TO UNDERSTANDING THE NOTION OF QUALITY OF LIFE

The manifestation or reality of a 'good life' or a decent quality of life can only be truly understood in the context of an individual's life. It is important to capture the essence of the individual's experience – in texts, in educational programmes, in research and as a reference point for human service programme changes. Clearly, each individual situation will have much to teach us and different individuals will provide different insights. It is therefore critical that we understand how quality of life is manifested in a number of different individuals' lives – in different countries, in different service models and in individuals with differing needs and competencies. In this way our learning can be enhanced and significant and positive changes can be made to improve the quality of life for individuals with a disability. Keeping a strong connection between the theoretical and the actuality of quality of life maintains the validity of the construct and ensures applicability.

It is within this context that Barry's 'story' is told. Both the problematic and satisfying aspects of Barry's life as seen from his perspective are described and discussed. This information was collected using qualitative research methods.

QUALITY OF LIFE AS AN INDIVIDUAL PHENOMENON

At the time of the study,* Barry was a 40-year-old man with a great sense of humour. He was totally blind and labelled as mentally retarded. It is important to note that in over 160 hours of interviews and participant observation with Barry, he did not once mention the term 'quality of life'. It is not a framework through which he saw his world. This is not to suggest that he could not discuss good or problematic aspects of his life but rather that his world was not ordered by such categories or distinctions. Quality of life is a theoretical construct developed by and for professionals. It is only useful in as far as it enhances our understanding of the lives of people with disabilities. With this understanding it is possible to improve services to enable the individual to experience a better quality of life. It is important to remind ourselves that the notion of quality of life is only a vehicle through which we can grasp at more elusive concepts – creating a 'good life', fulfilling one's potential and so forth.

ABOUT BARRY

Barry lived in a group home with seven other people, similarly labelled as mentally retarded and blind. His group home was a large house where staff provide 24-hour supervision (Barry's term). The residence was operated by a non-profit agency called Poulson Incorporated.

Poulson Incorporated also operated a supported employment programme that supported Barry to work at the Thompson Hotel which was a prestigious hotel located some distance from the group home. Poulson Incorporated employed a job coach to find the job for Barry. The job coach then trained Barry to do the work which was to fold the clean washing and to load and unload the washing and drying machines. Once Barry had learned the job, the job coach gradually withdrew her support. At the time of the study, Barry's job coach visited about once every one or two weeks. Barry was paid approximately $5 per hour which was above the minimum wage.

Church was very important to Barry and he attended the service on Sunday as well as other church activities such as social occasions or study groups. Barry also enjoyed doing courses, going out shopping, eating out or virtually any other activity that was offered that enabled him to be out in the community.

---

* The data collected for the study were the basis of the author's doctoral dissertation.

WHO IS BARRY?

This is Barry's own account of his background using his own words.

I was born in a hospital. I knew my parents and they took good care of me. When I was sick my mother took care of me. I had chicken pox and measles. My father went to work and brought money home to support us. Sometimes he worked a double shift. My mother stayed at home and cleaned house. She was a housewife. My brothers, Jack, Pat, Phillip, Joey, Eddy and Tony went to school. I had a twin sister Mildred. I remember I had speech problems when I was little, couldn't talk yet and had problems walking.

My mother got sick and couldn't take care of us no more. She had cancer of the liver and pneumonia. My dad was very sick. He had a bad heart attack. He did a lot of smoking and had high blood pressure. I was sent to Johnson (a residential institution) when my mother got sick and couldn't take care of us no more. We didn't want to go to Johnson, me and my sister cried.

Johnson was an institution, a state school. The staff there took me to the doctor. I kept getting sick. I met friends at Johnson. During the day I did occupational therapy and speech therapy. Occupational therapy is putting parts together. Speech therapy teaches you to talk slowly. I had a girlfriend there. I saw my parents once in a while, not a lot.

Then I moved to the Smithville Developmental Centre, 1963, May 10th because they thought I got too smart for it (Johnson) and they didn't have any programmes for me. They taught me a lot of things at Smithville; mobility, and how to prepare meals, how to tell time, tie shoe strings and zip my coat. I had speech therapy then and school. I worked on the Braille board. They didn't take the time to teach me Braille, they ran out of patience. I liked to play Braille cards. The staff encouraged me to talk slower. I had music class in the education building.

I liked it there because I could visit my sister whenever I wanted to. A lot of staff there were good. They gave me medicine when I was sick. Most residents were kind to me there, like Peggy. They worried about me when I got hurt.

I worked in the sheltered workshop. I did jumper cables and stuffing envelopes in books. Also did hockey games and gas pumps for toys. I counted five men and put a rubber band around them. I got paid every two weeks. I went clothes shopping with the money.

They gave me mellaril (psychotic drug) to calm me down. Got upset whenever I couldn't find something. Margaret Casety (doctor) had to put me on mellaril, thioridazine. They stopped me from scratching my chin, they said no. They had me on a behaviour programme. If I behaved I got a star to go out to lunch.

They took me to Niagara Falls, went out for rides in the van and out to dinner and breakfast. They took me bowling and swimming and they took me for a hair cut. They also took me outside and we sat on the swing. Sometimes we went to the canteen for lunch. They had volunteers for me too, Mr and Mrs Salter and another girl I had named Jodie. On my birthday they gave me a party, a celebration. They put me and my twin sister together. Then our parents would take us home every year.

I moved to Belltown because the social worker wanted me to try a different programme. I came to Belltown October 26, 1977. I was scared I wouldn't be able to visit my sister no more. The social worker said I can come and visit her. I didn't want to come to Belltown, but when I came here I made new friends. When I first came I cried.

HOW DOES QUALITATIVE RESEARCH ANSWER THE QUESTION: WHAT IS IMPORTANT IN BARRY'S QUALITY OF LIFE?

Although, as mentioned previously, the concept of quality of life was not a framework through which Barry saw his life, it was possible to capture that which was positive and important in his life and that which was problematic and then discuss this within the framework of the broader society. This information was collected in a number of ways.

DATA COLLECTION

Semistructured interviewing

Barry could answer simple and direct questions in a concrete way. His words above are an example of his response to the question: 'Let's pretend that you are going to meet my parents, what would you tell them about your life before you came to Belltown?'.

Informal interview/participant observation

Most of my understanding about Barry came from informal conversations conducted with him over a three-year period. Usually such conversations occurred over a meal. We would talk about what had happened during the week and often Barry had something important on his mind that he wanted to tell me. During the meal, Barry did most of the talking and I would prompt with questions about an event at work or church. I made a written record of our conversations as he spoke, which was possible because of Barry's slow rate of speech. This information was later analysed.

Participant observation

I was able to observe Barry in a variety of settings: at home, at work, at church, at classes, at parties and so forth. Usually in such settings I was an observer collecting information about Barry's behaviour. However, some settings demanded that I participate in the occasion at hand; for example, at church it would have looked obtrusive if I did not join in the rituals of kneeling and singing.

ANALYSIS

The information learned from Barry has been reorganized so that it is put into context and makes sense to the reader. The analysis presented below is selecting the best way to illuminate Barry's life, so that we can learn from it. As Emerson (1983) noted, the qualitative researcher 'organizes what might otherwise be irrelevant and unconnected events and features into some patterns' (p22).

Through using each of these techniques over a sustained period of time, I believe I developed a valid understanding about Barry's perception of what is good and what is problematic in his life. As a prelude to providing a 'second person' understanding, I would like to provide Barry's description of his life. This description is his response to the question, 'How would you describe yourself and your life to someone who didn't know you?'.

I have blue eyes, brown hair, am five foot six inches and weigh 315 pounds [his estimate of weight and height did not concur with my evaluation of him being approximately 6 foot tall and of average weight]. I have a problem with my eyes. I am a good worker, I do my work good and neat. I am punctual, have perfect attendance and come in when I am scheduled even though I don't like to get up (in the morning).

I live at 215 Lair Street with seven people. It is a nice home. I like the staff and the residents. The staff care and meet my needs. They give me a birthday party once a year.

I am a member of the church. I have a lot of friends even though I don't believe it (that I have a lot of friends). The staff (at the residence) and the pastor are trying to make me realize that people care. I disliked Lansen Avenue (former residence). I like to go to church on Sundays and Wednesdays. I like the pastor and I like the people at Belltown Assembly of God church. I have a lot of friends there. They gave me a birthday party and they invite me to their homes for holidays.

I like kids and I share my stuff with people when I have too much. I buy people birthday cards and presents. I like to go shopping and fishing. I also like to go out for dinner, breakfast, lunch and dessert. I like to make tapes and buy new clothes. I also help in the kitchen and keep my room neat. I empty my garbage can when it is full.

ACTIVITIES

Church

Barry actively and tenaciously pursued membership of a church. For Barry, as for many people, church was an important social activity. In his opinion a good church was one that had many social events and friendly people and particularly people who would invite him to their home during the religious holidays (Christmas and Easter).

Barry spoke of his 'church home' meaning a church where he felt he belonged. The quest for a 'church home' was a long one for Barry. Prior to the study, Barry had attended a Catholic church. At the beginning of the study Barry attended a Mennonite church. He had asked a staff member at his annual review meeting if he could attend. Barry said of this church, '[It was a] Good church, lets you get to know people. Catholic church you don't. People at the Catholic church ignore me'.

Barry also initiated his attendance at the weekly Bible study course by telling the staff member he wanted to attend. Through Bible study he met more people whom he called his friends. When asked why he wanted to attend Bible study, Barry replied, 'So I don't get bored'. It appeared that the act of going out and being busy was at least as important as the content of the event.

His closest church friend was Fred who picked him up each week to take him to church. Barry subsequently had long periods of time (five months) where he was required to work on Sundays. Although he was disgruntled at his inability to attend church, staff at the house and the supported employment agency did not see the issue as particularly important and Barry's discontent was dismissed. During this time Barry had an occasional weekend off but had difficulty contacting Fred.

Eventually, a new job coach assisted Barry to alter his work schedule to have Sunday off. With only intermittent contact with Fred, Barry started looking elsewhere for a 'church home'. Another church was found through Barry's housemate, who had been introduced to this church by a staff member of the sheltered workshop she attended. The first connection with this church was again made through the introduction of a client by a staff member.

Overall Barry was very content with his new church, the Belltown Assembly of God. It was considered by Barry to be a good church: it provided transportation on Sundays, there was a Sunday school, a music-filled church service and many other various church activities such as Wednesday evening worship, the men's retreat, men's breakfasts and a monthly singles' convention. Barry attended as many of the church activities as he could. The only limiting factors were finding transportation and his work commitments. Any special upcoming activities were spoken about at length as he anticipated what would happen. After the event he reminisced about what he had done and what people had said.

Barry participated in the church service that frequently lasted up to two hours. For at least half that time the congregation was actively involved by singing and clapping. Although Barry did not sing he had a good sense of rhythm and clapped along. It was a lively service with a large proportion of the time devoted to song. There was also an impressive orchestral accompaniment including piano, organ, trumpet, violin, tuba, drums, saxophone and clarinet. The music was supplemented by a technical sound system.

Barry was baptized and joined the church and he said that this meant he was 'not a Catholic any more, Pentecostal now'. Barry received his membership card and a membership letter in the mail and he proudly showed it to everyone. He had a staff member read the letter confirming his membership to his housemates. Barry announced that he had found his 'church home'.

Barry's church home was clearly a source of satisfaction and contributed greatly to his quality of life. Nevertheless, there were some areas of discontent. Church members were not always willing to invite Barry home for Christmas and Easter and this was a great source of anguish for him. Barry consistently asked his pastor to help him become 'more involved in church activities' although it was evident that he was already one of the more active members of the congregation. Barry frequently said he wanted to 'do more with my church friends'. He complained that few church members invited him to their homes. Barry reported, 'Pastor said ... [I] can't force them to open up homes to you ... but they love you. [They are] too busy working'.

Reflections about Barry's church experiences

Finding a good match between a person and an activity In my experience there is frequently careful planning to match a person with a disability to an interest. It could be locating a hockey club, a gym or fitness centre, a stamp-collecting club or a church, whatever reflects the person's interests. However, once a group is found, there is little evaluation of how well the particular group matches the needs and interests of the individual. Barry clearly demonstrates that not every church matches his idea of a 'church home'. For Barry, it was important to find a church where he would be welcomed and have an opportunity to participate in a range of activities. It took visits to many churches to find a better match. It was a long and active process.

Listening to what individuals say is important to them Although attendance at church was clearly significant for Barry and his quality of life, this was not recognized by the staff supporting him. For many months Barry clearly complained that he did not like to work on Sunday. He said this to his boss, his case manager, his counsellor, to the house staff and to his job coach. His complaints were not acted upon and Barry stated that people said 'lucky to have [a] job'. It was not until Barry's job coach changed and the new person negotiated with Barry's employer that he had Sundays rostered 'off'. This simple step of listening assumes that staff or support workers believe that people with disabilities have something important to say about how they wish to conduct their lives. Acting on Barry's expressed wishes made a huge impact upon Barry's lifestyle and psychological well-being.

The role of staff in making connections with the community For both churches that Barry attended, the initial connection was made through a human service worker. Because Barry had lived a very segregated lifestyle he had little interface with the broader community. The strongest connections Barry had with the community prior to his community-based employment was through human service workers. This situation was quite problematic because Barry's experience was that many 'staff' were unwilling to invite him into their personal domains, such as church and family life.

Good does not necessarily mean perfect Although a good match was found between Barry's needs and desires and his church, the situation was clearly not ideal. This is important to acknowledge because this meant that there may have existed possibilities or opportunities to improve Barry's church experience. Yet, with the structure of human services that supported Barry, the creation of a greater sense of belonging to his church home did not seem achievable. Human services, as constructed for Barry, appeared to have limited capacity to generate some of the 'good life' that he needed and wanted, such a feeling that he belonged to his church.

Subjective experiences are not always that obvious It is clear that church was a significant and positive component of Barry's quality of life. Many would make the assessment that Barry was very involved in his church community. He participated in the range of church activities, more than most of the congregation. At the minimum he would be involved in church-related activities twice a week. Yet for Barry, this was not enough; he clearly and repeatedly stated that he wanted to be more involved. Barry's subjective experience was in direct contrast to more typical perceptions or measurements of activity.

Work

Prior to working at the hotel, Barry worked in a sheltered workshop assembling pens. He received little remuneration for his work, the work was repetitive and when there was no work, which was quite frequent, the staff disassembled the pens that would be put together the next day. The workshop closed when Barry and the other employees were found employment in the community. Early in the study, on his rostered days off from the hotel, Barry liked to volunteer at the sheltered workshop. I believe this was because it provided more meaningful activity than being at home and that within such a setting he had positive social interactions with both the staff and other workers.

For most of the duration of the study Barry worked in the laundry of the housekeeping department at the prestigious Thompson Hotel. This was Barry's first job in the community and he was very proud of his work and his wage of $5 an hour. He also enjoyed the status of working. Barry attended all the official celebrations organized by the hotel such as the Christmas party, Valentine's party and employee acknowledgments. He was once awarded the 'employee of the month' and after two years of service, received a plaque at a special luncheon for him and a handful of other employees.

Intermittently, Barry spoke about changing his job, but the management at Thompson was very keen to keep him on. Throughout most of the research period he vacillated between staying and leaving the position. During an interview the manager said he was one of their most reliable workers: 'If he is rostered to work then he always shows up'.

Barry noted about work:

> Tina [supervisor] said, '[I am] Part of the family here. Don't want you to leave.' ... I don't want to [change jobs] ... [They] Give me what I want, Saturday, Sunday and Mondays off ... Tina talked to me about it before. If I go somewhere else, pay won't be as good. Have to learn it all over again. Won't have it as nice at another job. Told me a few months ago. I won't have it as good over there. [She] Said '[I am] Very lucky to take you in, hire you' ... Thursday get cheque every week, put in savings account, when weekends come, get plenty of rest ... money I get is to buy more stuff.

Julie was the laundry supervisor who was disliked by all of her co-workers, including Barry. By the end of the study, Barry called Julie his 'enemy'. Julie's manner was gruff and she discouraged social interaction in the laundry and reportedly yelled at people from time to time, including Barry. Barry's description captured the mood in the laundry: '[Julie] Says you guys [co-workers] should work instead of talking ... You guys drive me up the wall gabbing. She says it's all we do ... [I] Stayed out of it, kept working instead'.

However, Barry reported that he was also frequently a recipient of Julie's wrath and she frequently yelled at him. Everyone, including Barry, was far more easy-going and relaxed on Julie's days off. Some aspects of the social milieu of the work environment detracted from Barry's quality of life.

Clearly work was a significant aspect of Barry's quality of life. It gave him status and a role, something meaningful to do during the day and it provided a wage which enabled him to partake in many other activities such as holidays, dining out, shopping and so forth. Yet the social realm was problematic, to the extent that Barry was ambivalent about staying in the job.

Some reflections about Barry's work experience

Addressing the social aspects of work: match between work environment and the individual Although his contribution as a worker was acknowledged by his co-workers, Barry did not become part of the unofficial social network in the laundry. The work placement was a good match for Barry in terms of his competencies. He was given tasks that he could do as competently as the other staff. It was a compact environment in which he could find his way around and his contribution to the smooth running of the hotel was tangible. Having a wage also provided him with many material benefits, not previously accessible. However, apart from Julie's personality and gruff manner, the social environment at the Thompson Hotel was not a good one for Barry.

The noisy environment created by the washers and dryers was a deterrent to interaction with Barry. Although Barry could understand his co-workers who raised their voice over the noise, Barry spoke in a low drone and it was almost impossible to decipher what he was saying over the noise unless one was standing very close to him. Barry was able to hear, but unable to participate in many of the social interactions in the laundry.

Unlike the other workers, Barry primarily worked at a table by himself, sorting the linen and laying flat in neat piles the towels, bath mats, pillow cases and wash cloths. Although in a room with other people, he was usually socially and physically disconnected from them, within hearing distance of what others had to say, but not within talking distance. As a result, for a significant proportion of the time he worked alone.

Most of the social interaction occurred when people were folding sheets together, since it was a task that was shared. Some of his co-workers had developed quite warm friendships between each other and talked incessantly over the din during the folding of the sheets. Although Barry could fold sheets rather well and at a speed only marginally slower than his co-workers, he was not given this shared task as often as the other workers.

Barry's opportunities to develop social relationships were also significantly diminished with a change in the smoking rule. Barry did not smoke but most of his co-workers did. At the beginning of the study, employees were permitted to smoke cigarettes in the employee cafeteria during breaks. There were three work breaks: morning and afternoon breaks of 15 minutes each and a lunch break of 30 minutes. Barry was always accompanied by one of his co-workers to breaks, as he needed a guide through the busy and cluttered passageways. Barry and his co-workers sat together and enjoyed a conversation of which he was frequently a part.

When the non-smoking rule came into force, Barry's co-workers continued to take him to the cafeteria, but they quickly snatched a cup of coffee and a bite to eat and raced outside to enjoy a cigarette, where most of the social chatter took place. Although there were usually other people from other sections in the hotel in the cafeteria, Barry typically sat alone until one of his co-workers returned from their sojourn outside.

In conclusion, although Barry was immersed in a community setting, at work he remained relatively socially isolated. Even though the laundry was not a social place to work, other co-workers were able to forge friendships. Perhaps for some, other than Barry, social needs would be met in other life domains or perhaps some people need less interaction than others. However, Barry appeared to be very isolated and very lonely at work.

Barry's home

In many ways Barry enjoyed where he was living. He generally liked the staff and the people with whom he lived. He had a close relationship with Mark who had come from the same institution at about the same time Barry came to Belltown. Barry often invited Mark to breakfast with us. Barry had a room of his own and 24-hour staff supervision. Although I would not say that Barry had all or most of his social needs met in the house, he was never alone and this was important to him. Furthermore, the staff had his life well organized, attending regular dental and doctor appointments, weekly counselling, twice-yearly review meetings, house meetings once a week, taxis organized for work, bills paid, cash stored in the safe, weekly cooking rosters and menu planning, birthdays acknowledged, problems sorted out and so forth.

However, for all of the residents, including Barry, the house was not 'home'. At Christmas, Easter and Thanksgiving the house closed down and the residents went 'home' to their respective families. Barry had no sure place to go at these times and staying in an empty house had no appeal. He would frantically try to find a place to go during these times. Eventually, if the church was not forthcoming in offering somewhere, a staff member usually invited Barry to join their family at the last minute. For Barry the anticipation was excruciatingly painful: Where would he go, who would he be with? Again, the positive sits side by side with the problematic.

Staff were also keen that Barry move on to more 'independent living'. This means moving into an apartment without 24-hour staff supervision. This was discussed at every twice-yearly review meeting. However, Barry was adamant that this was not his desire and he was reluctant to participate in any programme that would improve his independent living skills, such as learning to cook a meal. I believe that Barry was afraid that in such a living arrangement, his social contacts would be severely diminished. In the way such arrangements were constructed, this is probably an accurate assessment. One resident had already made such a move and was a frequent visitor to the group home. She vividly described her loneliness and the fact that support staff were unreliable.

One of the most noticeable issues in Barry's house, from an observer's perspective, was the large turnover in staff: approximately 60 different staff in three years. I believed this must have had a big impact on Barry's quality of life, yet he seemed to accept such changes with equanimity. It would seem he had more important issues on his mind during our discussions.

Some reflections on Barry's home life

A home, not a house There is a very elusive and subtle difference between a house and a home. Capturing the qualitative essence of home would appear to be an important aspect of quality of life, at least for Barry. How to do this remains an unconquered challenge, at least in

Barry's life. There exist multiple dimensions to creating such intangibles and for Barry they include a sense of permanency, not being pushed into other residential settings and creating a place where one would enjoy celebrating the festive seasons with loved ones.

Ideologies may not take account of individuals' needs Although there are sound theoretical and values-based reasons to ensure that people with disability live as independently as possible, the way this was likely to have happened to Barry would have potentially diminished his quality of life. Within his current circumstances, Barry was already feeling lonely (see later section on friendships). An independent living situation would have meant less interaction with staff (because by definition it would have been less than 24-hour supervision) and fewer (or perhaps no) room mates. Given the large amount of time he spent at home, a reduction in staff and cohabitants would limit his social interactions even further. Any reduction in social interactions was perceived by Barry as negative.

On the other hand, undoubtedly Barry would learn new skills and abilities to cope without the full-time presence of staff. I am not advocating that people live in more restrictive settings, but rather suggesting services should look at identifying the barriers and obstacles for people to pursue a more independent lifestyle and then overcome them. For Barry the obstacle was social isolation.

ISSUES

There existed some unresolved issues in Barry's life that seemingly diminished his quality of life or sense of well-being. The problems revolved around being bored, the issue of friendship and not having a family.

BOREDOM

Doing nothing and boredom were constant themes in Barry's conversation. For Barry, being at home was 'boring'. When at home he sometimes listened to television, but noted he was 'not into television all the time'. He also had a 'read-out receiver' which was special radio equipment that had a transmission especially for people who were blind, but he noted, 'I don't use it much, it gets boring'. Barry also listened to a plethora of talking books (fiction transcribed to cassettes) borrowed from the library but he noted, 'Reading story books gets boring after a while'. Barry spent a significant proportion of his non-working hours at home, particularly on weekends, and these options did not adequately fill his hours or nourish his sense of well-being.

Barry was typically out four evenings a week, although during the summer it was less frequent. Staff at the house perceived this as a lot,

Barry perceived it as inadequate. This contrasts sharply with the words of the house manager, a mother of a four-year-old, who had chosen a very busy life for herself working full-time and a part-time graduate student:

> Barry does not like to stay home. It doesn't matter how much he goes out, he still complains that he doesn't go out enough. He always wants more. Keeping busy, keeping busy. Recreation. It drives me crazy. Keeping busy all the time. I don't know what it is. ... say to him you should have time just for you – leisure time – relaxation time instead of running around always doing something ... We have no idea what he thinks about when he has nothing to do. Barry viewed his social life as inadequate, but some staff at the group home had a different perspective.

Barry consistently and relentlessly raised the problem of boredom and lack of activity. He spoke out at the house meetings, at his biannual goal meetings, with his counsellor, with the house manager, with his pastor and his Sunday school teacher. When Barry interviewed the new house manager for the position, he asked, 'Do you plan recreation?'.

It appeared that Barry relied on staff to organize and pursue leisure activities. The problem regarding lack of activity was seen, by both Barry and the staff, as an issue of manpower; it was seen as strictly a lack of available staff to take Barry and the other residents out as much as they would like. The solution often touted, by Barry and the staff, was the acquisition of a volunteer, but one was not found for him.

Reflections on the issue of boredom

Staff perceptions may diverge from the perceptions of people with disabilities

This study was able to shed light on some reasons why this divergence emerged. First, being at home (for all except some of the staff in their 20s) meant time spent with spouse and/or family; that is, people whom one loved. For Barry, living in a group home lacked these emotional connections and, hence, it was not such a desirable place to be. Second, typically one spends a lot of time at home doing the chores of living: the constant cooking, cleaning, grocery shopping, paying bills, repairs and so forth. Barry had many of these chores of living provided for him by staff, giving him more time on his hands than most people would typically have. In particular, Saturdays and Mondays were virtually devoid of activity. Third, many people have a pastime. Some enjoy watching sport on television and others have a hobby or interest that sustains them. Barry had no real hobbies or interests. Fourth, the needs of staff sometimes conflicted with Barry's need for more social interactions. It is far easier for staff to manage the day-to-day running of a house for so many residents when people are content to sit at home. Searching with Barry for other social outlets was both challenging and time consuming.

Listening to and acting on Barry's stated wish for more activities

Again, it appeared that staff did not act on Barry's behalf to improve a very problematic aspect of his life. As noted previously, to address this issue would require staff and support workers to believe that Barry had something significant to say about his life and well-being. However, it is not clear from the data if this was the case. Alternative explanations about inaction are that staff may have been unable to (perhaps because of time) or did not have the expertise to assist Barry find more meaningful things to do to fill his time.

FAMILY

Barry did not have a 'significant other' whom he could call upon for support. At his first biannual review meeting, the first item of business was to identify a 'correspondent', described by the house manager as 'someone to notify if you were sick or something'. Barry suggested Mr and Mrs Salter whom he saw once a year. They lived about 200 miles away. Barry's caseworker whispered in an aside to the house manager, 'This is hard, Barry hasn't really got anyone'. A 'significant other' was usually a family member.

Barry's parents were apparently deceased and the whereabouts of his six brothers were unknown. Barry told me all his brothers had died. His twin sister, Mildred, was very important to him and was the primary reason he was reluctant to leave the institution. Mildred was described by Barry as 'retarded (because) she repeats everything you say'. She resided at the Smithville Developmental Centre where she had lived for the past 27 years. Barry visited her once a year. He remarked, 'Twin sister is [in the] same situation, no one [else] comes and visits her. Sad about [our] parents too, dead … [I am/She is] Only relative got left'.

Barry consistently noted, especially around the family occasions of Christmas, Easter and Thanksgiving, how hard it was for him not having a family. Barry frequently lamented the fact that he had no family and that he had no place where he belonged during these celebrations. When he first moved to Belltown, Barry returned to the institution for these occasions. The group home closed and everyone went 'home'. Barry's home was the Smithville Developmental Centre. Barry noted, '[I] Don't have family. Other people do … Angry I always have to run around on holidays. It's hard for me to cope with. … Bad moods around holiday time'.

Not only did Barry miss the experience of kin as a child belonging to a family, but also the opportunity that most of us have to create our own family as an adult. Marriage was not an expectation promoted by staff for people with disabilities, at least within the Poulson agency that supported Barry.

Reflections on the issue of family

When people with disabilities have lost their connections to family and loved ones, 'significant others' cannot be readily 'replaced' by the human service system. Perhaps this problem emphasizes the limitation of paid service and challenges us all to think of new paradigms in conceptualizing the way we construct services.

FRIENDSHIPS

Barry claimed friendships with 204 different people over the period of the research. This number was derived by asking Barry early in the research process to list his friends. This question was repeated intermittently and other people were added to the list as they arose in subsequent interviews. Of the 204, 87 were staff, 38 were other clients and 79 were community members (plus ten people whom I could not classify because Barry's descriptions were imprecise).

It would seem an incongruity that although Barry knew so many people, he frequently said he was lonely. He had no one on whom he could rely. Barry's perception of a friend was someone who did something for him. Barry noted that Stacey (one of his house managers) was his friend because 'she took me to get the bus'. Clare (Barry's job coach) was his friend because she 'found me a job'. Bill Bolst (a radio announcer) was his friend because he 'let me pick a song', following one visit to the radio station. Margaret Casety (the doctor at the institution) was his friend because she 'signed a paper saying I was blind'. It would seem that for Barry, a friend was somebody who acted in a friendly manner towards him or did something for him. Barry once noted that a friend was 'someone who comes up and says hello'.

It was in this way that Barry could cite 204 'friends'. This was not a case of Barry exaggerating his popularity, but a genuine difference in the way he defined friendship.

Reflections on the issue of friendships

The issue of loneliness would seem to relate to the absence of Barry's family, at least in part. However, it is also instructive to note that Barry is quite integrated, physically, in the community. Although perhaps his interactions were as frequent, as reflected by the number of people he knew, the depth and breadth of relationships appeared narrower than most ordinary citizens experience. Of special note is the absence of intense and intimate or very close friend types of relationship. Most of Barry's friendships would ordinarily be called acquaintanceships. This does not diminish the relationship that Barry has with his sister or with Mark (who moved with him from the institution), but is more a reflection of the cross-section of his relationships.

AN INTERESTING ABSENCE

Barry never spoke of his intellectual disability or his blindness as being a barrier or problem to his lifestyle or well-being. It was apparent from our conversations that from his perspective his disabilities *per se* were not an issue. The problems in Barry's life, as he saw them, were related to every-day living: his home, his work and his relationships. This is in direct con-trast to some of the writing in the field that implies that the major problem faced by people such as Barry is their disability. This research suggests this is not always the perspective of the person with a disability. Furthermore, this implies that the focus of many services should not be on the disability, but on other important life issues.

RESEARCHER BIASES

Given that Barry does not use a quality of life framework to reflect on his life, throughout this section I have in fact been an interpreter of Barry's quality of life. The assumption of such a role raises the thorny issues around validity discussed earlier in the chapter. In the introduction, four components were suggested as essential elements in considering quality of life issues for an individual. Given the duration of the research (three years) and the intensity of the data collection (weekly), I believe it is a reasonable assertion to say I have some knowledge of Barry, his circum-stances and how he perceives his circumstances. Furthermore, with this knowledge I am well placed to reflect on such experiences in the context of the wider society.

However, the issue of researcher bias is not so easily dismissed. As argued previously, one can at best hope to minimize such influences. It is useful for readers to understand the author's possible biases. I chose Barry as an informant because in comparison to other people with disabilities he had relatively frequent contact with the broader community, such as at work and church. I was interested in learning more about community integration. Yet at another level, my experiences as a professional working in the field were that, although services and support workers sometimes succeeded in facilitating physical integration, strong friendships, social participation and a real sense of belonging were frequently absent from the lives of people with disabilities. Indeed, this study confirmed that fact, at least for Barry. The reader must judge for themselves if the data convincingly fit the interpretation and how much of the interpretation has been invalidly driven (or enriched) by the researcher's preconceived ideas, experience and values.

RELEVANCE OF THIS RESEARCH PARADIGM FOR EVALUATION AND CHANGE

The implication of exploring quality of life issues for people with disabilities is that with our deeper understanding of the issues at stake, we are in a position to make changes that will enhance their lives. Potentially, our ever-growing understanding could be used to change the way we provide and deliver services. Because quality of life is such an individual phenomenon, clearly it is important that services evaluate how well they are serving their 'clientele'.

This chapter suggests that the first important criterion for evaluating the performance of an agency in creating positive life outcomes or a quality of life for people with disabilities is to involve the individual(s) concerned in the process. The qualitative methods of talking to individuals about their lives and coming to 'know' them and the context in which they live are central to any measurement (Goode & Hogg, 1994). This tenet appears to be generally accepted in the field, although for individuals with more severe disabilities the process of 'knowing' them can be a challenging one (Heal & Sigelman, 1990). Goode (1994) noted, 'Most believe that the collection of data reflecting how the individual sees his or her quality of life occupies an important and critical role in any research, evaluation, policy or programming using this concept (pvi)'.

The findings from this chapter also imply that if indeed services wish to focus on what is important to the person with a disability, then an in-depth understanding of that person is needed. The more we can understand about people in services, the more likely it is that we can come to know them and address their real needs (Klein, 1992). The methods used in this study suggest it is important to 'know' people in various settings: at home, at work, at church and so forth. The more we can come to know the individual being served, the more likely it is that our interpretations will be valid.

This study highlighted, at least in Barry's case, that service workers' understanding or perceptions of situations often differ considerably from those of the person being served. This suggests that it is important not to make assumptions about people with disabilities, including those who have been supported within an agency for a long period of time. Frequently, it would seem that the prism through which human service workers see the world is very different from the prism that colours the world for people with disabilities. Some of the methodologies discussed in this chapter suggest ways in which human service workers can see a person's situation in a different light. This would include trying to consciously articulate one's biases and assumptions.

Although the labels given to Barry by human services were not discussed in any detail in this chapter, it was evident that for Barry, such labels were not integral to his personal sense of identity or the way he saw his life. This finding is consistent with other quality of life-related studies that note that labels can be 'a barrier to understanding people on their own terms' (Taylor & Bogdan, 1990, p35). In order to conduct qualitative research it is important to put these labels aside. Klein (1992) argued that to provide good quality of life, people must receive support based on their individual needs rather than their labels.

This study reflected how complex the notion of quality of life is, even for one individual. Untangling the positive and problematic aspects of a person's life, when issues often do not lend themselves to categorizations of 'good' or 'bad', implies how important it is to have tools that can embrace the complexities and ambiguities of everyday life. Qualitative research and its methodologies have demonstrated in this study how such complexities can be understood, at least in part. Many researchers in the quality of life domains have noted how important it is to take a holistic approach (Brown, Brown & Bayer, 1994). Edgerton (1994) noted, 'Attempts to reduce the complex concept of life's quality to specific measures, scales or formulae are hazardous at best … one can hope that formulaic reductions of life to simplistic indices will be resisted (pii).' Related to this point is the sense gained from this study that many aspects of quality of life are not easily measured, but that insight and enlightenment are implicit in the descriptive nature of the information gathered.

Finally, this study identified and described some barriers Barry experienced in trying to move toward a better quality of life. Understanding such barriers is the first critical step needed before services can remove these obstacles so that people can continue to develop their potential.

CONCLUSION

In conclusion, it is argued that the lives of individuals can teach us much about service systems and the notion of quality of life. Knowledge of what contributes to and diminishes a person's well-being is a good foundation from which to implement service change, although I would recommend this be done in conjunction with value-based theories. Clearly, the understandings attained in this study are very person specific and yet there appear to be themes and issues that jump out in Barry's life, across a number of life domains.

Qualitative research is a powerful way to systematically gather information that enables us to understand the important aspects of someone's quality of life. Indeed, it is more than possible to make the leap from theory to practice through understanding the lives of individuals with a disability. Through understanding the problematic and satisfying in Barry's life, light has been shed on some of the service areas requiring rethinking. As Geertz (1983) noted, 'Where an interpretation comes from does not determine where it can be impelled to go. Small facts speak to large issues (p54)'.

REFERENCES

Becker, H. (1967) Whose side are we on? *Social Problems*, **14**, 239–47.

Bogdan, R. (1974) *Being Different*, John Wiley, New York.

Bogdan, R. and Biklen, S. (1982) *Qualitative Research for Education: An Introduction to Theory and Methods*, Allyn & Bacon, Boston, MA.

Brown, R., Bayer, M. and MacFarlane, C. (1989) *Rehabilitation Programs: Performance and Quality of Life of Adults with Developmental Handicaps*, Lugus, Toronto.

Brown, R., Brown, P. and Bayer, M. (1994) A quality of life model: new challenges arising from a six year study, in *Quality of Life for Persons with Disabilities*, (ed. D. Goode), Brookline Books, Cambridge, MA.

Donmeyer, R. (1990) Generalizability and the single-case study, in *Qualitative Inquiry in Education: The Continuing Debate*, (eds E. Eisner and A. Peskin), Columbia University Teachers College, New York, 175-200.

Edgerton, R. (1994) Foreword, in *Quality of Life for Persons with Disabilities*, (ed. D. Goode), Brookline Books, Cambridge, MA.

Eisner, E. (1981) On the difference between scientific and artistic approaches to qualitative research. *Educational Researcher*, **4**, 4–9.

Emerson, R. (1983) Introduction, in *Contemporary Field Research: A Collection of Readings*, (ed. R. Emerson), Waveland Press, IL.

Geertz, C. (1983) From the native's point of view: on the nature of anthropological understanding, in *Meaning of Anthropology*, (eds K. Basso and H. Selby), University of New Mexico Press, Albuquerque.

Glesne, C. and Peshkin, A. (1992) *Becoming Qualitative Researchers: An Introduction*, Longman, Harlow.

Goode, D. (1988) *On Understanding Without Words: Communication Between a Deaf Blind Child and Her Parents*, unpublished manuscript.

Goode, D. (1994) Editor's introduction, in *Quality of Life for Persons with Disabilities*, (ed. D. Goode), Brookline Books, Cambridge, MA.

Goode, D. and Hogg, J. (1994) Towards an understanding of holistic quality of life in people with profound intellectual and multiple disabilities, in *Quality of Life for Persons with Disabilities*, (ed. D. Goode), Brookline Books, Cambridge, MA.

Gouldner, A. (1970) *The Coming Crisis in Western Sociology*, Basic Books, New York.

Heal, L. and Sigelman, C. (1990) Methodological issues in measuring the quality of life of individuals with mental retardation, in *Quality of Life: Perspectives and Issues*, (ed. R. Schalock), American Association on Mental Retardation, Washington DC.

Heyl, A. (1979) *The Madam as Entrepreneur: Career Management in House Prostitution*, Transaction Books, New Jersey.

Kennedy, M. (1993) Turning the pages of life, in *Housing Support and Community: Choices and Strategies for Adults with Disabilities*, (eds J. Racino, S. Taylor, P. Walker and S. O'Connor), Brookes, Baltimore.

Klein, J. (1992) Get me the hell out of here: supporting people with disabilities to live in their own homes, in *Natural Supports in School, at Work, and in the Community for People with Severe Disabilities*, (ed. J. Nisbet), Brookes, Baltimore.

Klockars, C. (1975) *The Professional Fence*, Tavistock, London.

Lewis, O. (1959) *Five Families: Mexican Case Studies in the Culture of Poverty*, Basic Books, New York.

Lewis, O. (1961) *The Children of Sanchez: Autobiography of a Mexican American Family*, Random Books, New York.

Lewis, O. (1964) *Pedro Martinez: A Mexican Peasant and His Family*, Secker & Warburg, London.

Lewis, O. (1969) *Death in the Sanchez Family*, Random House, New York.

Martinez, C. (1990) A dream for myself, in *Quality of Life: Perspectives and Issues*, (ed. R. Schalock), American Association on Mental Retardation, Washington DC.

Phillips, D. (1990) Subjectivity and objectivity: an objective inquiry, in *Qualitative Inquiry in Education: The Continuing Debate*, (eds E. Eisner and A. Peshkin), Columbia University Teachers College, New York, 19–37.

Plummer, D. (1983) *Documents of Life*, George Allen & Unwin, London.

Rist, R. (1977) On the relations among educational research paradigms: from disdain to detente. *Anthropology and Education*, **8**, 42–9.

Schalock, R. (1994) The concept of quality of life and its current applications in the field of mental retardation/developmental disabilities, in *Quality of Life for Persons with Disabilities*, (ed. D. Goode), Brookline Books, Cambridge, MA.

Schofield, J. (1990) Increasing the generalizability of qualitative research, in *Qualitative Inquiry in Education: The Continuing Debate*, (eds E. Eisner and A. Peshkin), Columbia University Teachers College, New York, 201–32.

Scriven, M. (1972) Objectivity and subjectivity in educational research, in *Philosophical Redirection for Educational Research*, (eds H. Dunkel *et al.*), National Society for the Study of Education, Chicago.

Shaw, C. (1930) *The Jack Roller: A Delinquent Boy's Own Story*, University of Chicago Press, Chicago.

Shaw, C. (1931) *The Natural History of a Delinquent Career*, University of Chicago Press, Chicago.

Stensman, R. (1985) Severely mobility disabled people assess the quality of their lives. *Scandinavian Journal of Rehabilitation Medicine*, **17**(2), 87–99.

Taylor, S. (1994) In support of research on quality of life, but against QOL, in *Quality of Life for Persons with Disabilities*, (ed. D. Goode), Brookline Books, Cambridge, MA.

Taylor, S. and Bogdan, R. (1984) *Introduction to Qualitative Research Methods: The Search for Meaning*, John Wiley, New York.

Taylor, S. and Bogdan, R. (1990) Quality of life and the individual's perspective, in *Quality of Life: Perspectives and Issues*, (ed. R. Schalock), American Association on Mental Retardation, Washington DC.

Ward, N. (1990) Reflections on my quality of life: then and now, in *Quality of Life: Perspectives and Issues*, (ed. R. Schalock), American Association on Mental Retardation, Washington DC.

Wolfensberger, W. (1994) Let's hang up 'quality of life' as a hopeless term, in *Quality of Life for Persons with Disabilities*, (ed. D. Goode), Brookline Books, Cambridge, MA.

Quality of life: the scope of the term and its breadth of measurement

4

David Felce and Jonathan Perry

INTRODUCTION

Many measures have been developed to characterize the impact that services for people with pervasive disabilities have on the lives of those served. The service evaluation literature concerned with people with intellectual disabilities has broadened over time and an initial preoccupation with developmental growth as a principal outcome measure has been replaced by a willingness to explore the impact of care processes on a wide range of aspects relevant to people's day-to-day lives. Quality of life has emerged as a unifying concept. It may be defined to encapsulate developmental change in the individual and in their identity, the nature of their circumstances, experience and lifestyle and their perceptions about themselves and their circumstances.

QUALITY OF LIFE

The interest in quality of life in the learning disability literature has flourished since the 1980s (see Brown, 1988; Landesman, 1986; Schalock, 1990). Conceptualization has mirrored and drawn from quality of life assessment for the population as a whole (Andrews & Withey, 1976; Campbell, Converse & Rodgers, 1976). There is considerable agreement that the term refers to a concept which is multidimensional. Quality of life is concerned with intimate relationships, family life, friendships, standard of living, work, neighbourhood, city or town of residence, the state of the nation, housing, education, health and self (Campbell, 1981). We found considerable overlap between authors on what constituted relevant areas for assessment in a review which we undertook of fifteen conceptual papers on the subject taken from writing on the general population, intellectual disability, physical disability and mental health (Felce & Perry, 1995a).

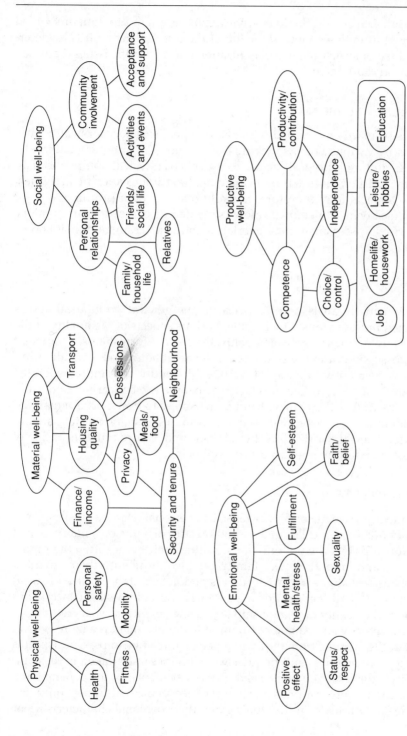

Fig. 4.1 Domains relevant to quality of life.

Figure 4.1 sets out the five-way categorization of life domains which emerged from this review of the literature. It is not an empirically determined factor structure but a classification into which the issues discussed by various authors fit.

PHYSICAL WELL-BEING

This is primarily concerned with health. Specific aspects of health mentioned by various writers include fitness, mobility and personal safety. Fitness and mobility both relate to aspects of physical ability and may be best defined as functional capacities relative to specific activities. These aspects may therefore partially overlap with productive well-being (see below). Personal safety is the degree of freedom from injury or harm; its assessment may overlap with the assessment of neighbourhood quality.

MATERIAL WELL-BEING

This is equally an issue of concern to the general population and is reflected most obviously by income. Various aspects of the quality of the living environment – housing quality, the level of furnishings, equipment and possessions and the character of the neighbourhood – are all intimately associated with material well-being. Tenure and, more generally, economic security reflect the fact that people are concerned about the future as well as their current situation. Access to transport is a material consideration associated with the opportunities a person has to maintain or extend social, work, educational, civic and leisure pursuits and may therefore underpin other aspects of well-being.

SOCIAL WELL-BEING

This includes two major dimensions: interpersonal relationships and community involvement. The quality and breadth of a person's interpersonal relationships include not only those within their home, often their most intimate and involving close family, but also those with their extended family and relatives and with friends and acquaintances. Size of social network or breadth of relationships is one aspect of possible concern, but so too is the quality of relationship (e.g. degree of intimacy, degree of support, reciprocity and equality). Community involvement is a more general facet of life, distinct from individual personal relationships. One aspect is reflected in the range and frequency of activities undertaken in the community – the use of amenities and services available for the general good of the community. Another is the level of acceptance or support provided by the community to individuals given their personal characteristics or circumstances, their aspirations and actual or potential requirements from the local infrastructure and inhabitants.

EMOTIONAL WELL-BEING

Emotional well-being includes affect, fulfilment, stress and mental state, self-esteem, status and respect, religious faith and sexuality. Fulfilment may overlap with achievement of social and functional pursuits. Degree of stress, which in this version replaces satisfaction included in our earlier framework (see Felce & Perry, 1995a),* reflects the conditions under which social and functional activities are pursued. Stress may affect the degree to which one derives satisfaction from life and is a factor which may contribute to or detract from emotional well-being.

PRODUCTIVE WELL-BEING

This is concerned with developmental growth and a person's ability to use time constructively according to their own tenets. Competence or the development of skills and experience is linked to self-determination – independence and the concomitant abilities to exercise choice or control – and contribution to self and others. All may be expressed through the pursuit of functional activities in different arenas such as home, work, leisure and education.

QUALITY OF LIFE THEMES IN EVALUATION

The validity of this multielement formulation of quality of life requires an empirical basis that has not been achieved here. However, support for the importance of the themes set out can be gained from evaluation practice.

Many of the domain areas, for example, are represented in British research on the deinstitutionalization of people with intellectual disabilities. Emerson & Hatton's (1994) review found attention being given to material standards, developing competence or adaptive behaviour, opportunities for choice, social relationships, extent of participation in activity, community involvement, acceptance by the community, social status and lifestyle satisfaction. Such scope is also to be found in some of the more comprehensive evaluation studies of services in our field on both sides of the Atlantic (Brown, Bayer & Brown, 1992; Burchard *et al.*, 1991; Conroy & Bradley, 1985; Felce, 1989; Lowe & de Paiva, 1991).

Health as an outcome has been given relatively little attention. The importance of health is reflected in studies of the primary health care status

* Satisfaction is used later in this chapter as a major dimension to include subjective appraisal across the content areas of all five domains. It is therefore redundant as an item to be considered within the categorization of life domains.

of people living in the community or in institutions (Beange & Bauman, 1990; Howells, 1986). Glossop *et al.* (1980) incorporated a health indicator – the annual number of morbidity episodes specified in terms of illness, injury and convulsion – in their matched-group evaluation of institutional and community residential services. Research has also investigated service usage and contact rates between individuals and health care professionals De Paiva & Lowe, 1992). Although the latter only provides an indirect x and there are considerable difficulties in using such information to ply anything about physical well-being, the fact that rate of professional nvolvement is of interest probably reflects an implicit concern for health as an important determinant of quality of life. Instruments exist to measure health status in the population generally and screening tools applicable to people with intellectual disabilities have been developed (e.g. Wilson & Hare, 1990).

Material well-being has been reflected in studies by reference to disposable income (Walker, Ryan & Walker, 1993), housing quality or the quality of the physical environment (Conneally, Boyle & Smyth, 1992; Rotegard, Hill & Bruininks, 1983) and the level of furnishings, equipment and possessions (Booth, Booth & Simons, 1990; Felce *et al.*, 1985). The character of the neighbourhood is represented in the Lifestyle Satisfaction Scale (Heal & Chadsey-Rusch, 1985) and Bellamy *et al.* (1990) include discussion of security, both in terms of housing tenure and the continuity of ties and other associations, as an important dimension of lifestyle quality.

Social well-being has received considerable attention (Felce, 1988; Romer & Heller, 1983). Direct observation of social interaction among people living in residential service settings and between residents and their carers has explored the quantity, quality and reciprocity of interaction within the home (Felce & Perry, 1995b; Landesman-Dwyer, Berkson & Romer, 1979). Rating scales have been developed to measure the 'social climate' of a setting (Moos, 1974) or the degree of 'social distance' between residents and staff (King, Raynes & Tizard, 1971; Pratt, Luszcz & Brown, 1980). The extensiveness and character of people's social networks and the frequency and nature of their social affiliations have been investigated using data from interviews or from the direct recording of social events (Felce, 1988; Knapp *et al.*, 1992). Family and friendship contact has been the subject of study (De Kock *et al.*, 1988), as has more general contact in the community (McConkey, Naughton & Nugent, 1983) and contact with neighbours (McConkey, Walsh & Conneally, 1993).

Community involvement has equally and frequently been the subject of assessment. The range and frequency of community activities undertaken by people with intellectual disabilities on a day-to-day basis have been measured through the use of questionnaires (Lowe & de Paiva, 1991) and rating scales (Raynes, Pratt & Roses, 1979) and through the direct recording and categorization of events (De Kock *et al.*, 1988).

Activity while using community amenities has been assessed by direct observation (Saxby *et al.*, 1986). Acceptance within the community has been explored in terms of community or neighbour attitudes to residential services (Lubin *et al.*, 1982, McConkey, Walsh & Conneally, 1993; Pittock & Potts, 1988) and by gaining the views of business proprietors, managers and staff of amenities frequented by people with intellectual disabilities (Saxby *et al.*, 1986). In addition, the direct experience of people with intellectual disabilities of the general public's reaction to them has been described (Close & Halpern, 1988; Flynn, 1989).

The measurement of developmental progress reflects the importance of developing competence and independence and service goals such as 'maximizing potential' (Close, 1977; Felce *et al.*, 1986; Hemming, Lavender & Pill, 1981). Such outcomes have been seen as some of the most consistently studied consequences of service arrangements. One aspect of independence is reflected by possession of adaptive behaviour skills, for which a range of alternative measures exists (Nihira, Leland & Lambert, 1993; Sparrow, Balla & Cicchetti, 1984). Another is the degree of autonomy or opportunities for control over day-to-day living. Various scales have been developed to address autonomy in this sense, including the Social Climate Scales referred to earlier, the Characteristics of the Treatment Environment Scale (Sutter & Mayeda, 1979), the Choice Making Scale (Conroy & Feinstein, 1986) and the Index of Adult Autonomy (Raynes *et al.*, 1994). Moreover, it would probably be more precise to conceive of the data measured by adaptive behaviour scales as representing a composite of two aspects: personal skills and the environmental opportunities available to use them (Emerson & Hatton, 1994; Schroeder & Henes, 1978).

The extent to which people engage or participate in the range of activities typical of ordinary living is a direct measure of environmental opportunity and the use of skills. It also corresponds to the notion of productivity. Research on activity patterns has been conducted by interview (Knapp, *et al.*, 1992; O'Neill *et al.*, 1981) and by direct observation (Felce, de Kock & Repp, 1986; Mansell *et al.*, 1984). Emerson & Hatton (1994) reported that directly observed engagement in activity has been the most frequently used outcome measure in British deinstitutionalization research.

Evaluation of emotional well-being is represented in the general literature on quality of life (e.g. Andrews & Withey, 1976) but relatively neglected in the intellectual disability literature (Emerson & Hatton, 1994). The potential exists for using measures developed for general application, such as the Perceived Quality of Life Scale (Andrews & Withey, 1976) and the Positive and Negative Affect Scales (Bradburn, 1969). Psychiatric screening instruments have been developed for people with intellectual disabilities to reflect problems in mental state (Matson,

1988; Reiss, 1988). Scales of life stress are prevalent and general measures may be adapted for use with people with intellectual disabilities (Bramston, 1994). Similarly, research on self-concept or self-identity may follow application of general approaches (Gowans & Hulbert, 1983), as in the use of repertory grid technique (Oliver, 1986). Cummins (1993) has included consideration of intimacy in the general and the disability versions of his quality of life scale, an aspect of life which may be closely associated with self-esteem, understanding of sexuality and general emotional well-being.

OBJECTIVE OR SUBJECTIVE APPRAISAL?

Much of the research cited above has involved objective measurement. However, it is a very common view that personal satisfaction with lifestyle is the ultimate criterion. People differ in what they prefer, in their priorities and values and how they choose to lead their lives. Taylor & Bogdan (1990) argue that the quality of life concept has no meaning apart from what a person feels and experiences. It is a question of what an individual thinks about their life, not what others attribute to it. Emerson (1985) identified resident satisfaction as one of the under-researched areas in the intellectual disability deinstitutionalization literature. Consequently, the development of quality of life scales which reflect the user perspective has been a growth area, despite the problems in understanding and communication inherent in intellectual disabilities (Brown & Bayer, 1992; Cummins, 1993; Heal & Chadsey-Rusch, 1985; Schalock, Keith & Hoffman, 1990).

However, there is considerable uncertainty as to whether quality of life is wholly synonymous with personal satisfaction (Landesman, 1986). Borthwick-Duffy (1992) presented three perspectives, with quality of life being defined as the quality of the conditions experienced in life, as the degree of satisfaction with life or as a combination of the two. Subjective appraisal has been a cornerstone of research on the quality of life of the general population. The individual's personal autonomy to maintain or change their quality of life is seen as a paramount consideration. Yet, the primacy of expressed satisfaction as a commentary on the acceptability of the life conditions experienced relies on assumptions about freedom of choice which may be unrealistic. Reports of well-being may well themselves be shaped by experience. Experience may teach a person that they have a choice and that change is possible. Low satisfaction under these circumstances may indicate that a desired circumstance has not been achieved; high satisfaction, that it has. However, experience may also teach that desired change is rarely achieved. Expressions of satisfaction may be bounded by pervasive life conditions which are typical for the individual and their class or peer group. Under such circumstances, expressions of satisfaction may adjust to habitual life conditions even if those conditions are towards the least favoured end of the distribution for the population as a whole.

The ability to change life conditions in line with personal preference is not universally found. Many societal groups are disadvantaged economically, educationally or by class, racial origin or other factors. The autonomy to maintain or change life conditions in line with subjective appraisal is restricted and, for some groups, atypically so. Most people with intellectual disabilities lack independence and experience constrained opportunities and autonomy, a combination which frequently results in them inhabiting worlds of other people's construction. Research of people with intellectual disabilities living relatively independently has provided a picture consistent with low expectation; individuals say they are satisfied despite experiencing many adverse conditions including: poverty, poor housing, threats to health, threats to safety, victimization, social isolation, experience of loss and failure to gain or retain employment (Close & Halpern, 1988; Edgerton, Bollinger & Herr, 1984; Flynn, 1989). At this extreme, one cannot conclude that lifestyle necessarily reflects personal choice or that satisfaction is an adequate measure of quality of life.

However, the fact that personal appraisal has a validity for which there is no substitute if one person's values are not to be imposed on another does imply that the assessment of quality of life should take account of subjective viewpoints. A number of quality of life scales combine both objective and subjective considerations (e.g. Schalock, Keith & Hoffman, 1990). Cummins (1993) has also suggested that the conceptualization of quality of life should take account of individual value structures so as to accommodate the relative importance an individual may place on competing concerns. This approach is consistent with the notion that well-being stems from the degree of fit between an individual's perception of their situation and their needs, aspirations or values (Andrews & Withey, 1976; Campbell, Converse & Rodgers, 1976). It provides a model whereby objectively assessable aspects of lifestyle, as well as subjective appraisals of satisfaction across the range of possible lifestyle domains, are summed to form a single personalized index of quality of life according to the weight a person gives to the constituent concerns. In this way, the imperative that only individuals can decide the trade-off between competing aspects of their own personal welfare is met.

QUALITY OF LIFE: A MULTIDIMENSIONAL, MULTIELEMENT FRAMEWORK

Figure 4.2 illustrates such a model. Quality of life constitutes a general well-being influenced by objective circumstances and subjective perceptions across a variety of life domain issues. Individual difference is not

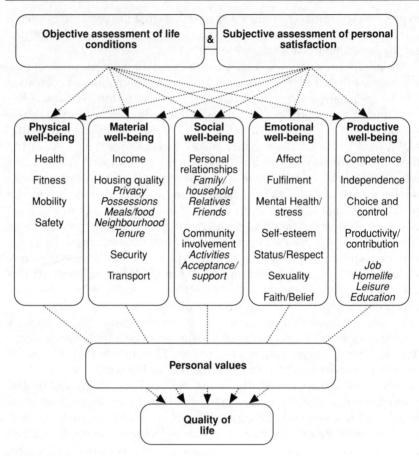

Fig. 4.2 Framework for exploring quality of life.

only reflected in the element of subjective appraisal, but also in the fact that such appraisals and the person's objective circumstances are weighted in ratio to the values which the person holds. Hence, size of social network may count more for a more gregarious person and income for a more materialistic person. Relative weightings will inevitably differ across individuals and life domain concerns.

The three major dimensions – objective circumstances, subjective appraisal of circumstance and personal values – are potentially inter-dependent at all times. A change on one dimension may affect another. For example, experience of increasing wealth and satisfaction with the lifestyle opportunities income brings may alter a person's appreciation of the importance of income. It may also lead to greater satisfaction with income *per se* and to a revision of the person's values with respect to material well-being. Alternatively, a deteriorating sense of satisfaction with lifestyle despite increasing income may prompt a change in values in the opposite direction. This may then lead to revised priorities and precipitate changes in objective circumstances. For example, a person may come to believe in a non-materialist way of life as a better mode of existence, become less satisfied with their range of functional pursuits, change their job and lower their material standards. The important corollary to this analysis is that the relationships between the three elements which interact to form an individual's quality of life are neither static nor uniform. Knowledge of one set cannot predict another.

LANGUAGE UNDERSTANDING AND SUBJECTIVE ASSESSMENT BY PEOPLE WITH INTELLECTUAL DISABILITIES

Up to this point, although the illustrations of evaluation practice cited come from the field of intellectual disabilities, there is nothing about the quality of life model described which is specific to this group of people. Indeed, the importance of the ability to compare the situation for a particular group with that for society as a whole implies the desirability of general rather than specific definitions of the quality of life concept. However, language proficiency is a particular concern with respect to people with intellectual disabilities. Great progress has been made in considering people with intellectual disabilities as capable of taking reasonable control over life decisions (Brown, Bayer & Brown, 1992). There has been a concomitant growth in self-advocacy groups, by which people with intellectual disabilities draw collective strength to express their opinions, and in the attention being given to individual preferences and choices in day-to-day living and in service planning reviews. Research has also sought the views of people with intellectual disabilities: both qualitative accounts (Edgerton, Bollinger & Herr, 1984; Flynn, 1989) and their response to structured interviews (Knapp *et al.*, 1992). In addition, a number of quality of life scales have been developed to reflect service user perspectives, including the Lifestyle Satisfaction Scale (Heal & Chadsey-Rusch, 1985), the Quality of Life Questionnaire (Schalock, Keith & Hoffman, 1990) and the ComQoL–ID version (Cummins, 1993).

However, it is also true that gaining ratings of satisfaction from people with poor receptive and expressive language is associated with special problems of inconsistent reliability and uncertain validity. There is a tremendous range in understanding and communicative competency among people with intellectual disabilities, ranging from a level of comprehension and articulation equal to some people not so labelled through to virtually no understanding of language or means of expression. Sigelman *et al.* (1981) demonstrated that it was not possible to gain a response to even simple questions from some people with severe intellectual disabilities and most people with profound intellectual disabilities.

Moreover, inconsistency, inaccuracy and the tendencies to acquiesce and choose the last of a possible range of responses offered were other problems encountered. Such problems tended to increase with greater severity of intellectual disability, but evidence also suggested that they were found in some people with only mild or moderate intellectual disabilities too.

Validity also needs to be addressed; in particular, the extent to which people with intellectual disabilities have the same conception of terms as others with more developed language. In order to boost responsiveness and consistency, investigators have often adopted relatively simple response formats, supported by pictures and line drawings, and used scales with few points so that the discrimination required is kept to the most basic level. While such strategies may acknowledge and compensate for difficulties in expressive communication, what assumptions are being made about the understanding of the conceptual issues addressed? It seems inconsistent to recognize language limitations in producing a response to questions but not to recognize equal limitations in understanding the terms in which they are posed.

Whatever the precise extent of the problem, cognitive and language limitations among people with intellectual disabilities will imply that the ability to gain their subjective views and personal values structures will be severely constrained for a significant proportion. A rational approach will need to be taken to the interpretation of objective data on quality of life under these circumstances. One obvious possibility would be to compare the objectively assessable situation of people with intellectual disabilities as a class with the distribution of similar data for society as a whole. One may be unable to take a definitive view about individual welfare without subjective appraisal by the individual, but the relative disadvantage or advantage in life conditions compared to the general public can be established.

APPLICATION OF QUALITY OF LIFE MEASUREMENT

Such an application for quality of life data provides a reminder that the origins of the quality of life concept are to be found in the concern to encapsulate the well-being of populations rather than individuals (Wolfensberger, 1994). Whereas an individual focus brings with it attendant concerns that quality of life, once operationalized, will be imposed without regard to individual difference, there is an obvious objection to an externally imposed quality of life framework replacing personal autonomy as a mechanism for making choices and determining personal circumstances. Quality of life data at the aggregate level may have considerable use in monitoring social inequality and shaping social policy. In general, a view that an acceptable quality of life had been achieved would require that both expressed satisfaction with various aspects of life and objective descriptors of those aspects were in keeping with, or at least not inferior to, what was typical for society as a whole, bearing in mind the relative personal values of population members. Where subjective assessment is not possible, the range and distribution of life conditions in the population as a whole can be taken to reflect personal differences. Aggregated objective data may therefore be compared as if they already embody subjective viewpoints. The situation of a societal subgroup can be established if one can make the *a priori* assumption that variation due to individual difference will be similar to that in the total population.

If cultural norms and ranges are to provide a standard of reference for a defined group of interest, it is clear that any conceptualization of quality of life must not be limited to a particular vulnerable or devalued societal subgroup, but be generally applicable to the population as a whole. The five domains suggested here to categorize the content areas relevant to quality of life are all of a general nature and, indeed, reflect the scope of quality of life assessment as applied to the general population. This is clearly desirable from the perspective of developing a quality of life measurement system which has broad utility. The adequacy of the scope of the items needs to be examined by research which establishes which indicators of quality of life are sufficient to reflect the range of public concerns. Once established, the task of defining a range of measures should not be too difficult. The scope of the quality of life concept is broad, but the earlier brief review of measurement applications demonstrates that research has also adopted a wide-ranging focus.

CONCLUSIONS

The development of a common approach to quality of life applicable across societal groups and to the total population is vital if information regarding one section of society is to be interpreted with confidence. Such an approach will need to be multidimensional and reflect varying aspects of the complex lives of human beings. A framework based on common ground is described here which, as well as classifying potential issues of concern in five domain areas, suggests that measurement of life conditions, subjective assessments about life and personal values are all relevant. People differ in what they like and what they think is important. Problems in inferring what alternative quality of life might be reasonable in the individual case are compounded by the fact that life conditions and satisfaction with life inevitably vary across individuals in all groups within society. Aggregate comparisons may provide a surer footing. Data for a defined group of interest, compared to the statistical distribution for the population as a whole, can be used to reflect whether life conditions and satisfaction in various domains are typical of the general pattern or have a significantly different profile. Social policy may then respond to conspicuous inequality.

REFERENCES

Andrews, F.M. and Withey, S.B. (1976) *Social Indicators of Well-being: Americans' Perceptions of Life Quality*, Plenum Press, New York.

Beange, H. and Bauman, A. (1990) Health care for the developmentally disabled. Is it necessary? in *Key Issues in Mental Retardation Research*, (ed. W. Fraser), Routledge, London.

Bellamy, G.T., Newton, J.S., LeBaron, N.M. and Horner, R.H. (1990) Quality of lifestyle outcomes: a challenge for residential programs, in *Quality of Life: Perspectives and Issues*, (ed. R. Schalock), American Association on Mental Retardation, Washington DC.

Booth, W., Booth, T. and Simons, K. (1990) Return journey: the relocation of adults from long-stay hospital into hostel accommodation. *British Journal of Mental Subnormality*, **36**, 87–97.

Borthwick-Duffy, S.A. (1992) Quality of life and quality of care in mental retardation, in *Mental Retardation in the Year 2000*, (ed. L. Rowitz), Springer-Verlag, Berlin.

Bradburn, N.M. (1969) *The Structure of Psychological Well-being*, Aldine, Chicago.

Bramston, P. (1994) *Lifestress Test Manual*, University of Southern Queensland Psychology Department, Toowoomba, Queensland.

Brown, R.I. (1988) *Quality of Life for Handicapped People*, Croom Helm, London.

Brown, R.I. and Bayer, M.B. (1992) *Rehabilitation Questionnaire Manual: A Personal Guide to the Individual's Quality of Life*, Captus Press, Ontario.

Brown, R.I., Bayer, M.B. and Brown, P.M. (1992) *Empowerment and Developmental Handicaps: Choices and Quality of Life*, Chapman & Hall, London.

Burchard, S.N., Hasazi, J.S., Gordon, L.R. and Yoe, J. (1991) An examination of lifestyles and adjustment in three community residential alternatives. *Research in Developmental Disabilities*, **12**, 127–42.

Campbell, A. (1981) *The Sense of Well-being in America*, McGraw-Hill, New York.

Campbell, A., Converse, P.E. and Rodgers, W.L. (1976) *The Quality of American Life: Perceptions, Evaluation and Satisfaction*, Russell Sage Foundation, New York.

Close, D.W. (1977) Community living for severely and profoundly retarded adults: a group home study. *Education and Training of the Mentally Retarded*, **12**, 256–62.

Close, D.W. and Halpern, A.S. (1988) Transitions to supported living, in *Community Residences for Persons with Developmental Disabilities: Here to Stay*, (eds M.P. Janicki, M.W. Krauss and M.M. Seltzer), Brookes, Baltimore.

Conneally, S., Boyle, G. and Smyth, F. (1992) An evaluation of the use of small group homes for adults with a severe and profound mental handicap. *Mental Handicap Research*, **5**, 146–68.

Conroy, J.W. and Bradley, V.J. (1985) *The Pennhurst Longitudinal Study: A Report of Five Years Research and Analysis*, Temple University Developmental Disabilities Center, Philadelphia.

Conroy, J. W. and Feinstein, C. (1986) *The Choice Making Scale*, Conroy & Feinstein Associates, Philadelphia.

Cummins, R.A. (1993) *Comprehensive Quality of Life Scale-Intellectual Disability*, 4th edn, Psychology Research Centre, Melbourne.

De Kock, U., Saxby, H., Thomas, M. and Felce, D. (1988) Community and family contact: an evaluation of small community homes for adults. *Mental Handicap Research*, **1**, 127–40.

De Paiva, S. and Lowe, K (1992) Service change: changes over five years in a total population sample. *Mental Handicap Research*, **5**, 33–8.

Edgerton, R.B., Bollinger, M. and Herr, B. (1984) The cloak of competence: after two decades. *American Journal of Mental Deficiency*, **88**, 345–51.

Emerson, E.B. (1985) Evaluating the impact of deinstitutionalisation on the lives of mentally retarded people. *American Journal of Mental Deficiency*, **90**, 277–88.

Emerson, E. and Hatton, C. (1994) *Moving Out: Relocation from Hospital to Community*, HMSO, London.

Felce, D. (1988) Evaluating the extent of community integration following the provision of staffed residential alternatives to institutional care. *Irish Journal of Psychology*, **9**, 346–60.

Felce, D. (1989) *Staffed Housing for Adults with Severe and Profound Mental Handicaps: the Andover Project*, BIMH Publications, Kidderminster.

Felce, D. and Perry, J. (1995a) Quality of life: its definition and measurement. *Research in Developmental Disabilities*, **16**, 51–74.

Felce, D. and Perry, J. (1995b) The extent of support for ordinary living provided in staffed housing: the relationship between staffing levels, resident dependency, staff:resident interactions and resident activity patterns. *Social Science and Medicine*, **40**, 799–810.

Felce, D., Thomas, M., de Kock, U., Saxby, H. and Repp, A. (1985) An ecological comparison of small community-based houses and traditional institutions for severely and profoundly mentally handicapped adults: II Physical settings and the use of opportunities. *Behaviour Research and Therapy*, **23**, 337–48.

Felce, D., de Kock, U. and Repp, A.C. (1986) An eco-behavioural comparison of small home and institutional settings for severely and profoundly mentally handicapped adults. *Applied Research in Mental Retardation*, **2**, 393–408.

Felce, D., de Kock, U., Thomas, M. and Saxby, H. (1986) Change in adaptive behaviour of severely and profoundly mentally handicapped adults in different residential settings. *British Journal of Psychology*, **7**, 489–501.

Flynn, M. (1989) *Independent Living for Adults with a Mental Handicap: A Place of My Own*, Cassell, London.

Glossop, C., Felce, D., Smith, J. and Kushlick, A. (1980) Evaluation of alternative residential facilities for the severely mentally handicapped in Wessex: contact by professionals and client morbidity. *Advances in Behaviour Research and Therapy*, **3**, 37–42.

Gowans, F. and Hulbert, C. (1983) Self-concept assessment of mentally retarded adults. *Mental Handicap*, **11**, 121–3.

Heal, L.W. and Chadsey-Rusch, J. (1985) The Lifestyle Satisfaction Scale (LSS): assessing individuals' satisfaction with residence, community setting and associated services. *Applied Research in Mental Retardation*, **6**, 475–90.

Hemming, H., Lavender, T. and Pill, R. (1981) Quality of life of mentally retarded adults transferred from large institutions to new small units. *American Journal of Mental Deficiency*, **86**, 157–69.

Howells, G. (1986) Are the medical needs of mentally handicapped adults being met? *Journal of the Royal College of General Practitioners*, **36**, 449–53.

King, R., Raynes, N. and Tizard, J. (1971) *Patterns of Residential Care*, Routledge & Kegan Paul, London.

Knapp, M., Cambridge, P., Thomason, C. *et al.* (1992) *Care in the Community: Challenge and Demonstration*, Ashgate, Aldershot.

Landesman, S. (1986) Quality of life and personal life satisfaction: definition and measurement issues. *Mental Retardation*, **24**, 141–3.

Landesman-Dwyer, S., Berkson, G. and Romer, D. (1979) Affiliation and friendship of mentally retarded residents in group homes. *American Journal of Mental Deficiency*, **83**, 571–80.

Lowe, K. and de Paiva, S. (1991) NIMROD: an overview. HMSO, London.

Lubin, R. A., Schwartz, A.A., Zigman, W.B. and Janicki, M.P. (1982) Community acceptance of residential programs for developmentally disabled persons. *Applied Research in Mental Retardation*, **3**, 191–200.

Mansell, J., Jenkins, J., Felce, D. and de Kock, U. (1984) Measuring the activity of severely and profoundly mentally handicapped adults in ordinary housing. *Behaviour Research and Therapy*, **22**, 23–9.

Matson, J. L. (1988) *The Psychopathology Instrument for Mentally Retarded Adults*, International Diagnostic Systems, Orland Park, IL.

McConkey, R., Naughton, M. and Nugent, U. (1983) Community contacts of adults who are mentally handicapped. *Mental Handicap*, **11**, 57–9.

McConkey, R., Walsh, P.N. and Conneally, S. (1993) Neighbours' reactions to community services: contrasts before and after services open in their locality. *Mental Handicap Research*, **6**, 131–41.

Moos, R. (1974) *The Social Climate Scales: An Overview*, Consulting Psychologists Press, Palo Alto.

Nihira, K., Leland, H. and Lambert, N. (1993) *AAMR Adaptive Behavior Scale – Residential and Community*, 2nd edn, PRO-ED, Austin, Texas.

Oliver, C. (1986) Self-concept assessment. *Mental Handicap*, **14**, 24–5.

O'Neill, J., Brown, M., Gordon, W., Schonhorn, R. and Greer, E. (1981) Activity patterns of mentally retarded adults in institutions and communities: a longitudinal study. *Applied Research in Mental Retardation*, **2**, 367–79.

Pittock, F. and Potts, M. (1988) Neighbourhood attitudes to people with a mental handicap: a comparative study. *British Journal of Mental Subnormality*, **34**, 35–46.

Pratt, M.W., Luszcz, M.A. and Brown, M.E. (1980) Measuring dimensions of the quality of care in small community residences. *American Journal of Mental Deficiency*, **85**, 188–94.

Raynes N.V., Pratt, M.W. and Roses, S. (1979) *Organisational Structure and the Care of the Mentally Retarded*, Croom Helm, London.

Raynes, N.V., Wright, K., Shiell, A. and Pettipher, C. (1994) *The Cost and Quality of Community Residential Care*, David Fulton, London.

Reiss, S. (1988) *Test Manual for the Reiss Screen for Maladaptive Behavior*, International Diagnostic Systems, Orland Park, IL.

Romer, D. and Heller, T. (1983) Social adaptation of mentally retarded adults in community settings: a social-ecological approach. *Applied Research in Mental Retardation*, **4**, 303–14.

Rotegard, L.L., Hill, B.K. and Bruininks, R.H. (1983) Environmental characteristics of residential facilities for mentally retarded persons in the United States. *American Journal of Mental Deficiency*, **88**, 49–56.

Saxby, H., Thomas, M., Felce, D. and de Kock, U. (1986) The use of shops, cafes and public houses by severely and profoundly mentally handicapped adults. *British Journal of Mental Subnormality*, **32**, 69–81.

Schalock, R.L. (1990) *Quality of Life: Perspectives and Issues*, American Association on Mental Retardation, Washington, DC.

Schalock, R.L., Keith, K.D. and Hoffman, K. (1990) *Quality of Life Questionnaire: Standardization Manual*, Mid-Nebraska Mental Retardation Services, Hastings, NE.

Schroeder, S. and Henes, C. (1978) Assessment of progress of institutionalized and deinstitutionalized retarded adults: a matched-control comparison. *Mental Retardation*, **16**, 147–8.

Sigelman, C.K., Schoenrock, C.J., Winer, J.L. *et al*. (1981) Issues in interviewing mentally retarded persons: an empirical study, in *Deinstitutionalization and Community Adjustment of Mentally Retarded Persons*, (eds R.H. Bruininks, C.E. Meyers, B.B. Sigford and K.C. Lakin), American Association on Mental Deficiency, Washington DC.

Sparrow, S.S., Balla, D.A. and Cicchetti, D.V. (1984) *Vineland Adaptive Behavior Scale*, American Guidance Service, Circle Pines, MN.

Sutter, P. and Meyeda, T. (1979) *Characteristics of the Treatment Environment: MR/DD Community Home Manual*, Lantermann Developmental Center, Pomona, California.

Taylor, S.J. and Bogdan, R. (1990) Quality of life and the individual's perspective, in *Quality of Life: Perspectives and Issues*, (ed. R.L. Schalock), American Association on Mental Retardation, Washington DC.

Walker, C., Ryan, T. and Walker, A. (1993) *Quality of Life after Resettlement for People with Learning Disabilities*. Summary of the report to the North West Regional Health Authority. Sheffield University Department of Sociological Studies, Sheffield.

Wilson, D. and Hare, A. (1990) Health care screening for people with mental handicap living in the community. *British Medical Journal*, **301**, 1379–80.

Wolfensberger, W. (1994) Let's hang up 'quality of life' as a hopeless term, in *Quality of Life for Persons with Disabilities: International Perspectives and Issues*, (ed. D. Goode), Brookline Books, Cambridge, MA.

Assessing the quality of life of adults with profound disabilities*

5

David Goode

INTRODUCTION

As the title suggests, this chapter explores the current status of quality of life assessment of persons with profound disabilities. That this is the topic of the chapter is itself a remarkable matter since just a few years ago the idea that, for example, persons with profound mental retardation had and could experience a quality of life would have been 'scientifically' suspect. Sadly, in the 1970s when I worked on a state hospital ward with children born deaf, blind and retarded, this was the prevailing attitude among the professional staff. As I relate in my book *A World Without Words: The Social Construction of Children Born Deaf-Blind*, when I suggested to the research staff that my research project was to focus in on the life-world of one child in order to attempt to empathize and discover how she experiences the world, I was passed an anonymous note reading: 'You should see a psychiatrist'. I and my work were literally the laughing stock of the empiricist researchers and even some of the professional staff that worked at State Hospital. Thus, the background assumptions of this writing, that persons with profound disabilities experience a quality of life and that this experience is 'valid', propositions which I believe are today probably shared by most readers of this book in a relatively non-problematic way, are testament to how substantially values and ideas in our field have changed over the past two decades.

The chapter has four sections: the first describes what is meant by the term quality of life, the next presents an overview of the current

* This chapter includes excerpts reproduced with permission from Goode & Hogg, 1994. The basic conceptual frame, referred to as a 'holistic' assessment of quality of life, emerged from our reading of Parin A. Dossa's (1989) work and our own experiences in the field of disabilities.

methodological thinking about investigating quality of life, the third specifically focuses on assessing quality of life of persons with profound mental and communicative disability, and finally there is a summary and discussion.

WHAT IS MEANT BY QUALITY OF LIFE?

Before we can discuss the assessment of the quality of life of persons with profound intellectual disabilities we must have some sense of what we mean by the term quality of life and how it might be applied to the disability field. While I and others have reviewed various definitions of the term and discussed the dangers of defining quality of life (see below), I have argued for the following provisional definition of quality of life policy (Goode, 1994c).

By 'quality of life policy' is meant the use of quality of life (an emphasis on promoting general feelings or perception of well-being, opportunities to fulfil potentials and feelings of positive social involvement) as a guide, common denominator or core principle with respect to decision making in services/supports for persons (requiring special supports). Such a policy would direct itself at minimizing the discrepancies between individuals' perceived and desired conditions of life. Research on or assessment or evaluation of quality of life, done under such a policy, would be ultimately aimed at understanding the individual's perspective about their life and then to gain knowledge that would minimize these perceived discrepancies. Thus, some of what is currently done in research and assessment would be subsumed under this policy. Note that this provisional definition does not include all uses within the literature of the term quality of life; for example, it would exclude the kind of work done by Shaw (1977) that uses quality of life as a way to grant or deny neonatal services to infants with disability, thus distinguishing itself from the quality of life research literature (see especially Wolfensberger, 1994). In addition, some people with disability and some researchers have objected to the exclusive equation of a good quality of life with feelings of happiness or pleasure. The National Institute of Disability and Rehabilitation Research's (NIDRR) suggested definition is specifically formulated to allow '… for individuals to rate quality of life high in spite of pain or dissatisfaction when they see it as leading toward growth'. I have heard this same sentiment from people with disabilities in Sweden, Finland and Denmark. Minimally, this aspect of 'satisfaction' and 'well-being' associated with many definitions of quality of life in our field will need to be examined more closely.

There appears to be some consensus that discussions of quality of life for persons with disabilities should not be divorced from discussions about quality of life for people without disabilities (Goode, 1994b; Holm et al., 1994; Schalock et al., 1990; Woodill et al., 1994). This is also explicit in the Helios Program and the UN's Standard Rules on the Equalization of Opportunities for Disabled Persons in which it is argued that disability policy should be part of member nations' national policies and in the latter in Rule 14: 'The needs and concerns of persons with disabilities should be incorporated into general development plans and not be treated separately' (p21). This connection can be argued on a value or moral basis (i.e. quality of life should not be different for persons with or without disability), according to the research literature (the logic and relationships of quality of life for persons with disabilities are no different from those of persons without disabilities) or on policy basis (for political or ethical reasons, we want to produce a society in which there is no difference in quality of life for persons on the basis of disability). Thus, the concept of quality of life is generic, not particular to people with disability at all.

As part of a more general trend in social policy (see Goode & Hogg, 1994) there appears in current thinking in the field a belief that people with disabilities themselves ought to be greatly involved in the creation of policies and programmes aimed at bettering their quality of life. Generally, people with disabilities are seen as persons who should assume as much control as possible over the processes affecting their life, whether this be disability policy, quality of life assessment, service evaluation, planning or so on.

Thus, quality of life is a term that is generic and not at all specific to disabilities. It focuses us on the individual's perspective of their life and upon discrepancies between what is and what is desired. It commits one to involving persons with disability in quality of life discussions, research and assessment in the strongest possible way.

Without having described the kind of persons who will be described as 'profoundly disabled' in this chapter, one can already intuitively anticipate how such an orientation might prove problematic when employed with such persons.

METHODOLOGY AND ASSESSMENT OF QUALITY OF LIFE*

Before we discuss the assessment of the quality of life of people with profound disability *per se*, we should examine the current status of the assessment of quality of life more generally. In this section I will look at the current status of quality of life methodology, measurement and assessment and describe some of the key issues.

The state of quality of life assessment reflects a definitional ambiguity that is itself probably part of a difference in researchers' world views. On

---

* In this section I rely upon text prepared for the 1994 Conference on Quality of Life for People with Special Needs, Copenhagen, Denmark, December 10-14 (Goode, 1994c).

the one hand, there are researchers who maintain that quality of life can be validly measured objectively and subjectively. In a book I edited, *Quality of Life for Persons with Disabilities: International Issues and Perspectives* (QOLPD) (Goode, 1994b), this kind of work is best exemplified in the chapter by Schalock, an early pioneer of quality of life measurement in the field, whose chapter in QOLPD I rely upon in explicating the current state of the art in quality of life measurement. Then there are researchers who believe that quality of life cannot be measured and that it is best to conceive of quality of life as a 'sensitizing concept' that cannot be precisely defined or measured. In QOLPD this position is explicated most fully in the chapter by Steve Taylor. Despite their apparent contradiction, I believe that there is merit in both these conceptions of quality of life. Hence both these conceptions should have methodological implications for quality of life research.

Because the research literature has traditionally reported a lack of correlation between objective assessments of quality of life and subjective ones, the above situation takes on an added significance. It means that any assessment of quality of life of an individual must contain subjective and objective elements and that there may be differences between these.

I argue that quality of life assessment should also have a relational or social component, that is neither 'objective' or 'subjective' but a reflection of the individual as embedded in social relationships. I also argue that all 'subjective' data about persons who cannot express themselves in formal languages are inferential, since the individual cannot be asked in so many words 'How do you feel about. ...?'. In some sense, all subjective data about any person are inferential, since even the answers to such questions are only indirect indices of how the respondent indicates 'an internal or subjective state'. In order to distinguish between 'real' subjective data, or self-report, and subjective data inferred by the observer, I refer to the latter as 'reputational data'. That is, when the rater or assessor uses their opinion about how the person with disabilities feels in order to assign 'a subjective state' based upon their observations or empathic responses. Ultimately the difference between reputational data and subjective data is a matter of degree and not quality. Both represent inferences made by hearers, signers or readers on the one hand and observers on the other.

Figure 5.1 overviews the current methodologies employed in quality of life research, quantitative and qualitative. It shows the logic of each position and suggests a co-operative relationship should be established on the level of application.

I will briefly review each position and its current state of development.

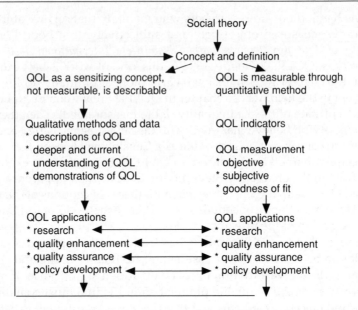

Fig. 5.1 Conceptual overview of QOL research (modified from Schalock, 1994).

QUALITY OF LIFE IS A USEFUL BUT NOT MEASURABLE CONCEPT

As far as I am aware, the first person in our field who maintained that quality of life was essentially unmeasurable because it was too subjective and complex was Dick Scheerenberger in the mid-1970s. Edgerton also expressed and later published this sentiment (personal communication and 1990) and was the first person to sensitize me to the possible tyrannical outcomes to quality of life definitions and measurement. But the most eloquent and substantial argument against quality of life operationalization and measurement is in the work of Steve Taylor (1994) and Robert Bogdan (Taylor & Bogdan, 1990). Here it is argued that quality of life is not by nature operationalizable, but is useful primarily as a 'sensitizing concept'. A sensitizing concept is one that lacks definitive characteristics and benchmarks and:

> …consequently it does not enable the user to move directly to the instance and its relevant content. Instead, it gives the user a general sense of reference and guidance in approaching empirical instances. Whereas definitive concepts provide prescriptions as what to see, sensitizing concepts merely suggest directions along which to look.
>
> (Blumer as cited by Taylor, 1994, p261)

Under such a conception quality of life is not something that can be measured, since it lacks definitive characteristics and benchmarks, but is better used to get 'looking directions'. That is, quality of life is a matter that may be described and discussed and perhaps even inductively understood on some level. But quality of life will ultimately, as Taylor & Bogdan argue, remain so open to such cultural, historical and personal variance that it is essentially uncodifiable and not measurable against some general standard. Attempts to do so violate this essential truth about it.

The argument made by these thinkers is not that quality of life should not be used in the field of disability, but rather that it should be used in primarily a descriptive rather than an evaluative or even prescriptive way. None of the authors cited above are against studying someone's, or some set of persons, quality of life as they see it. In fact, these authors are generally in favour of descriptive, ethnographic studies of the everyday lives of people with disabilities and how they experience them. Theirs is a serious argument that needs to be considered by our field. Taylor shorthands this logic by saying he is 'in support of research on quality of life but against QOL'.

Their observation that we need better descriptions of the lives of people (with disabilities) in order to better understand their quality of life is certainly grounded. There are indeed many aspects of people's lives, and particularly the lives of people with disabilities, that are not understood on the descriptive level – perhaps even the most important things about their lives – and without being adequately described, those who argue against quantification might say that it makes little sense to run around and measure the degree to which poor descriptions are correlated or distributed (I have referred to this as a kind of 'measurement madness'). Qualitative studies of the lives of people with disabilities reveal data and results that are simply unavailable to, and perhaps at odds with, the measurement approach. If one looks at my recently published (Goode, 1994a) ethnomethodological study of deaf and blind children with rubella syndrome, *A World Without Words*, one can see that the research would fit under the policy guidelines of quality of life research (that is, concerned with people's perceptions of well-being, social connectedness, opportunities to fulfil potentials and with the discrepancy between what is perceived as desirable and what exists). The study utilizes participant observation and ethnomethodological techniques that recover data about the everyday social lives of these children and how they experience them. These data simply cannot and will not be captured in studies employing quantitative analyses of their quality of life. The data and the sociological discussions they underwrite are essential to any understanding of quality of life for persons like Christina and Bianca, the two children about whom I write. On the one hand, this is true perhaps because qualitative methods are suited to capturing certain kinds of phenomena, for example, subjective ones without clear benchmarks or definitive characteristics (this would follow Taylor & Bogdan's argument). On the other hand, and my own work would be an example of this, qualitative methods can produce some fairly demonstrable, definitive or hard sociological results. I would hold up the discussion of the social construction of the deaf-blind children in a state hospital and those in a family as examples of what I mean by this. The social logic of these case studies, the sociology which they help discover and to which they point, extend far beyond themselves and are actually paradigmatic analyses for a sociology of disability generally. This was put to me most clearly in the late 1980s by Lars Kebbon who, after hearing me claim that my case studies tell us nothing more than what they say about that case and that case only, came up to me afterwards and asked half-jokingly, 'You are not serious about that?'. In a few succinct comments he convinced me that I was not. While one wants to have some humility about one's work, the experience I have had with respect to these case studies is that they represent many general processes in disability that transcend their existence in these particular studies. The relationship between the particular and general, written about, intriguingly, by Mao Tse-Tung in the 1930s, is also a preoccupation of many social sciences today. Certainly in ethnomethodology, structures of everyday life are seen as emerging out of deep, punctilious analyses of incidents. My own work is not at all unique with an increasing number of qualitative research works appearing in the disability field. Many of these would also fit within the general parameters of 'quality of life research' and provide invaluable and deep insight to the worlds of people with disabilities, insight that cannot be gained through behavioural research and questionnaires.

Thus, while not all qualitative methods are 'of a piece', generally qualitative studies of quality of life provide certain kinds of data and insight that cannot be obtained through census and survey type data. Qualitative methods are uniquely suited to discover the subjective viewpoints of actors under study, which as stated above can often be in contradiction to objective assessment of their quality of life. Because qualitative methods can involve long-term and intimate association between subject and researcher, these methods produce relatively valid reputational data about how subjects view their own quality of life. These methods are also able to address questions of a hermaneutical nature – to ask questions about 'world constitution', as Habermas puts it. They are discovery oriented and concerned with how things are described in the most basic sense, rather than concerned with the distribution of things already well defined (as in the quantificationist model). Such methods tolerate ambiguity and paradox well (which are unknown to the quantificationist methods), that may be key features of the everyday lives of people (with disabilities). As Mannheim would say, qualitative methods can 'deepen one's understanding' of the thing in question (for detailed discussion, see Pollner & Goode, 1990, and Goode, 1991).

QUALITY OF LIFE CAN BE OPERATIONALLY DEFINED AND MEASURED

Much like Thomas Szasz's denial of the existence of mental illness, when the above writers maintain that quality of life cannot be measured they do not mean this in an existential sense. Even a cursory reading of the quality of life literature indicates that the bulk of quality of life research has been primarily quantitative and that much is known about quality of life as operationally defined and measured. Quality of life has been measured on almost every level – individual, organizational, community and national. Measurement devices have been based on a variety of theories and definitions of quality of life and sometimes (unfortunately) no theory or explicit definition. The vast bulk of the research has had very little to do with disabilities or disability issues, although this is changing over the past few years.

In his chapter in this volume, Cummins refers to over 100 scales measuring quality of life currently employed. Some of these devices are based in explicit conceptual quality of life frameworks and were developed with psychometric sophistication. They often measure both subjective and objective components of quality of life. The most common factors assessed in quality of life scales are: home and community living; financial (employment/possessions); social integration (family, friends, natural supports); health status/safety; and personal control and decision making (Schalock, 1994). Depending on the way one discusses validity, several of these scales have various forms of validity to varying degrees. Some research addresses critical problem areas of quality of life assessment – for example, the discrepancy between objective and subjective quality of life assessment. There is some very good work being done in making our subjective quantitative data of better quality. The work of Roy Brown and colleagues (Brown, Brown & Bayer, 1994) and Bob Cummins (1993) and Laird Heal's work (Heal *et al.*, 1993) on the Lifestyle Satisfaction Scale are notable examples.

I will not undertake either a critical review of these scales or general discussion of what advantages being able to operationally define and measure concepts has for researchers. It is clear that this kind of assessment can perform important functions for researchers and other actors in the disability field, including possibly in the long run people with disabilities. The major applications of social science research – applied research, evaluation, policy and quality assurance – are usually done employing quantitative methods and measures. Thus quantitation of quality of life is both practically necessary and, if done with sufficient quality, of potential benefit to people with disabilities. And, while one would want to forcefully point out the dangers that go along with this way of studying people with disability and perhaps even suggest that certain kinds of quantitation should not be done, I do not want to advocate ceasing these kinds of studies entirely, as a practical and political matter.

What appears to make sense in the case of quality of life assessment is a serious attempt by these two sets of researchers, qualitative and quantitative, to work with one another on a commonly defined domain with mutually disclosed and understood methodological procedures. This is what is indicated in Figure 5.1 by the arrows at the bottom that link the applications of quality of life research. This kind of co-operation is what is suggested in the QOLPD chapter by Goode & Hogg (1994) concerning the holistic quality of life assessment of people with profound mental disability. And while co-operation always sounds like a good idea, 'the devil is in the details'.

QUALITY OF LIFE AND PROFOUND DISABILITY*

ASSESSMENT OF SUBJECTIVE PERCEPTION OF QUALITY OF LIFE

It is now possible to proceed to a discussion of the specific case of quality of life assessment and persons with profound disability.

If quality of life is to be assessed subjectively at the individual level and if persons with disability are to participate in the assessment process and implementation of agency policy, then it is no accident that quality of life projects all over the world are wrestling with how to achieve these ends with persons who have profound communication and/or cognitive disabilities. The problem is mostly a technical one with persons who are cognitively intact but have problems expressing their understanding (e.g. persons who are paralysed or who otherwise cannot speak but who do not have intellectual disability). What is usually required in such cases is some form of technology. When dealing with persons who have profound intellectual disability or who have autism or who experience severe forms of emotional disability, however, the problems of achieving a 'subjective' understanding of quality of life and of involving the individual in the conduct of quality of life assessment become more complex, especially if the individual in question does not participate in formal language systems.

When I write 'persons with severe disabilities', what kinds of persons do I mean? The range of communicative abilities in people with 'profound intellectual disability' and those with additional physical and/or sensory impairments is wide. At one extreme we find the adult characterized as having profound intellectual disability who 'has [a] speaking vocabulary of over 300 to 400 words and uses grammatically correct sentences. If nonverbal ... may use many gestures for communication.

---

* This section of writing expands upon the ideas presented in Goode & Hogg, 1994.

Understands simple verbal communications, including directives and questions ... Relates experiences in simple language' (Grossman, 1983). In contrast, other individuals with profound mental retardation may lack any formal symbolic vocal or gestural language. Communication may be presymbolic or action based (see Goode, 1994a), idiosyncratic and, from the perspective of carers, entirely absent (see Hogg & Lambe, 1988). Paralleling this extreme range in communicative ability is the diversity of such persons' cognitive development (see Hogg & Sebba, 1986). This state of affairs will clearly influence the nature and complexity of understanding that, regardless of communicative development, will affect the person's experience of what determines their quality of life.

It is not surprising that the subjective perception of quality of life adopted within this communicative-cognitive state will depend upon the individual's condition and experiences in life.

Quality of life assessment also depends on the experiences and perceptions of the person(s) designing and performing the assessment as much as it does upon those of the person being assessed. One of the major problems with this population is that the assessors (scientists and human service professionals) and those being assessed (people with profound intellectual and related disabilities) may not share experiences that are similar enough to assume a 'reciprocity of perspectives'. Thus we do not wish to give the impression in this discussion that the only relevant factors in understanding how a person with such profound intellectual disability perceives their own quality of life are their experiences and countenance. What 'we' find out in our enquiries is also clearly a reflection of our own experiences and ways of being in the world. This is not to say that scientists/professionals and people with profound intellectual handicaps do not share a great deal, because they do. But there are also very real, sometimes even insurmountable differences – for example, being a symbolic language user or not. Experience of the individual who is disabled is important because implicit in the concept of subjective quality of life is not only the contemporary experience of personal status, but its implications for future selection from options, i.e. choice. Choice has become a central tenet of policy in the field of disability and is as relevant for the person with profound disabilities as any user of a human service. With persons who have profound disabilities, choice and experience may be, however, inextricably bound up in ways that are difficult to assess. Bannerman *et al.* (1990) have emphasized that the ability to make choices is dependent upon experience of choice and that learning choice making should be part of the wider curriculum. This is important because such a view treats choice not as an absolute but as an inherent part of the person's history. It implies a time course in coming to the state of being able to make informed choices that are responsible and within the person's competencies. If we assume the possibility of choice making when the person has limited experiences or has even been subjected to highly insulting and hurtful life events, with the attendant difficulty of understanding and codifying experiences of life, then any assessment of quality of life is further complicated (see Coulter, 1990). Acknowledging this minimizes the danger to the person with profound disabilities that any behaviour they display is taken at face value as being a choice. The claim that someone should be allowed to continue in self-injurious behaviour, 'because he is choosing to do so' is too simplistic and while this may be a choice existentially speaking, it may be so constrained by lack of experience and/or pathological experience that it is more of a compulsion than real selection among options. Clearly there are dangers here. Many non-disabled people, rightly or wrongly from some abstract standard, actually live their lives with 'self-abuse' (drugs, alcohol, dangerous and unhealthy eating, remaining in punishing and negative psychological situations, etc.) built into their work, recreational or even family life. Are they 'free' to choose to do so? We are as yet poor judges of what might constitute informed or uninformed choice or even choice behaviour from communicative expressions not indicative of choice, or for that matter what constitutes free or real choice behaviour.

Nevertheless, choice is not expressed in a vacuum and people with profound cognitive disabilities clearly make choices. These will be related to perceived available options and will be expressed vocally, gesturally, motorically or through some affective expression, conventional or idiosyncratic. With persons who cannot communicate through conventional symbol systems, it is the understanding of both the environment that offers options and its relation to the mode of expression that is critical. Through such an appreciation, subjective quality of life in people with profound intellectual disabilities may be made more understandable. While such matters are sometimes well understood and anecdotally described by the 'direct care personnel' who take care of persons with profound disability, there is little systematic research in this area. Several projects directed to this issue are at present being undertaken, e.g. Chauvie, Iribagiza & Musitelli (1992) in Switzerland and Hogg (1992a) in Great Britain. In the latter work, carers and staff define for the research team behaviours that from their perspective are indicative of the way in which a person with profound disability expresses preference and engages sensorily with the environment. The profile for an individual is then validated through direct observation by both researchers and service providers and will in due course be used to evaluate subjective response to various elements of service provision and community experience. Other approaches involving observation or videotaping are suggested in Goode, 1983; Holm *et al.*, 1994; Taylor, 1994; Taylor & Bogdan, 1990.

Related to direct observational approaches has been the use of what in sociology is referred to as 'reputational data'. Here a surrogate or surrogates complete standardized assessment instruments (Holm *et al.*, 1994; Schalock, 1994; Woodill *et al.*, 1994). Such approaches are practical and efficient, but present very basic methodological and epistemological problems. Simply put, people are so surprising and complex that as well as we might know one another, it is always possible to profoundly misread the other's thoughts and feelings. All of us have probably had this experience at some time with close relatives and friends. And this situation is only compounded when one cannot question the other or obtain direct verbal indications of their feelings. Thus, while surrogate-based questionnaires for determining subjective quality of life of people with severe intellectual disabilities may be the only practical option in many agencies, they pose the risk of creating a 'tyranny of quality', a phrase coined while discussing surrogate or committee determination of quality of life for people with disabilities with the Danish contributors to QOLPD. The term points to the possibility of quality of life assessment becoming something that does not reflect the viewpoint or perspective of the individual being assessed. In the same way that normalization, albeit highly misinterpreted, became the basis for a kind of 'tyranny of the normal', a standard by which people were judged independent of whether they agreed with the elements of PASSING, so, too, could quality of life end up being a criterion or standard by which people were measured whether or not they agreed with that standard.

This danger exists for any quality of life assessment, but especially those involving surrogate or objective indicators of quality of life. The danger of the 'tyranny of quality' is present whether the individual is profoundly retarded or not but it is especially potent when we are talking about persons with highly unusual countenance and experience and with whom formal communication may be impossible. This is not to deny the importance or desirability of objective and reputational quality of life data, but rather to point to an inherent problem in their use.

Related to surrogate quality of life assessment is the concept of life sharing that has been advocated by Goode and others (for example, by John O'Brien and Connie Lyle of Responsive Systems Associates in Georgia) in approaching the quality of life orientation with service agencies. A life-sharing approach involves the intentional sharing of life histories (biographies and autobiographies) of persons involved in agency life (both 'clients' and staff), e.g. the writing of a biography of a person with profound intellectual disability by a staff member that would be published in the agency newsletter or helping a citizen-user who has marginal language skills to write their autobiography. While life sharing does not precisely meet the definition of quality of life-oriented policy presented at the start of this chapter, it nonetheless creates an atmosphere in agencies that enhances information about and understanding of the lives of people with severe disabilities.

OBJECTIVE QUALITY OF LIFE ASSESSMENT AND PROFOUND DISABILITY

There are many reasons why it would not be justifiable to develop a service within the exclusive context of subjective quality of life indices within the adult population of people with profound disability, even if they prove to be sensitive and discriminating with respect to both environmental variation and the subtlety of subjective response. That this would be irresponsible and incorrect has to do with the limited intellectual comprehension of some persons. For example, with respect to health care, among those with profound and multiple disabilities development is inherently slow and the presence of additional medical conditions prevalent. Yet, they may be entirely unaware of either their slow development or additional medical conditions. Indeed, they may even lack any comprehension whatsoever of what a disease is. From the perspective of those providing services and indeed from that of the wider society, a failure to intervene would and should be regarded as culpable. Educational and medical intervention is called for, respectively to enhance physical and social interactions in order to extend options for choice, but also to maintain and/or improve functioning and reduce physical distress. These are, of course, important parts of a person's quality of life.

Once we admit to this, there are additional complications that arise. With regard to adult education, for example, not all educational efforts with adults with profound disabilities are appreciated by them. Even in a curriculum that most would agree benefits the individual, we can find examples of persons who do not subjectively appreciate this and who may actively resist our efforts, which might be regarded by the adult with profound disabilities as not enhancing their subjective quality of life. How long do we persist with such educational intervention? To what extent are the subjective indices noted above to be taken as rejection of what is on offer, even where progress is being made with respect to cognitive, communicative, social and adaptive skills? This is an essential and challenging question if we are to admit a holistic view of quality of life. Perhaps one answer might be a procedure that continues to explore the area in question so that subjective and objective indices can be brought into harmony. Here we are dealing with clinical questions that require the exercise of clinical judgement. In the absence of any carefully evaluated attempts to explore the interaction of subjective and objective indicators of quality of life, it is premature to attempt an *a priori* and possibly hypothetical resolution of this tension.

Are the same issues raised in relation to the assessment of health-related quality of life of people with profound disabilities? Professional staff will typically wish to follow practices that maintain good health or deal with evidence of illness or conditions such as epilepsy. For many people with profound and multiple disabilities, informed consent for serious medical interventions, (e.g. surgical procedures) will not be possible. It would be ingenuous, however, to assume that all medical interventions are benign or incontrovertibly for the best. This point can be illustrated with respect to the prevalence of hysterectomies in women in this group (e.g. Kaunitz, Thompson & Kaunitz, 1986), the removal of all teeth to prevent self-mutilation (e.g. Watts *et al.*, 1974) or excessive polypharmacy (Hogg, 1992b). While indications of the subjective response to treatment would remain central to any holistic approach to medical treatment, the role of an independent and informed advocate operating within the existing legal framework will be central to much of the decision making in this area. While such a view is threatening to the medical profession, calling into question their clinical judgement, there is sufficient controversy regarding medical treatment of this group and its adverse impact on quality of life to indicate the importance of an independent advocate. It is my experience that often direct care staff who care for the individual in question can be good sources of information about how the person might feel about risks and benefits in medical procedures. As a case in point, I was once involved in a medical decision regarding life-threatening surgery to a young woman who had been born with very severe facial anomaly. After finding out about the surgery and its risks, I went to several of the nursing staff who had worked with Vicki for many years. I discussed the situation with them individually and asked each 'What would Vicki say if we could ask her?'. Each staff member answered without hesitation, 'She would have it done'. When we assembled in a team meeting later that week, it was understood already what was going to happen. All those people loved Vicki and wanted her life to be a better one. And while that decision was fraught with the danger of misreading Vicki, this is about the best that we have in human services today. Luckily Vicki had several nursing staff who cared very much for her and who had known her for many years.

It is clear from earlier studies of quality of life in people with developmental disabilities (Goode, 1988a,b), however, that the domains that require consideration, from both subjective and objective perspectives, are far more extensive than health and education. Housing, with its close links to social life (including family relationships, neighbourhood involvement and natural environment features), mobility, friendship, leisure, religion, work, etc. may all occupy central importance in an individual's experience of quality of life. In principle, the same general challenges and arguments relating to subjective and objective quality of life apply in these domains. The critical issues remain the manner in which we assess the former and then harmonize this information with the assessment of housing and social work department staff, supported by whatever specialized assessments are deemed administratively necessary.

DISCUSSION

The initial discussion of Figure 5.1 was methodological and not specific-ally linked into an explication of quality of life assessment of persons with profound disabilities *per se*. The reader may now see how that methodological discussion parallels the more clinical one in the previous section. On the right side of the figure are those who will assess the qual-ity of life of persons with profound disability through some process of quantitation of behaviour, disposition and/or environment. These evaluations, as discussed by Schalock, can be both objective and 'subjec-tive' (reputational). When dealing specifically with persons who cannot give clear and unambiguous communication about choices or viewpoint on their quality of life, all data are either objective or reputational in a strict sense, since we cannot get direct (i.e. self-reported) indications of subjectivity. Subjectivity is inferrable, perhaps even strongly so in certain kinds of methods, but only inferrable. Invariably, no matter how sophisticated or complex the scale, what is produced is a rating that reflects the observer's impression of the individual's subjectivity.

On the left side of the figure are those who will describe the quality of life of persons with profound disability and who will produce data that are both reputational (i.e. their observations of the individual's subjectiv-ity and emotional disposition) and sociological or relational (for example, in my own work, how children were socially constructed). These qualita-tive methods can produce data that reveal the subjective viewpoint of the person being studied. Qualitative methods allow the researcher or qual-ity of life assessor to get relatively close to the everyday life of the person being assessed. Clearly such intimacy is an advantage when trying to understand persons with profound disability.

The figure illustrates co-operation between these two sets of researchers at the level of application. This kind of arrangement is neces-sary because of the mentioned disjuncture between subjective and objec-tive quality of life indices. Given the political climate today, both styles of quality of life assessment are supposed to be done with the input and involvement of persons with disabilities. Just how co-operation is to work or how people are to be involved must be worked out now in detail. I am confident that these are the correct questions, even if I am not suggesting specific answers to them in this chapter.

On the right side of Figure 5.1 are those who use scales to assess the subjective (i.e. reputational) and objective aspects of quality of life. When it comes to quality of life assessment of persons with profound disability, and certainly if we are dealing with a person with a 300–400-word vocabulary, there are now direct question protocols being developed that allow for quality of life assessment with some psychometric validity. If we are talking about people who cannot communicate normally or who even lack language systems, then the surrogate approach must be relied upon. Surrogate quality of life assessment can use either or both of the approaches in Figure 5.1. Thus, two staff filling out Schalock's Quality of Life Questionnaire and my own descriptions of a deaf-blind child's perception of her life on the ward are both examples of surrogate quality of life assessment. Through different methodologies we speak for, on behalf of, the individual who cannot directly represent their own opinions on the matter.

Direct and detailed observation of the lives of persons with profound disabilities should be resonant with quantitative assessments of these lives. For example, if a population is studied with an instrument that quantitates their quality of life, then a subsample of individuals studied through direct observation should yield consistent results. I argued above that qualitative methods are suited to retrieve the 'subjective' view of the individual. They can get close to the lives in question and yield data that reflect this closeness and familiarity. They are also ways to discover the relational or sociological aspects of these lives. Thus if such methods produce results that are in contradiction to quantitative measures, the difference(s) must be understood.

There are many reasons why a holistic approach to the assessment of quality of life of people with profound intellectual disabilities may be an important development in their future welfare. Such an assessment will be developed, but because of the complexity of the issues involved this may take a long time to do validly and correctly. I suspect that many of the issues that have been raised will not be quickly resolved.

Hogg and I suggested that subjective quality of life data (the opinions and perspective of the person in question) or reputational quality of life data (the opinions of others, or surrogates, about the viewpoint of the person in question) and objective quality of life data (clinical and behavioural about the persons and environments in question) have their place in assessing quality of life. Admittedly, the harmonization of these data may not be easy but the knowledge gained from the experimental and exploratory research going on in Scotland, Switzerland, Denmark, the United States and other countries is important for the development of quality of life assessment for this population. We need to develop more systematic ways of recognizing the prelinguistic ways in which persons without formal language communicate their preferences, ideas, reactions and feelings.

But quality of life assessment of people with profound intellectual disability will, I suspect, never qualify as a hard science. More probably, the scientific knowledge we will gain in the study of quality of life for these individuals will always be employed in ways similar to how knowledge is employed in an art or a craft. Due to the complexity of quality of life and especially due to the differences in countenance and experience between the assessors and those being assessed, determining the quality of life for people with profound cognitive disability will probably always rely on very fine judgements and forms of empathy, things not easily operationalized and put to paper. But also like artists and craftsmen, those in charge of the quality of life assessment may develop a facility in doing it over time.

Enhancing the quality of life of people with profound disabilities needs to be our primary goal in providing them with supports and services. Part of doing this is assessing quality of life and therefore, despite the dangers inherent in defining and measuring quality of life described above, I am advocating that such protocols of quality of life assessment be designed and put into place with great care. There are many potential benefits if the process can safeguard against the 'tyranny of quality'. This can only be achieved if subjective data (or reputational approximations of them) are seriously incorporated into the process and if any harmonization of these different forms of quality of life data respects first and foremost the viewpoint of the individual in question. Without glorifying subjectivity, ignoring the problems and limitations inherent in subjective quality of life data discussed above or suggesting that clinical and other objective data are not relevant to the assessment process, the respect for the individual's viewpoint is the necessary condition for quality of life assessment of any person, with or without disability, and no matter what the degree or quality of disability. This statement is perhaps the most fitting conclusion to a chapter titled as this one is.

REFERENCES

Bannerman, D., Sheldon, J.B., Sherman, J.A. and Harchik, A.E. (1990) Balancing the right to habilitation with the right to disabilities to eat too many doughnuts and take a nap. *Journal of Applied Behavior Analysis*, **23**, 79–89.

Brown, R., Brown, P.M. and Bayer, M.B. (1994) A quality of life model: new challenges resulting from a six year study, in *Quality of Life for Persons with Disabilities: International Perspectives and Issues*, (ed. D. Goode), Brookline Books, Cambridge, MA.

Chauvie, J-M., Iribagiza, R. and Musitelli, T. (1992) *Contribution du Groupe Romand sur le Polyhandicap Profond*. Seminaire d'Octobre 1992 du Reseau Europeen d'Echanges sur le Polyhandicap, Consacre au Theme de La Communication.

Coulter, D. (1990) Home is the place: quality of life for young children with developmental disabilities, in *Quality of Life: Issues and Perspectives*, (ed. R. Schalock), American Association on Mental Retardation, Washington DC.

Cummins, R.A. (1993) *Comprehensive Quality of Life Scale: Intellectual Disability*, 4th edn (ComQol-ID4), Deakin University, Burwood, Victoria, Australia.

Dossa, P.A. (1989) Quality of life: individualism or holism? A critical review of the literature. *International Journal of Rehabilitation Research*, **12**(2), 121–36.

Edgerton, R.B. (1990) Quality of life from a longitudinal research perspective, in *Quality of Life: Perspectives and Issues*, (ed. R. Schalock), American Association on Mental Retardation, Washington DC.

Goode, D.A. (1983) Who is Bobby? in *Health Through Occupation*, (ed. G. Kielhofner), F.A. Davis, Philadelphia, PA.

Goode, D.A. (1988a) *Quality of Life for Persons with Disabilities: A Review and Synthesis of the Literature*, Mental Retardation Institute/UAP, Valhalla, New York.

Goode, D.A. (1988b) *Discussing Quality of Life*, Mental Retardation Institute/UAP, Valhalla, New York.

Goode, D.A. (1994a) *A World without Words: The Social Construction of Children Born Deaf-Blind*, Temple University Press, Philadelphia.

Goode, D.A. (ed.) (1994b) *Quality of Life for Persons with Disabilities: International Perspectives and Issues*, Brookline Books, Cambridge, MA.

Goode, D.A. (1994c) *Quality of Life and International Disability Policy*. Paper presented at the First European Quality of Life Conference on People with Special Needs, Copenhagen, Denmark, December 10–14.

Goode, D.A. and Hogg, J. (1994) Towards an understanding of holistic quality of life in people with profound intellectual and multiple disabilities, in *Quality of Life for Persons with Disabilities: International Perspectives and Issues*, (ed. D. Goode), Brookline Books, Cambridge, MA.

Grossman, H.J. (1983) *Classification in Mental Retardation*, American Association on Mental Retardation, Washington DC.

Heal, L., Harner, C.J., Amado, A.R.N. and Chadsey-Rusch, J. (1993) *Lifestyle Satisfaction Scale*, IDS Publishing, Worthington, OH.

Hogg, J. (1992a) *Behavioural State and Affective Communication in People with Profound Intellectual and Multiple Disabilities as Indicators of Their Response to Service Provision*. Grant application submitted to the Scottish Office Home and Health Department, White Top Research Unit, Dundee University.

Hogg, J. (1992b) The administration of psychotropic and anticonvulsant drugs to children and adults with profound intellectual disability and multiple impairments. *Journal of Intellectual Disability Research*, **36**, 472–88.

Hogg, J. and Lambe, L.J. (1988) *Sons and Daughters with Profound Retardation and Multiple Handicaps Attending Schools and Social Education Centres: Final Report*, Royal Society of Mentally Handicapped Children and Adults, London.

Hogg, J. and Sebba, J. (1986) *Profound Retardation and Multiple Impairment. Volume 1: Development and Training*, Croom Helm, London.

Holm, P., Holst, J. and Perlt, B. (1994) Co-write your own life: quality of life as discussed in the Danish context, in *Quality of Life for Persons with Disabilities: International Perspectives and Issues*, (ed. D. Goode), Brookline Books, Cambridge, MA.

Kaunitz, A.M. Thompson, R.J. and Kaunitz, K.K. (1986) Mental retardation: a controversial indication for hysterectomy. *Obstetrics and Gynecology Annual*, **68**, 436–8.

National Institute of Disability and Rehabilitation Research (1993) *Quality-of-life Research in Rehabilitation*, Rehab Brief *II*, (1), 10–15.

Pollner, M. and Goode, D. (1990) Ethnomethodology and person centered practices. *Journal of Person-Centered Review*, **5**(6), 203–20.

Schalock, R.L. (1994) The concept of quality of life and its current applications in the field of mental retardation/developmental disabilities, in *Quality of Life for Persons with Disabilities: International Perspectives and Issues*, (ed. D. Goode), Brookline Books, Cambridge, MA.

Schalock, R.L., Bartnik, E., Wu, F. *et al.* (1990) *An International Perspective in Quality of Life: Measurement and Use.* Paper presented at the 114th Annual Meeting of the American Association on Mental Retardation, Atlanta, Georgia.

Shaw, A. (1977) Defining the quality of life. *Hastings Center Reports*, 7(5), 11.

Taylor, S.J. (1994) In support of research on quality of life, but against quality of life, in *Quality of Life for Persons with Disabilities: International Perspectives and Issues*, (ed. D. Goode), Brookline Books, Cambridge, MA.

Taylor, S.J. and Bogdan, R. (1990). Quality of life and the individual's perspective, in *Quality of Life: Perspectives and Issues*, (ed. R. Schalock), American Association on Mental Retardation, Washington DC.

United Nations (1994) Standard Rules on the Equalization of Opportunities for Persons with Disabilities, *A/RES/48/96*.

Watts, R.W.E., McKeran, R.O., Brown, E., Andrews, T.M. and Griffiths, M. (1974) Clinical and biomedical studies on treatment of Lesch-Nyhan syndrome. *Archives of Disease in Childhood*, **49**, 693.

Woodill, G., Renwick, R., Brown, I. and Raphael, D. (1994) Being, belonging and becoming: an approach to the quality of life of persons with developmental disabilities, in *Quality of Life for Persons with Disabilities: International Perspectives and Issues*, (ed. D. Goode), Brookline Books, Cambridge, MA.

Wolfensberger, W. (1994) Let's hang up 'quality of life' as a hopeless term, in *Quality of Life for Persons With Disabilities: International Perspectives and Issues*, (ed. D. Goode), Brookline Books, Cambridge MA.

An analysis of the dimensions of quality of life

6

Trevor Parmenter and Michelle Donelly

INTRODUCTION

The emergence of quality of life as an index of the outcomes of disability programmes in the Western world over the last decade has generated a significant body of theoretical and empirical literature. Opinions on the utility of this construct have ranged from the warmly supportive (Brown, Bayer & MacFarlane, 1989; Schalock, 1990) to those who are concerned we may be fostering a 'tyranny of quality' (Goode, 1990) or perpetuating 'a hopeless term' (Wolfensberger, 1994).

While quality of life is a relatively recent area of study in the disability field, it has had a long history in the health field and in the study of the quality of life of communities. Organizations such as the World Health Organization (Orley & Kuyken, 1994), OECD (1976) and UNESCO (Solomon *et al.*, 1980) have sponsored major studies. Many of the early national studies of quality of life and well-being were conducted in the Nordic countries in the 1970s (cf. Nussbaum & Sen, 1993).

Early support for the utility of quality of life assessments as a means of evaluating both the processes and outcomes of disability programmes came from writers such as Brown, Bayer & MacFarlane (1989), Brown, Bayer & Brown (1992), Edgerton (1975), Emerson (1985), Landesman-Dwyer (1981, 1985) and Schalock (Schalock, 1990; Schalock & Lilley, 1986). The 1990s have seen an increasing emphasis upon programme standards and outcome-based evaluation in a period Schalock (1995) has described as an 'era of accountability' (pvii).

As with health and urban studies, quality of life is increasingly being used as a social indicator for purposes of policy development in the disability service area. However, the history of social indicator research and its impact on social policy has not always produced auspicious results

(Parmenter, 1996). In its quest for objective and quantifiable data social indicators research often resorted to very simplistic indices of rather complex constructs. Nowhere is this more the case than in quality of life research.

In much of the health field, and more recently the disability field, instruments purporting to assess 'quality of life' have been developed. In much of this development there has been an emphasis upon the achievement of a 'gold standard' against which quality of life could be assessed. Missing from many of these developments has been the direct involvement of the people under study.

A major issue that has been debated concerning quality of life is the dichotomy between objective and subjective measures, with most commentators agreeing that it is necessary to include aspects of both if one is to obtain a comprehensive picture of a person's quality of life. In terms of measurement the functional paradigm has been dominant, with the search for assessment instruments which will capture the essential ingredients while at the same time conforming to established psychometric principles. But is it realistic to imagine that one can devise an instrument which will capture the elusive qualities which make up such a complex construct? Basically, a person's view of their life quality is subject to myriad factors – some may be quite static, but in the main the major determinant is the person's value system. In other words, what do they see as important in contributing to their life satisfaction? This may change over time as a person's life situations change. On objective measures an outsider may assess a person's quality of life as being extremely poor, but the person's own assessment may be quite different. The reverse can also be true.

This paradox was discussed by Zapf et al. (1987) who referred to it as the 'paradox of satisfaction'. Bowles (1995), in her study of people with spina bifida, found that Zapf et al.'s suggestions were supported. Despite relatively poorer quality of life on objective measures when compared to a non-disabled contrast group, the sample of people with spina bifida suggested their quality of life was satisfactory. In Australia, governments are endeavouring to ensure that basic objective factors are available to people with a disability through various human rights legislation and the enforcement of programme standards in services they fund. Obviously, these initiatives may be *necessary* conditions for supporting life quality, but it is doubtful if they are *sufficient* conditions. The latter are integral to the processes and outcomes of programmes, rather than the legislative mandates which surround the programmes.

We are also witnessing a paradigm shift from the delivery of programmes and services to people with disabilities driven by government imperatives to a situation where these people are demanding more say in and power over the decisions which are made in their lives (Knox *et al.*,

1995). There is a fine line to be drawn between social justice principles forming the basic philosophical underpinnings of disability services and the possibility of a bureaucratization of values by those who are called to administer the financial supports (Blatt, 1979).

Perhaps in our efforts to provide better programme outcomes for people with disabilities, we have ignored Knoll's (1990) suggestion that 'the definition of programme standards and quality is a process that transcends empiricism. This process ultimately appeals to the fundamental values of society' (p235). It might be added that the ultimate index is the value system of the individual but of course, as we have seen from Bowles' study, the individual's expectations are influenced by societal factors.

TOWARDS A THEORETICAL BASE FOR QUALITY OF LIFE

In tracing the history of the quality of life phenomenon it was apparent that much of the work lacked an adequate theoretical base, especially in the area of disability research. The social indicator movement had placed much emphasis upon quantifiable measures. Carley (1981) has explained that social indicators are both *surrogates* and *measures*. As *surrogates* they do not stand alone; they take quite abstract and intrinsically measurable concepts and translate them into operational terms. Thus they act as a proxy for an unmeasurable concept. Owing to the intrinsic difficulties in assessing these unmeasurable concepts, we resort to indirect measures, often drawing inferences from the resulting quantifiable data.

INDEPENDENT LIVING MOVEMENT

Another factor overlooked in the context of disability research was the intrinsic measurement of 'disability'. One of the first to address this issue was De Jong (1981) who used the concept of 'independent living' as an analytical tool. De Jong suggested that the anomalous situation of people with severe physical disabilities achieving independence without the benefit of professional rehabilitation services served as the impetus for the shift from a rehabilitation paradigm, characterized by professional control, to the independent living paradigm, characterized by consumer control. The former paradigm, he suggested, saw the problems residing in the individual, whereas for the emerging independent living paradigm, 'the locus of the problem is not the individual but the environment that includes not only the rehabilitation process, but also the physical environment and social control mechanisms in society-at-large' (De Jong, 1981, p29). These views have been echoed more recently by several writers including Barton (1989), Fulcher (1989) and Oliver (1989). There was a distinct shift from the basic functional measures of independence to a more qualitative assessment. For instance, Zola (1993) suggested that 'it is not the quantity of tasks we can perform without assistance, but the quality of life we can live without help' (p10).

While De Jong's approach signalled a watershed in the notion of independence, his approach to assessment was still overly narrow. Williams (1983) pointed out that De Jong's analysis assumed a one-way causal relationship between environmental contingencies and individual states and ignored the mediating effects of symbols and contexts of social life (p1009). Similarly, his model severely limited the influence individual personality characteristics and personal choice may have upon defining outcomes. For instance, the question of whether 'living alone' should be seen as a desirable outcome or not depends, in part, upon the personality and value system of the individual and the value they place upon social relationships and privacy.

De Jong, coming from a physical rehabilitation background, may have overlooked the broader sociological impacts of disability, especially the way society has exerted influence on how disability is viewed in the social context. Bogdan & Kugelmass (1984) pointed out that the word 'disability' is not a symbol for a condition that is already there in advance. Paradoxically, disability is part of the mechanism whereby the condition is created. Taking a symbolic interactionist view, it is suggested that human experiences are mediated by interpretation. The development of a self-identity arises and is maintained in a symbolic and interactive context.

A SYMBOLIC INTERACTIONIST APPROACH

Physical and/or psychological impairments set the parameters in which the definitions develop, but the way in which people determine their definitions depends upon a variety of factors including personal and community attitudes toward people who appear different. As we live in a society where diversity is not valued or even tolerated (Kalantis, 1989), people with disabilities are conditioned by negative stereotypes from early childhood.

COLLECTIVE RULE MAKING

Scott (1972), in his analysis of the symbolic nature of rule making, has argued that this dimension of the social order is the most important one for understanding deviance. Society develops a view of reality which attempts to bring order and meaning to an otherwise random universe through the construction of a system for classifying human existence. In operational terms this results in objects, events and people having to conform to the class or category to which they have been assigned. It also requires that there are simple means available for discriminating among the classes of things. However, people with disabilities are seen as anomalous in this view of the social order. Consequently, viewed from the perspective of a symbolic universe, the property of deviance is assigned to these anomalous individuals.

THE AREA OF INTERPERSONAL RELATIONS

The development of social identity or stereotyping has particular relevance for the study of deviance. McCall & Simmons (1978) have suggested that identification of persons and of other 'things' is the key to symbolic interaction, for once things are identified and their meanings for us established, we can get on with our individual pursuits. Once we categorize or place a person in a particular 'box', we know how to behave towards that person. But Schur (1971) has noted that this is a two-way process: 'Just as the individual constantly "types" other people, so he is constantly typed by others and indeed also by himself' (p41). For people without disabilities stereotyping obviously simplifies their interaction with people who have disabilities, but this tends to limit their perception of the individual so that relationships seldom develop beyond a superficial level.

For the person with a disability there is often a lack of congruence between their desired personal identity and their assigned social identity. Hurst (1984) has commented that stereotypes focus upon generalities. This is supported by Scott's (1972) observation that society has ascribed to people with visual disabilities the attributes of 'helplessness, dependency, melancholy, docility, gravity of inner thought, (and) aestheticism', all traits, he has suggested, 'that common sense views tell us to expect of the blind' (p4). The effects of this role-making process are such that the person with a disability will often struggle to develop an authentic identity. Unfortunately people who have been assigned an identity or role in society may ultimately fulfil the expectations others have of them, thus reinforcing in the eyes of others the validity of their assessments.

The closer the perceptions of self by the person with a disability come to those ascribed by society, the greater is the chance that secondary deviance or career disability will emerge as the major form of role adaptation. Burback (1981), in distinguishing between primary and secondary deviance, has suggested that people with 'primary' deviance do not see their 'differentness' as defining them as a person, whereas people with 'secondary' deviance see their 'differentness' as the crucial defining element in their concept of self. In this respect career disability has been a major focus of attention of a number of writers in the field of rehabilitation (De Jong, 1979, 1981; Finkelstein, 1980; Stoddard, 1978). For instance, in his analysis of attitudes and disabled people, Finkelstein (1980) has indicted professional groups as having contributed significantly to the social oppression of people with disabilities, a view consistent with writers such as Barton (1989) and Oliver (1989).

THE IMPLICATIONS OF LABELLING FOR THE QUALITY OF LIFE
QUESTION

In his illuminating analysis of the labelling issue, Burback (1981) has suggested that it is a superficial question to ask whether we should or should not label anomalous individuals. He pointed out that labelling and categorizing people is a normal process of apprehending and organizing our world. Of more importance is '*how* we label (people) and *with* what *consequences*' (Burback, 1981, p376). Burback's contention is that people with a disability are in a double bind situation. In addressing the issue of what it means to be disabled, they are confronted by two messages. One comes from outside and proceeds from the social order. The other, however, comes from within and relates to what they know they can or cannot do. Thus they have to deal with the negative aspects of their personal condition and at the same time cope with the negative effects of stigmatization and stereotyping. From a philosophical point of view there is a conflict between the existential nature of the person and the social nature of human experience.

It may be prudent, however, not to overgeneralize these issues, for some people with a disability are able to assert their personal identities, despite the negative stereotypes society often ascribes to them. The factors that contribute to variance in this population in this respect require further empirical investigation in the context of the general population and other marginalized social groups.

In trying to establish a coherent meaning for life as well as creating and maintaining self-esteem, the conflict between the messages the person with a disability receives often presents insuperable problems. On the one hand the person can live in a cocoon-like existence built on socially invalidated meanings or, on the other, they can conform to the patterns of behaviour that are expected of them by society generally. Neither of these approaches leads to a satisfactory explanation of how they define their own meanings. Here, it is proposed, lies the hub of the quality of life issue. Quality of life represents the degree to which an individual has met their needs to create their own meanings so the individual can establish and sustain a viable self in the social world. The resolution proffered by Burback draws upon the basic principles of symbolic interactions. That is, there is a need for *consensuality* whereby humans help each other unfold and establish contact and unity in their social existence.

COMMUNITY LIVING

In examining the outcomes of community or independent living pro-grammes for people with disabilities, a crucial element to be examined is the degree to which they are *of* rather than simply *in* a community. A measure of this will undoubtedly be the quality of their interpersonal relationships with others within their community. Here the sociological concepts of *Gemeinschaft* and *Gesellschaft* are useful analytical tools. *Gemeinschaft* refers to a community of spirit whereas *Gesellschaft* describes a community organized on a formal or contractual basis where relation-ships are impersonal. Neither necessarily specifies a geographical or physical entity, but from the above discussion of the development of self, it is appreciated that simply observing the superficial and outward characteristics of a community-based facility does not indicate whether it has *Gemeinschaft*. This reinforces the earlier discussion on the inade-quacies of many outcome studies which, it is suggested, have ignored the quality of life dimension.

While not without its critics (e.g. Sharp & Green, 1975), the symbolic interaction theory has usefully contributed to our understanding of aspects of the social situation of people with disabilities. Barton & Tomlinson (1984) have suggested that this approach has at least two strengths. First, it emphasizes the viewpoint of the participants in social interaction and second, the perspective explores aspects of social life which have historically either been taken for granted or ignored. Other sociological approaches might emphasize economic considerations and the distribution of resources in the society (e.g. structuralist neo-Marxism) or use the traditional Marxist class conflict model to explore the imbalance of power between disabled and non-disabled groups in society. These theories may not be mutually exclusive, for in the context of quality of life it is suggested that the consciousness of self and social identity, status and social role are obviously preconditions for political activism and social change.

DEVELOPMENT OF A MODEL OF QUALITY OF LIFE

In the first edition of this book, a multidimensional interactive model of quality of life was proposed which incorporated aspects of a person's functional behaviours, variables associated with the 'self' and societal influences which impacted upon the person (Parmenter, 1988) (see Fig. 6.1). Underpinning the model was the importance of the development of one's 'identity' as an authentic person. The sociological concept of sym-bolic interactionism provided a useful theoretical base upon which the development of 'identity' could be explored.

Within the three components of the model, the list of subcomponents is presently tentative but, from an examination of the research literature,

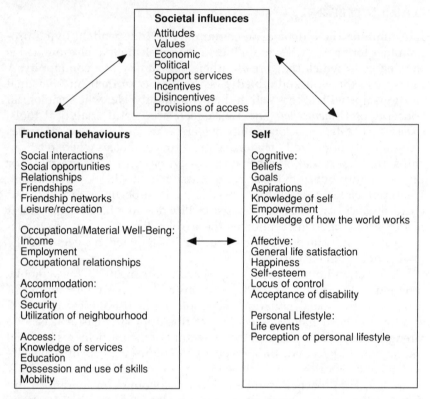

Fig. 6.1 A model of quality of life for people with disabilities (Parmenter, 1988).

together with the issues explored under the symbolic interactionist rubric, it would appear they represent important elements. This model has some parallels to the model *Having, Loving, Being*, developed by the Finnish sociologist Erik Allardt (1975, 1993).

APPLICATION OF THE MODEL

The remainder of this chapter will use the model as a framework for examining the quality of life of a group of people with a physical disability, half of whom decided to move from a large nursing home into community-based accommodation and half who decided to remain.

In 1993 people living in a large-scale supported accommodation service were asked whether or not they wished to move to a smaller accommodation service running on a group home model. Some people agreed to move while others opted to stay. The study explored the factors relating to quality of life which were considered by individuals in making their decision. Nine months after the changes in their accommodation had occurred, each person's views of the factors affecting their quality of life were again examined.

METHOD

In order to ensure that issues of concern to residents were canvassed, focus groups were formed among residents including people who were to move and those who had elected to stay. The focus groups identified factors which residents considered to be important in determining their quality of life, in addition to issues which they felt must be addressed in both congregate and community care facilities. Factors nominated by people in the focus group meetings as important in determining quality of life and/or of concern to them at the present time included: personal, physical and financial security; choice over whom you would live with; choice about who would provide you with personal care; control over hiring and firing staff; choice of doctor; and opportunity to keep in contact with friends and family.

Information identified in the focus groups, as well as in the literature, was used to generate questions and topics which would be discussed with residents. Semistructured, open-ended interviews were conducted with each of the nine people who had elected to move out of the facility. The study included people with severe disabilities who required total assistance with eating, drinking, dressing, toiletting and mobility due to physical and/or sensory and/or cognitive impairments and people with moderate disabilities who did not require assistance with any of these tasks but who nevertheless required accommodation support due to sensory and/or physical and/or cognitive disabilities. Two people had developmental disabilities, the remainder acquired their disability later in life. In addition, they had resided in the congregate care facility for from two to 25 years. Of the residents who had elected to remain, nine people, who matched the group leaving in terms of background, gender and aspects of functional performance, were selected to form a contrast group. They also participated in semistructured, open-ended interviews.

Nine months after changes in their accommodation had occurred, each of the 18 people's views of the factors affecting their quality of life were re-examined. The 36 interviews ranged from 1.5 to 3.5 hours in duration. This interview time may seem excessive, but most of the residents maintained a lively interest in the issues being discussed. This highlighted the advantages of having the residents determine the areas to be explored. Initial data analysis using open coding of qualitative data transcribed from audiotapes of the interviews and crosstabulation of more structured items revealed a wide range of factors identified by participants as influencing their decision making and their life satisfaction.

RESULTS

In terms of the multidimensional model of quality of life, responses of the residents were interesting. The majority of their responses related to issues subsumed under 'self' and 'societal influences'. These may be respectively grouped under factors which provided them with power to make decisions about their lives and the level of support they needed to enable them to exist in a less restricted environment.

Table 6.1 Comparison of the level of support required for the performance of daily living tasks by people who chose to move and people who chose to stay, before and after moving

% Task completed	Residents who moved (N=9)		Residents who stayed (N=9)	
	Before	After	Before	After
Completed independently	31	39	34	33
Completed with assistance	22	28	24	23
Completed by others	47	33	42	44
	100	100	100	100

DAILY LIVING TASKS

It is interesting to note that there were only minor differences in terms of the support required to perform daily living tasks between the people who chose to stay in the nursing home and those who chose to move.

An inspection of Table 6.1 reveals that the levels of support the two groups required were very similar and for the group which moved, their support levels were little changed after the move. This is not surprising as the majority of the residents had quite high personal support needs because of the nature of their impairments. Thus, the notion of physical independence did not appear to be a factor in their perception of their life satisfaction. Indeed, a critical concern for both groups was the availability of support to assist them with their daily living tasks. The key factor which appeared to affect a person's decision to move or stay was their perception of the support they would receive after the move. There was a strong suspicion by many who chose to stay that the necessary support would not be available outside the nursing home.

Don's and Laura's comments illustrate the apprehension some residents had about a move into community-based accommodation (note that all names used are pseudonyms).

> *Don*: There are people here staffing 24 hours a day … if anything happens … you know I never even thought about it, just the thought of getting out of here, oh heaven … but when we started talking about it … living out in the community you have to rely on the person getting there in time … I have lived out in the community, I know what it is like, it's not easy … there are a lot of health reasons to why we thought about this, the more we spoke about it the more frightened I got.
>
> *Laura*: You would be more institutionalized – e.g. out in the community – because you would have to be home by a certain time to be put to bed before your carer went home … whereas here, you can be put to bed anytime because you know, you've got someone there to help at all times.

However, while these natural fears significantly influenced their decision to stay in the nursing home, the contrast group still expressed a high degree of dissatisfaction with their current living arrangements. Typical comments included the following:

> *Bill*: Things grow legs in this place, you have to keep stuff locked up and carry a key to the cupboard around or they will go into your cupboard and knock off everything of value.
>
> *Vivienne*: I am sharing a room with a person with whom I have nothing in common. The person can scream for up two hours at a time and talk right through the night.
>
> *Dianne*: If you go out you miss out on a shower altogether. Have to stick to a routine all the time, no flexibility. That really upsets me.
>
> *Nancy*: Lots of sleepless nights you have because you know who is getting you up in the morning and they are not an appropriate person to be on staff here. But you don't have any say in who will do what for you and you can't say what you want to say because there are repercussions.
>
> *Paul*: Agency nurses often don't know what to do and won't listen, it's so frustrating. I need very specialized assistance and they ignore what l say, even though I have been training staff to be able to help me for years and years. A few weeks ago I waited three and a half hours and asked five people before I got help to get to the toilet. People just don't know what it is like. When you tell the management, they just won't believe you. I've always believed you have to listen to people to ask them to give me a hand when they're finished

> what they are doing. People tell me I'm too nice and I think I'll have to change, just can't keep waiting but don't want to be like that.
> *Betty*: Some of the staff are very good, other staff treat you as a child, as if you don't know your own mind. I don't like people running my life.
> *Mary*: They make decisions above your head and tell you … I like to be consulted before appointments are made.

These comments illustrate very clearly the critical role support staff play in the lives of these people, especially because of the very personal help they provide to the person with the disability. Lack of privacy and personal space in the nursing home environment was a frequent comment from both groups. One of the most frequently mentioned issues was the need for consistency in personnel who attended to the very personal aspects of a person's life, as evidenced by Nancy's and Paul's comments above. Two aspects are involved here. One is purely technical, in that the person with the disability has a preferred way certain procedures should be performed, while the second relates to the very intimate nature of these procedures.

In both cases stability of staffing was a very important issue. Unfortunately, in neither accommodation option was this stability guaranteed. Staff turnover, especially in the group home model, is a recurring issue which is endemic to most Western countries. One wonders whether quality of life for staff has been examined with the same vigour as it is being explored for the person with the disability. It would seem the two are related (Brown, Bayer & McFarlane, 1989).

When reinterviewed nine months after some people had moved out, the people who had chosen to stay had become more dissatisfied.

> *Bob*: … used to be quite tolerant of behavioural things, but it gets me down now, just don't know what to do. People have behavioural problems because of frustration.
> *Nancy*: It's not their fault but they are extremely hard to live with and I admit that I don't have the patience I did a decade ago.
> *Tom*: No one is here out of choice but out of necessity. You don't come here because you like to live here but out of necessity. The place is far too institutionalized and you keep waiting for changes and improvements but they just haven't happened. I haven't lived in a lot of other places and if I had I might think that this place was better than it is. Because I came from home, I realize that this place could be a lot better than it is.

> *Betty*: There is a lack of communication between residents and staff, the behaviour of residents is stirred up by staff. Things have changed a great deal in the last two years. I have been reassured by staff that it is going to get better. I tell them, you can resign tomorrow.

These comments can be attributed, in part, to two factors. First, there was a noticeable change in the nature of the residents who were being moved into the surplus space available in the nursing home. Many of the newer residents were suffering the effects of head injury and a number experienced quite severe behavioural problems. Their presence was causing significant levels of dissatisfaction among those who had lived for some years in the nursing home. They felt their 'home' was being taken over by people they had no say in choosing. Second, the departure of the group of nine resulted in a breakdown of friendships and further exacerbated feelings of isolation and loneliness among those who remained.

The following comments illustrate the sense of responsibility residents felt for each other:

> *Julie*: I just can't cut myself off from people who have been with me all these years, especially people I speak up for. It's got to the stage where I am an advocate for them because their families are away and I watch out for them.
> *Sue*: I worry about what's going to happen to the ones who are left behind. Who is going to protect them, who is going to keep an eye on the staff?

Some residents also appeared to have analysed the options and expressed a degree of distrust that a move would, in fact, enhance their life quality. These views are reflected in the following comments:

> *Tim*: I would love to be in my own home, I have always said I wanted to, but I see the obstacles, whereas the first group (of people who chose to move out) can't see the obstacles for themselves.
> *Ron*: What would be the point of moving out if you don't get the choice of staff and the people that I live with and at the homes they are not getting the choice of staff even though they were told they would, the first house did not get the choice of people they live with. ... What worries me if you move out of here is you have to place a lot more trust in your staff because there is no one looking over their shoulder supervising them.

Some residents, however, had a rich network of friends in the wider community. They perceived that the nursing home provided them with a base from which they could venture into the wider world.

> *Julie*: I still think I live in the community, I can't see any difference, I think it is just what you make of your life. I mean if you live in an institution, you just make that institution your whole world, going out and doing things and enjoying yourself once you leave the front door you leave that world behind. So I consider myself to be in the community.

Not all people expressed dissatisfaction with the nursing home environment. For some, community was perceived as the network they had within the nursing home.

> *Bill*: I'm quite happy here. Get well taken care of. Get your meals cooked for you and your washing done for you. You can come and go when you like.
> *Vivienne*: There are some good staff here. There are a few good things, I do have friends here, we stick together and look out for each other all the time. The best thing is my friendships.
> *Elizabeth*: I like the people, all the nurses are very nice. I'm satisfied.

Interestingly, when the contrast group was interviewed for the second time, a number commented how the decrease in support levels following the departure of their friends, had reduced their quality of care. In particular, waiting time for assistance increased and the time available for staff to provide assistance was reduced.

> *Mary*: Things are getting worse here, we are losing all our good nurses. Last weekend my family came to visit me on Sunday afternoon, I was still in bed, they thought I must have been sick to be still in bed. They knew we were short of nurses but only then did they really get the message.

People in the contrast group found this extremely disturbing and it had a big impact on their perception of the organization. A number of people in the contrast group changed their mind about staying in the nursing home. Despite their concerns about the level of support available to people who had moved out, their concern about deteriorating conditions in the congregate care facility and the capacity of the organization to support them in the community convinced them that, comparatively, they were more likely to be able to influence the quality of care by living in the community. When this occurred there was remarkable similarity between the groups in terms of their views of the organization and what had prompted them to consider an alternative. For example:

> *Interviewer*: What will be different about living in a group home from living here?
>
> *Richard*: I'll be able to eat what I like – be able to go out, hopefully, control my finances. Here you are told what to do and when to do it. In a house, I will be consulted, we will have to agree. Looking forward to it.
>
> *Don*: Here it is an institution, a gaol. In your home you are running the ship, no one else is running it, you're working for me and you will do what I tell you. No back stabbing, you work together.
>
> *Julie*: It will be a smaller place, we can help one another prepare meals, you can make up your own times when you eat, get up, go to bed, things like that, you are not locked into a routine.

It is illuminating to contrast these comments of Don and Julie with those they made earlier.

WHAT IS THE IDEAL HOUSEHOLD?

People were asked what would be the ideal or perfect household for them. Prior to the move out, they focused on an 'ordinary home' where people were compatible, 'there were no fights' and 'people had respect for each other's privacy' and there was the 'freedom to choose what to do and where to go'.

People who chose to stay in the large-scale accommodation service mentioned similar themes and also wanted the opportunity to choose the people they would live with and the people who would look after them. These themes were consistent at the interviews nine months later.

DECISION MAKING

A consistent theme in the comments from both groups was the prominence they gave to decision making and control over their lives. Examples are as follows:

Nina: Decisions are made for you here … what time you eat, what time I go to bed, what time I get up, it is all made for me here … living in the community you make your own … more geared to my needs. The wardsman takes me to the toilet at 1pm and if I don't go, he won't toilet me at any other time. But I don't always feel like going at 1pm but at 2pm, I might. Then he says no you didn't go at one, now you can wait till three.

Derek: … there will be less people to be taken care of and we won't be told what to do, we will be asked if we want to do it …

Bill: … there will be more challenges and opportunities and support to use your brains and to show initiative …

Sue: Will be able to make, to take control, life control, control of my own life.

These quotes indicate that the possibility of exercising more freedom, autonomy and decision making were important, especially for those participants who decided to move from the congregate care facility. This is further corroborated in the responses of participants to questions about opportunities for decision making surrounding a wide range of daily living tasks.

Table 6.2 summarizes the results to questions raised with participants about who makes decisions and who does the planning related to a wide variety of daily living tasks. Tasks included eating, drinking, dressing, bathing, toiletting, grooming, cooking, mealtimes, shopping, housework, gardening and moving house. Responses were totalled for each group, resulting in the percentages in each cell of the table. Each numeral refers to the total percentages of decision-making tasks performed by all the members of that group of people at that particular time, either independently, shared or made by others.

Table 6.2 Comparison of participation in decision making affecting daily living tasks by people who chose to move and people who chose to stay, before and after moving

% of Decision making	Residents who moved (N=9)		Residents who stayed (N=9)	
	Before	After	Before	After
All decisions by residents	26	43	44	41
All decisions by others	65	22	42	42
Shared decision making	6	30	14	17
No opportunity/not relevant	3	5	0	0
	100	100	100	100

Table 6.2 shows a marked difference between the two groups in terms of their participation in decisions which affected their daily living tasks. Before the move, it appears that the group who had decided to move made relatively fewer decisions about these activities than did the contrast group. However, nine months after the move, those who had moved reported a much higher degree of control over decisions while the contrast group remained unchanged. It is interesting to note that there was a marked increase in shared decision making by the group who moved, indicating the positive effects of sharing a house rather than a nursing home ward.

OTHER VIEWS ON THE EFFECTS OF THE MOVE

In addition to greater satisfaction concerning decision making, residents expressed pleasure in having their own bed, the peacefulness, the availability of support, greater freedom and being able to do more for oneself. They also indicated that they would like to have more room for wheelchair access, additional toilets and showers and low bench tops and drawers which they could reach from a wheelchair. A number commented that they would prefer to own their own home. Views include the following:

> *Cecily*: It's better so far, it makes you feel human. The staff here view you like a person, they are not so rushed. There is more time to get to talk and know each other. It is not as frightening as I thought it would be, but I am disappointed that we can't choose the staff, as was first proposed. We also didn't get a choice about whom we would live with. I'm learning to live with people. At the large-scale accommodation service, I shared a room with half a dozen others, but didn't learn to live with people. Here people talk to me.
> *Rebecca*: Yes, I made the right decision, it's tons better. I can do anything, it's a home. I'm happy with the level of support.
> *Nancy*: Place still operates on the same principles as the large-scale service except I have my own room. It's still not possible to have a sexual relationship.

VIEWS ON SELF

Cecily's comments indicate that she has felt a change in her identity. Other comments concerning their views on their disability were: 'No, I'm just a normal person with a disability'; 'Don't like unpleasantness – always try to keep out of it. I'm not good at handling that. Rather not say too much';

'Would like to think they wouldn't see me as disabled. There are a lot of things I can do, you are also able'; 'Believe in themselves, believe in what they feel is right'. These feelings of self indicate that societal attitudes may have an influence on the way the person's identity is shaped. Despite the negative attitudes these people have experienced they show a resilience and a belief in themselves.

One resident addressed the question of his disability by responding that he would prefer to be alive than to have the alternative.

> Seeing I am a disabled person, I am thankful I was born like it rather than having it taken away from me. I consider I accept my disability very well, but I consider it would be so much hardship if I had a normal life and had it taken away from me (i.e. by an accident or illness). Even though I admit I'm going to die wondering what it would be like to do all the normal things.

His response provides support for the view that disability should not always be perceived as a negative and suffering condition. The publication *Just Technology: From Principles to Practice in Bio-ethical Issues* (ILSPMH, 1994), covers this issue in detail.

Another resident spoke of the importance the attitudes of other people have upon their quality of life. She commented that:

> There's nothing worse than having someone coming in who is young enough to be your grandchild and ordering you around. Having control is important. Some people think that because you are in a wheelchair that what comes out of your mouth is wrong. I tell them I'm a professional chronic invalid – I know more than they do sometimes.

VIEWS ON QUALITY OF LIFE

The following comments on their perceptions of quality of life indicated that control over their own lives is one of the paramount characteristics.

> *Denis*: Reasonable freedom; choice to do what you want to do; enough things to keep your mind active; to know about work in which I could help others; to be able to help other disabled people. I went through a very difficult time where I couldn't get any help or information. I would like to help other people through this!

Harry: Money.
Felicity: Have a place to live.
Sue: To move out of here, be in a home. Being happy doing the things and where you want to go.
Denis: The freedom to choose and the choice of living standards. Generally, just being in control. Adequate finances and assistance physically and spiritually. Don't give up, keep fighting, keep determined; fight to achieve and you will achieve more. You must have determination and force to achieve. If you wish to achieve anything, you can.
Sue: Try and try and try and try. Try to be better, try to get something better.
Mary: Think about it, when you have thought about it, act.
Julie: Don't be afraid, take a deep breath and go for it. There's nothing like living in a house. It's smaller, quiet and people listen to you.
Henry: To be able to do what I want to do when I want to do it. To be able to go out a lot more socially and feel freer to make our own decisions. Being able to choose the staff and the people I want to live with.
Nora: Enjoy what you are doing – being able to communicate with other people, being able to go out, not being locked up in four walls. Having a good family and friends.
Nancy: Shopping, I just love it.
Tom: Being fed and cared for, being able to have enough money to make life comfortable. To be interested in things, know people, things become more interesting.

These comments indicate that, in addition to a strong desire for control over their lives and the opportunity to exercise choice, many residents revealed characteristics which are consistent with the concepts of *Having, Loving, Being* (Allardt, 1993).

ADVICE ON HOW TO ACHIEVE A GOOD QUALITY OF LIFE

A final question asked the residents what advice they might offer to someone about achieving a good quality of life.

Greg: I don't know how to achieve that. How do you achieve that? I've been trying to achieve quality of life as addict and motor bike rider and living in hospitals for seven years. How could I get a quality of life after doing all that shit?

> *Julie*: Believe in themselves, believe in what they feel is right.
> *Jean*: Work together.
> *Nancy*: If there is something worrying you, you would want to talk to someone about it.

SUMMARY OF RESULTS

In summary, the following conclusions may be drawn from the views expressed by the residents who chose to move into community-based accommodation and the contrast group who initially chose to remain in the nursing home.

- There was little difference in the level of physical support each group required to perform daily living tasks. For the group which moved, individual residents appeared to require less support than the contrast.
- A major determinant in making a decision to move was the perception that adequate support would be available in the community house.
- While many residents saw that the community-based home would provide them with greater freedom, a number who decided to remain in the nursing home expressed the view that they already had a rich community life, with friends both within and without the home.
- Comments on the ideal household related to issues of compatibility, choice and freedom to go out.
- Freedom to make one's own decisions featured prominently in the comments of both groups. This characteristic appeared to be a central theme in the views of those who chose to move. In analysing the exercise of choice, the group which moved made significantly more decisions after the move than before it. There was no change in the levels of independent decision making by the contrast group. The difference seemed all the more marked when it was observed that the group which moved appeared to have less control over their decisions on daily living tasks than did the contrast group before the move. This may indicate that the group which moved had a much higher level of dissatisfaction with the nursing home environment.
- Other views on the effects of the move reflected a change in their perceptions of themselves: 'It makes you feel human'. At the same time, they were looking for ways to improve their lifestyle further.
- Views on their identity reflected a deep belief in their own ability to take control of their lives. They saw support people as a necessary provision to enable them to lead a normal lifestyle. They did not see this in terms of psychological dependency. However, it is suggested that societal attitudes played a role in forming their identity as a person.

DISCUSSION

The results of the interviews have a number of implications for the development of a theoretical model of quality of life. First, it would appear that the basic functional area of the individual's response to ecological domains was not the most pressing issue in their lives. They did not see themselves developing additional 'independent living' skills in the community setting. Rather, they asserted their needs for adequate support mechanisms in the areas of personal care and basic living skills. They stressed the need for comfort and security, but these they could obtain to some degree within the institutional setting. A number of residents indicated that the nursing home gave them a base from which they could have social opportunities, develop relationships and have friendship networks. Others suggested that the community setting afforded them a greater opportunity for extending their social networks as long as physical supports were supplied, especially transport.

The residents' responses in both groups, however, basically centred upon issues related to the self component of the model. All residents emphasized the need for greater psychological independence, including opportunities to make personal decisions about their lives. They wished to determine with whom they would live and whom they would employ as personal assistants. There was deep resentment that opportunities did not exist for them to exercise choices and decision making within the nursing home environment. Others were disappointed, too, that they still had limited control over these basic decisions in the community setting.

Despite the restricted environment in the nursing home, the group which initially chose to move into the community setting demonstrated a deep capacity for influencing events concerning their lives. They had developed a strong positive locus of control and a belief that they could effect changes in their lives. They were prepared to take risks to enhance their lifestyle. This fact was possibly influenced by the strong advocacy skills a number of residents had developed over the long periods many had spent in the nursing home. A number of responses portrayed individuals with a strong resilience and a determination to fight adversity.

The range of responses suggested that it is unwise to make too many generalizations about the factors which people value in their lives. It also supports the principle that questions concerning quality of life issues are specific to individuals and casts doubt upon the wisdom of using standardized global instruments to 'measure' quality of life.

This finding supports the contention by Brown, Bayer & McFarlane (1989) that quality of life is:

> the interaction between the individual and the environment. It can be described in terms of personal control by the individual over the environment. It must be assessed by consulting the individual directly.
>
> (p57)

The area of self-identity is more complex. Earlier discussion suggested that community stereotypes of people with disability severely influenced their development of a self-identity. A number of residents confirmed that the move to a community residence enhanced their self-identity. Others agreed that societal attitudes did affect the way they saw themselves, but they still had a strong belief in themselves. There is little doubt that the experience of disability contributed to their self-identity, but it did not seem to be the dominant factor.

A consistent theme throughout the interviews was the notion of empowerment, not being empowered by an external agent, but being empowered from within. Donelly & Parmenter (1995) have suggested that it is important not to decontextualize quality of life research. Decontextualization occurs when politicized needs and processes are translated into administrable needs and processes, typically in the service of established social organizations. In the case of the present study, the decision to follow the 'group home' model was largely predetermined by the organization and other options were not explored with the same vigour. Services are usually predicated in the context of the needs of the service organization and not sufficiently on the needs of individuals requiring support. The paradigm shift from a professionally dominated rehabilitation model to one where the autonomy of the individual with the disability is paramount is evolving very slowly.

Future developments in deriving a useful theoretical model with which to analyse the life quality of persons with a disability may be supported by the work of Amantyne Sen (1993) and Erik Allardt (1993). Sen, influenced to an extent by the Aristotelian concept of *eudaimonia*, has stressed the notion of capability and well-being as a basis for examining quality of life. His approach is 'based on a view of living as a combination of various "doings and beings", with quality of life to be assessed in terms of the capability to achieve valuable functionings' (p31). Ostenfeld (1994) has explained *eudaimonia* as living well and doing well. He suggested that 'It is not just a subjective experience, but also a realization of the person's mental potential, feelings as well as intellect' (p22). He further noted that it is:

an optimal mental activity according to our special human capabilities ... the working and self-realization of the human being, which is the good for man, the most satisfactory, desirable highest good or value.

(p30)

This framework, which is somewhat similar to the self component of the model proposed earlier, finds some support from the interviews conducted in this study. It was not the physical capabilities of the residents *per se* but their determination to achieve a level of well-being beyond that possible in the nursing home which was the driving force in their quest for the good life, particularly for those who chose to move.

An alternative approach, and one that is also multidimensional, is Allardt's (1993) model of *Having, Loving, Being*. Rather than using the term 'functional', as in Parmenter's (1988) model, Allardt proposed *Having*, which includes economic resources, housing conditions, employment, health and education. *Loving* stands for the need to relate to other people and to form social identities and may include attachments and contacts in the local community, attachments to family and active patterns of friendship with workmates. *Being* stands for the need for integration into society and to live in harmony with nature. Indicators may measure the extent to which persons can participate in decisions and activities influencing their lives.

It would appear that a basic theme underlying each of these analytical approaches is the self-actualization of the person. A person does need to address who they are and to have the opportunity to exercise choice in how they might achieve their life goals. In essence the sense of achievement of the good life is an amalgam of both feelings and intellect.

Those residents who elected to move from the nursing home environment wanted the freedom to grow as individuals, to set life goals, to exercise choice and possibly the freedom to fail in trying to achieve some of their goals along the way. Above all, they wanted the excitement of 'having a go'.

REFERENCES

Allardt, E. (1975) *Having, Loving, Being: On Welfare in the Nordic Countries*, Argos, Borgholm.

Allardt, E. (1993) Having, loving, being: an alternative to the Swedish model of welfare research, in *The Quality of Life*, (eds M. Nussbaum and A. Sen), Clarendon Press, Oxford.

Barton, L. (ed.) (1989) *Disability and Dependency*, Falmer Press, London.

Barton, L. and Tomlinson, S. (eds) (1984) *Special Education and Social Interests*, Croom Helm, London.

Blatt, B. (1979) *In and Out of Mental Retardation: Essays on Educability, Disability, and Human Policy*, University Park Press, Baltimore.

Bogdan, R. and Kugelmass, S. (1984) Case studies of mainstreaming: a symbolic interactionist approach to special schooling, in *Special Education and Social Interests*, (eds L. Barton and S. Tomlinson), Croom Helm, London.

Bowles, W. (1995) *Quality of Life of Adults with Spina Bifida in New South Wales: Perspectives of People with Spina Bifida*. 8th International Conference on Spina Bifida and Hydrocephalus, Sydney.

Brown, R.I., Bayer, M.B. and MacFarlane, C. (1989) *Rehabilitation Programmes: Performance and Quality of Life of Adults with Developmental Handicaps*, Lugus, Toronto.

Brown, R.I., Bayer, M.B. and Brown, P.M. (1992) *Empowerment and Developmental Handicaps: Choices and Quality of Life*, Captus Press, Toronto.

Burback, H.J. (1981) The labeling process: a sociological analysis, in *Handbook of Special Education*, (eds J.M. Kauffman and D.P. Hallahan), Prentice-Hall, Englewood Cliffs, NJ.

Carley, M. (1981) *Social Measurement and Social Indicators*, Allen & Unwin, London.

De Jong, G. (1979) *The Movement for Independent Living: Origins, Ideology and Implications for Disability Policy and Research*, Michigan State University, University Center for International Rehabilitation.

De Jong, G. (1981) *Environmental Accessibility and Independent Living Outcomes: Directions for Disability Policy and Research*, Michigan State University, University Center for International Rehabilitation.

Donelly, M. and Parmenter, T.R. (1995) Approaches to the measurement of quality of life. Paper presented to the 12th World Congress of the International Federation of Physical Medicine and Rehabilitation, Sydney.

Edgerton, R.B. (1975) Issues relating to the quality of life among mentally retarded persons, in *The Mentally Retarded and Society*, (eds M.S. Begab and S.A. Richardson), University Park Press, Baltimore.

Emerson. E.B. (1985) Evaluating the impact of deinstitutionalization on the lives of mentally retarded people. *American Journal of Mental Deficiency*, **90**, 277–88.

Finkelstein, V. (1980) *Attitudes and Disabled People: Issues for Discussion*, World Rehabilitation Fund, New York.

Fulcher, G. (1989) *Disabling Policies? A Comparative Approach to Education Policy and Disability*, Falmer Press, London.

Goode, D.A. (1990) Thinking about and discussing quality of life, in *Quality of Life: Perspectives and Issues*, (ed. R.L. Schalock), American Association on Mental Retardation, Washington DC.

Hurst, A. (1984) Adolescence and physical impairment: an interactionist view, in *Special Education and Social Interests*, (eds L. Barton and S. Tomlinson), Croom Helm, London.

International League of Societies for Persons with Mental Handicap (1994) *Just Technology: From Principle to Practice in Bio-ethical Issues*, Roeher Institute, Toronto.

Kalantis, M. (1989) Ethnicity meets gender, meets class in Australia, in *Australian Feminist Interventions*, (ed. S. Watson), Allen & Unwin, Sydney.

Knoll, J.A. (1990) Defining quality in residential services, in *Quality Assurance for Individuals with Developmental Disabilities: It's Everybody's Business*, (eds V.J. Bradley and H.A. Bersani), Brookes, Baltimore.

Knox, M., Parmenter, T.R., Atkinson, N. *et al.* (1995) *If Only They would Listen to Us*, Macquarie University, Sydney.

Landesman-Dwyer, S. (1981) Living in the community. *American Journal of Mental Deficiency*, **86**, 223–34.

Landesman-Dwyer, S. (1985) Describing and evaluating residential environments, in *Living and Learning in the Least Restrictive Environment*, (eds R.H. Bruininks and K.C. Laken), Brookes, Baltimore.

McCall, G.J. and Simmons, J.L. (1978) *Identities and Interactions: An Examination of Human Association in Everyday Life*, Free Press, New York.

Nussbaum, M. and Sen, A. (eds) (1993) *The Quality of Life*, Clarendon Press, Oxford.

Oliver, M. (1989) The social and political context of educational policy: the case of special needs, in *The Politics of Special Education Needs*, (ed. L. Barton), Falmer Press, London.

Organization for Economic and Co-operative Development (OECD) (1976) *Measuring Well-being*, Springer-Verlag, New York.

Orley, J. and Kuyken, W. (eds) (1994) *Quality of Life Assessment: International Perspectives*, Springer-Verlag, New York.

Ostenfeld, E. (1994) Aristotle on the good life and quality of life, in *Concepts and Measurement of Quality of Life in Health Care*, (ed. L. Nordenfelt), Kluwer, Dordrecht.

Parmenter, T.R. (1988) An analysis of the dimensions of quality of life for people with physical disabilities, in *Quality of Life for Handicapped People*, (ed. R. Brown), Croom Helm, London.

Parmenter, T.R. (1996) The utility of quality of life as a construct for social and health policy development., in *Quality of Life in Health Promotion and Rehabilitation: Conceptual Approach, Issues and Applications*, (eds R. Renwick, I. Brown and M. Nagler), Sage, New York.

Schalock, R.L. (ed.) (1990) *Quality of Life: Perspectives and Issues*, American Association on Mental Retardation, Washington DC.

Schalock, R.L. (1995) *Outcome-based Evaluation*, Plenum, New York.

Schalock, R.L. and Lilley, M.A. (1986) Placement from community-based mental retardation programmes: how well do clients do after 8 to 10 years? *American Journal of Mental Deficiency*, **90**, 669–76.

Schur, E.M. (1971) *Labeling and Deviant Behavior: Its Sociological Implications*, Harper & Row, New York.

Scott, R.A. (1972) A proposed framework for analyzing deviance as a property of social order, in *Theoretical Perspectives on Deviance*, (eds R.A. Scott and J.D. Douglas), Basic Books, New York.

Sen, A. (1993) Capability and well-being, in *The Quality of Life*, (eds M. Nussbaum and A. Sen), Clarendon Press, Oxford.

Sharp, R. and Green, A. (1975) *Education and Social Control*, Routledge & Kegan Paul, London.

Solomon, E.S., Denisov, V., Hankins, E., Mallmann, C.A. and Milbrath, L.W. (1980) UNESCO's policy – relevant quality of life research program, in *The Quality of Life: Comparative Studies*, (eds A. Szalai and F.M. Andrews), Sage Publications, Beverly Hills, CA.

Stoddard, S. (1978) Independent living, concepts and programmes. *American Rehabilitation*, **3**, 2–5.

Williams, G.H. (1983) The movement for independent living: an evaluation and critique. *Social Science and Medicine*, **17**, 1003–10.

Wolfensberger, W. (1994) Let's hang up 'quality of life' as a hopeless term, in *Quality of Life for Persons with Disabilities*, (ed. D. Goode), Brookline Books, Cambridge, MA.

Zapf, W., Glatzer, W., Noll, H.H. *et al.* (1987) German social report. Living conditions and subjective well-being, 1978–1984. *Social Indicators Research*, **19**, 3–171.

Zola, I.K. (1983) Defining independence, in *International Perspectives about Independent Living*, (eds D.G. Tate and L.M. Chadderdon), Michigan State University, University Center for International Rehabilitation.

Assessing quality of life 7

Robert A Cummins

INTRODUCTION

The title of this book could give the impression that there is something different about quality of life for people with disabilities when compared with the general population. This, indeed, is the central issue for quality of life researchers as they attempt to define and measure the life quality of population subgroups. Should the obvious limitations imposed by disability mean the expectation of a life quality that is lower than normal? Should life quality be measured in ways different from the general population? Should we accept the views of such people on their own quality of life or should we seek the vicarious views of their non-disabled helpers and friends?

The answers to such questions are not clearcut for two main reasons. First, the field of quality of life is young and little data can be regarded as reliable empirical anchors to test theory. Second, the conceptual framework within which questions are asked strongly influences the answers. Thus, researchers who are immersed in the area of disability are likely to view life quality within a different conceptual framework from researchers who deal exclusively with general population surveys. Because of these two factors, views on such fundamental issues relating to life quality for people with disabilities differ markedly from one author to another, as the chapters in this book attest.

My purpose is to examine issues related to quality of life assessment both for people with and for people without a disability. This examination will be in terms of the contemporary theoretical and empirical support from the literature. Our journey will proceed through a discussion of eight propositions related to the definition of life quality and will end with a brief description and evaluation of those quality of life instruments that have been devised for people with a cognitive impairment.

ISSUES OF DEFINITIONAL AGREEMENT

The literature on quality of life contains well in excess of 100 definitions and models. Some relate specifically to disability, others to the general adult population. An analysis of these varying conceptions provides a means for studying the influence that various frames of reference have had on the concept of life quality and, in turn, the manner in which such conceptions become operationalized as tools for assessment.

It is neither practical nor necessary to list all of these approaches; some are clearly representative of others while some are cast in such vague or inclusive terminology that their heuristic value approaches zero. What follows are some of the ideas and definitions that have clear operational implications for the measurement of life quality.

OBJECTIVE VS SUBJECTIVE

The conception of life quality in its modern form was first articulated in the early 1960s. Prior to this time, national and international measures of population well-being had used 'social indicators' defined, for example, by the US Department of Health, Education and Welfare (1969) as 'statistics of direct normative interest which facilitate concise, comprehensive and balanced judgements about the condition of a major aspect of society' (p97). The number of such indicators is virtually unlimited and they include such measures as gross national product, cost of housing, rate of unemployment, etc. Such measures have two important characteristics: they are objectively measured and they are normative to a population or group.

What distinguished the new conception of life quality was a focus at the level of the individual. As reported by Flanagan (1982), this was first indicated within the Report of President Eisenhower's Commission on National Goals, published in 1960, which included a concern with individual views on such issues as health and welfare. Then, in 1964, Lyndon B. Johnson made a speech which both coined the term 'quality of life' and made clear the separation of its objective and subjective components. According to Bech (1993), he stated: '... goals cannot be measured in the size of our bank balance. They can only be measured in the quality of the lives that our people lead ...'.

And so it gradually came about that people, from political commentators to human welfare researchers, began to think about life quality for the individual as distinct from the global population measurements yielded by social indicators. Indeed, people began to argue that such measures were morally required for any assessment of the human condition (Shea, 1976). So, slowly, the quality of life literature, embodying this new interest in individual, personal values, began to emerge. Spitzer (1987) states that only four papers had quality of life in their titles between 1966 and 1970, while this applied to 33 papers over the next five years (1970–1974). This exponential rate of increase has been maintained to the present time where the term has become a political and media catchphrase. The literature is now too vast for any individual researcher to fully assimilate.

How, then, has all of this impacted on the area of disability? One answer is ... very slowly. Borthwick-Duffy (1992) has noted that a monograph of the American Association on Mental Retardation (Meyers, 1978) entitled 'Quality of life in severely and profoundly mentally retarded people: Research foundations for improvement' did not, in fact, contain any reference to quality of life and focused on such topics as reducing behaviour problems and teaching techniques. In that same year, Butler & Bjaanes (1978) referred to the 'quality of life' of people with intellectual disability living in the community. They seem, however, to have considered quality of life as equivalent to normalization and report only objective measures. This unfortunate misconception as to what constitutes life quality for people who are disabled continues to be reflected by a substantial proportion of the literature.

When Nirje (1976) and Wolfensberger (1972) established the basis for normalization, their goals were clearly directed at remedying the gross discrepancies between people with intellectual disabilities living in institutions and the living standards of the general population. Consequently, the measurement tools that were developed to demonstrate such disparities (PASS and PASSING) only measured objective variables (Wolfensberger & Glenn, 1975; Wolfensberger & Thomas, 1983). It is important to realize, therefore, that while such measurements have utility within the framework for which they were devised, they do not measure subjective quality of life. They do not measure the levels of satisfaction, happiness, life fulfilment, etc. that are currently accepted as essential to any statement of life quality for people in the general community.

There is now general agreement that the term 'quality of life' implies some combination of objective and subjective variables. In a census of the quality of life definitions reviewed for this chapter, it was found that around 80% incorporate both 'axes' of the construct, with the remainder restricting their attention to the subjective quality of life axis only. Thus, three general propositions that seem to have general acceptance in relation to a quality of life definition that can be applied to all people are as follows:

Proposition 1: The term 'quality of life' refers to both the objective and subjective axes of human existence.
Proposition 2: The objective axis incorporates norm-referenced measures of well-being.
Proposition 3: The subjective axis incorporates measures of perceived well-being. This axis is also frequently referred to in the literature as 'subjective well-being'.

QUALITY OF LIFE DOMAINS

There are two basic approaches to quality of life definition and measurement: either to regard quality of life as a single, unitary entity or to regard it as being composed of discrete 'domains'.

An example of the former approach has been provided by Zautra & Goodhart (1979) who state that quality of life pertains to the 'goodness' of life and that this goodness 'resides in the quality of the life experience, both as subjectively evaluated and as objectively determined by an assessment of external conditions' (p1).

In relation to the subjective axis, this idea of some perceived Gestalt has been incorporated into one of the most popular measurement instruments. Devised by Andrews & Withey (1976), it consists of the single question 'How do you feel about your life as a whole?' with the respondent using a Likert scale of life satisfaction/dissatisfaction. Used on a population basis, this form of measurement has been shown to produce remarkably consistent data, forming, indeed, one of the few empirical benchmarks for life quality (Cummins, 1995a).

This approach also suffers from two obvious limitations. It cannot be applied to measurements on the objective axis and it yields only a crude measure of perceived well-being. Consequently, the great majority of definitions, models and instruments have attempted to break down the quality of life construct into its constituent domains. However, there is little agreement regarding either the number or the scope of such domains; an issue of considerable relevance to the other quality of life measurement scales reviewed later in this chapter.

Notwithstanding the wide diversity of opinion on this issue, the available empirical data can be used to deduce the most likely constituent domains. These are presented in the following proposition which is numbered to follow on from those in the previous section.

Proposition 4: At least five separate quality of life domains can be identified as emotional well-being, health, social/family connections, material wealth or well-being, and work or other form of productive activity.

Of the 27 definitions located that attempt to identify the quality of life domains, 85% include emotional well-being (Emotion) in some form (satisfaction, happiness, self-esteem, etc.), 70% include health, 70% social and family connections (Intimacy), 59% material wealth or well-being (Material) and 56% work or other form of productive activity (Productivity). Thus, it may be concluded that there is at least a majority opinion that these five domains should be included in any definition of quality of life.

Further empirical support for the inclusion of these five domains is provided by data from surveys which asked respondents to indicate whether various domains of life are important to them. Four large population surveys have been located that provide relevant data. The earliest is Abrams (1973) who found that the top four ranked domains were Health, Intimacy, Material and Productivity. No domain directly relevant to Emotion was included. In 1976, Campbell, Converse & Rodgers asked people to rate domain importance on a five-point scale. Expressed as a percentage of the maximum scale score of importance, items relevant to the domains scored Health 91%, Intimacy 89%, Material 73%, Productivity 70%. Again, no domain directly relevant to Emotion was included. Finally, Flanagan (1978) and Krupinski (1980) both asked respondents to rate domain importance. The percentage of people who ranked items relevant to each domain in the top two categories (very/extremely important; important/very important) were respectively: Health (97, –), Intimacy (81, 80), Emotion (86, 73), Material (83, 70) and Productivity (78, 55). From these data it can be safely concluded that the five domains are regarded as very important aspects of their lives by a large majority of people.

Other data that can be brought to bear on the relevance of these five domains are the amount of variance they explain in measures of subjective well-being or life satisfaction. Some representative findings are as follows:

- *Material*: Both Spreitzer & Snyder (1974) and Headey (1981) found indicators of perceived material well-being to be significant predictors of global life satisfaction.
- *Health*: Fernandez & Kulik (1981) entered 15 variables against global life satisfaction and found that perceived health correlated the highest. Woodruff & Conway (1992) found self-assessed health to explain 17% of the variance in subjective well-being.
- *Productivity*: In terms of zero order correlation, the relationship between job satisfaction and subjective well-being has been found consistently to be positive (e.g. $r=.35$, Headey, Holmstrom & Wearing, 1984; $r=.49$, Evans *et al.*, 1993).
- *Intimacy*: Global life satisfaction has consistently been found to be predicted by such variables as satisfaction with social contacts (e.g. Bowling, Farquhar & Browne, 1991) and intrafamily support (e.g. Dunst, Leet & Trivette, 1988).
- *Emotional*: Headey (1981) found global life satisfaction to be significantly predicted by perceived fun/enjoyment from life, while Fehring, Brennan & Keller (1987) reported subjective well-being to be significantly negatively predicted by depression.

These cited data are merely illustrative of the very large number of studies that have included variables related to these domains. However, the weight of this extended literature is consistent with these cited studies and provides further evidence that these five domains are all very relevant to subjective well-being. Of course, it would be highly desirable to know much more about these domains: about the extent to which they independently contribute to life quality and share variance among themselves. While scattered data are available in relation to these matters they are not yet sufficient to be able to make any strong statements; that is a task for the future. What can be stated with some conviction is that these five domains, at least, should be included in any definition or model of life quality. An argument for the inclusion of two additional domains will be made under Proposition 8.

DOMAINS SHOULD ENCOMPASS LIFE QUALITY

Proposition 5: The domains, in aggregate, should cover the entire spectrum of life quality.

Very few definitions or models attempt to meet this necessary and logical requirement. Of the 27 definitions referred to in the previous section, only two include each of the five domains that have been proposed. Stark & Goldsbury (1990) propose seven domains, with the additional two being living environment and education. In addition, Felce & Perry (1993) propose six domains, with the addition of personal development.

The definition by Felce & Perry (1993) is the only one that fulfils all of the requirements to this point. It states:

Quality of life is defined as an overall general well-being which comprises objective descriptors and subjective evaluations of physical, material, social and emotional well-being together with the extent of personal development and purposeful activity all weighted by a personal set of values.

(p11)

The suggested incorporation of an individual weighting system leads to the next proposition.

NORMATIVE VS INDIVIDUAL VALUES

Proposition 6: The objective axis should reflect normative values. The subjective axis should reflect the values of the individual respondent.

It has already been documented that normative data underpinned the measurement philosophy of social indicators and it seems reasonable to consider that the objective axis of life quality would also contain variables that are norm-referrable. But what of the subjective axis? Here the situation is not so clear. If a respondent to a quality of life scale does not regard one or more of the domains as having much relevance to their personal situation, then it does not matter how satisfied or dissatisfied they are with domains that contribute little to the individual's life. If, on the other hand, a respondent regards strong links with their family and friends as integral to their life quality, then their level of satisfaction with such a domain is of paramount relevance. This introduces the idea that the subjective axis should be measured using a scale which reflects individual differences in domain relevance.

There is, of course, abundant evidence that people do apply different degrees of relevance to the domains of their lives, as can be seen from data generated from the studies of domain importance cited earlier. In addition, evidence is available to indicate that the hierarchy of domain relevance varies across groups according to gender and age (Flanagan, 1978), level of education (Krupinski, 1980), race (Lang et al., 1982) and high versus low levels of overall life satisfaction (Yetim, 1993).

So, in order to be able to make meaningful comparisons across populations and subpopulations, some weighting system is required that results in the final subjective quality of life score reflecting the level of satisfaction with personally relevant domains. Various schemes have been proposed to achieve this end, but all use the level of perceived domain importance as the weighting factor.

Guyatt et al. (1987) used the product of item importance and satisfaction, but determined the importance metric by average across-group data. This approach misses the point. In order for importance to be useful as a weighting device, it must be calculated on an individual basis.

This latter approach has been adopted by both Ferrans & Powers (1985) and Cummins (1993a), each of whom have proposed different arithmetical procedures for combining importance and satisfaction. While the merits of each approach have been argued in Cummins (1993a), each yields a single metric for each domain which reflects the degree of satisfaction weighted by its level of perceived importance.

To summarize the argument to this point, it has been proposed that a majority opinion, derived from the literature, holds that life quality can be described on both an objective and a subjective axis. While the former reflects culturally normative values, the latter should reflect satisfaction with life domains weighted in accordance with their value to the individual. It has also been proposed that a majority view can be deduced for the existence of five life domains as material well-being, health, productivity, intimacy and emotional well-being. Later in this chapter an argument will be put to extend this number of domains to seven, but before this it is necessary to consider whether the agreed domains of life quality for the general population should be different for people who are disabled.

DEFINITIONS RESTRICTED TO POPULATION SUBGROUPS

Proposition 7: Global definitions and models of life quality must be equally relevant to both the general population and all defined subgroups.

People with an intellectual disability

Since most minority groups have a lower standard of living than the general population, there is a great danger of defining quality of life for such people in terms that seem appropriate for minority groups, but which would be unacceptable to the majority of people. This problem can be readily exemplified by analysing some of the quality of life definitions that have been devised specifically for people with an intellectual disability.

Quality of life is '... a multi-dimensional construct [whose] dimensions include normalized and decent living conditions, some degree of autonomy, opportunities for personal growth, and general happiness' (Vitello, 1984, p348). From this it may be deduced that a high quality of life is consistent with living like ordinary folk and having just a modicum of autonomy. Ordinary folk would probably disagree. The definition has restricted the vision of what constitutes a high quality life by focusing on the low subgroup baseline.

> ... the same four dimensions – residential environment, interpersonal relationships, activities/community involvement, and stability – seem adequate to describe the major aspects of a quality of life model, regardless of intelligence level.
>
> (Borthwick-Duffy, 1990, p178)

On the contrary, while a concentration on these four domains may seem to have relevance when the view is restricted to people with an intellectual disability, they are certainly not adequate to represent life quality when viewed against quality of life literature as a whole, as was argued under proposition four.

All such definitions indicate how a view limited to a population subgroup can restrict the view of what might constitute a high life quality for its members. Such definitions are shaped by the deficits of the groups to which they refer and, as a consequence, have been downgraded to reflect the assumption of a lower life quality than normal. Such assumptions, however, are likely to be invalid. The huge literature on positive and negative affect (e.g. Watson & Pennebaker, 1989) is consistent in its appreciation that each is independent of the other, such that people with serious disabilities may nevertheless describe themselves as happy, enthusiastic and excited about life. Moreover, and consistent with this understanding,

Cummins *et al.* (1997) have demonstrated no differences in quality of life between college students, adolescents attending high school and people with intellectual disabilities, despite gross differences in objective life quality between these groups.

Medical quality of life definitions

As a further example of the dangers inherent in targeting population sub-groups, a wide range of definitions have been produced from the medical perspective which attempt to define life quality for people who have some form of physical illness or disability. The following are some examples.

Schipper, Clinch & Powell (1990) define quality of life functionally, by considering patients' perception of performance in four areas: physical and occupational ('strength, energy and the ability to carry on expected normal activities'); psychologic ('the most studied are anxiety, depression and fear'); social interaction ('ability to carry on the person-to-person interactions that form the core of communal living'); and somatic sensation ('The ... unpleasant physical feelings which may detract from someone's quality of life').

The problem here is confusion as to what might constitute a reasonable set of dependent variables to measure medical outcome and quality of life. All variables are referenced either to what is 'normal' or to pathology and one half of the quality of life construct is defined through medically related measurement. An even more extreme example of such thinking is provided by Wiklund, Lindvall & Swedberg (1986) who distinguish three major components of quality of life in clinical medical settings as: functional capacity, subjective perceptions and symptoms and their consequences. In this scheme attention is restricted almost totally to medical parameters.

A formalization of this approach has appeared in the literature recently, in the form of a construct called 'health-related' quality of life. For example:

> [Quality of life is defined] ... as a broad range of physical and psychological characteristics and limitations which describe an individual's ability to function and derive satisfaction from so doing. ... However, with regard to measuring the benefits of medicines, health related quality of life is probably the key term and this is defined as the level of well-being and satisfaction associated with an individual's life and how this is affected by disease, accidents and treatment.
>
> (Walker, 1992, p265)

Just as was demonstrated for definitions concerned exclusively with the quality of life for people with intellectual disabilities, so too is this definition concerned exclusively with limitations to functioning and a life quality that is expected to be less than normal. It does not easily embrace the idea that people may be medically or physically compromised and yet enjoy a life quality higher than that of the non-disabled general population.

> [Quality of life] ... is an organizing concept that brings together a set of domains related to the physical, functional, psychological, and social health of the individual. When used in this context it is often referred to as 'health-related quality of life' ... Health-related quality of life involves the five broad dimensions of opportunity, health perceptions, functional status, morbidity or impairment, and mortality.
>
> (Testa & Nackley, 1994, p537)

This definition exemplifies all of the concerns previously expressed. It is a narrowly based, medically dominated conception that focuses exclusively on pathology. Presumably the mortality dimension would be operationalized as a dichotomous variable with absolute predictive certainty, at least in this life.

In summary, health-referenced quality of life definitions impose an overly restricted view of the construct. They tend to produce self-fulfilling prophecies by concentrating on the negative aspects of disease and injury. In contrast, broader approaches to measurement allow for a much more positive view. For example, data cited by Cummins (1995a) indicate that, using such broader forms of measurement, people with a physical disability, an intellectual disability or people who have survived an organ transplantation can register a level of subjective well-being as high or higher than the normal range for the population.

Quality adjusted life years

One final abuse of the quality of life definitional structure must be mentioned. This is the generation of 'utility' or 'trade-off' quality of life models which give rise to the metric called a Quality Adjusted Life Year (QALY). A huge literature pertains to the methodology of calculating QALYs (for reviews see Feeny, Labelle & Torrance, 1990; Revicki & Kaplan, 1993) and such measures are taken very seriously indeed by economists and members of the medical fraternity who are concerned with cost–benefit analyses. In truth, however, the QALY is a bizarre notion that is based on invalid psychometric assumptions.

There are several methods for calculating a QALY but all rest on the idea that someone in good health is able to make a valid judgement about how it would feel, as a hypothetical exercise, to have various kinds of disabling conditions. To take a simple example: the healthy respondent is asked to choose between (a) living as a diabetic for 20 years or (b) living in perfect health for 20 years. The latter is obviously preferred. The respondent is then asked to choose between (a) and (c) living in perfect health for 15 years; then 10 years and so on until the respondent is indifferent to the two alternatives. Then, if it is determined that this point of indifference lies at the choice of five years in perfect health, the QALY can be calculated as 5/20 or .25. In other words, one year living as a diabetic is 'equivalent' to 0.25 Quality Adjusted Life Years.

While the above description is certainly a simplification of the actual QALY methodology, its logic is accurately represented. Moreover, the QALY methodology is complete nonsense in that it implies any relationship with subjective quality of life. No one can validly respond to such hypothetical situations, as a number of authors have pointed out (e.g. Ferrans, 1990; Goodinson & Singleton, 1989). There are several reasons. Perhaps the most salient is that they ignore the processes of adaptation so vividly portrayed by Brickman, Coates & Janoff-Bulman (1978). These authors compared major lottery winners, people who had been rendered paraplegic through an accident and no-event controls. Within an interval that was generally less than one year following the event, the groups showed a remarkable similarity in their level of professed happiness. While this study certainly contained various methodological weaknesses (see Headey & Wearing, 1989), its result has been very widely cited both because of its radical comparisons and because it is an interesting, but not entirely surprising finding, for theorists who espouse Adaptation Level Theory (Helson, 1964). In this view the adaptation level of a person at any instant is a weighted geometric mean of all relevant stimuli past and present. Thus, adaptation level will be constantly changing as new stimuli are experienced and, as this occurs, the judgement of what constitutes a 'neutral' stimulus will also change. For example, since an event of extreme good fortune constitutes a highly positive comparison point, it will result in an upward shift of adaptation level and, as a consequence, many of the ordinary life pleasures will seem more neutral. The reverse also applies. Highly negative events cause a downward shift in adaptation level with the result that previously neutral experiences now seem pleasurable.

This is a powerful conception which has been widely employed to account for changed perceptions over time, but it is not the only mechanism that has been proposed to explain the recovery of perceived well-being following a traumatic event. Brickman & Campbell (1971) have discussed changing levels of aspiration, while Tversky & Griffin (1991) have pointed to changes in the comparison group, i.e. people who have become disabled start to compare their lives with others who are disabled rather than against the non-disabled population. Taylor, Wood & Lichtman (1983) have suggested yet other mechanisms, such as selected focus on personal attributes, that make the person seem advantaged ('brain is more important than brawn'), creating hypothetical worse worlds, construing benefit from the event and manufacturing normative standards of adjust-ment that make their own adjustment appear exceptional. And so on. Undoubtedly this list of adaptive mechanisms is incomplete, but it serves to indicate a crucial characteristic of human experience: people adapt to their circumstances, such that the level of subjective well-being reported by people with spinal cord injury (Schulz & Decker, 1985), congenital neuromuscular/skeletal disorders (Parmenter, 1988), intellectual disability (Barlow & Kirby, 1991) or cancer (Muthny, Koch & Stump, 1990) may be little different from that of the general population.

So how does all of this fit with the idea that people can validly report on the vicarious experience of disability? Of course it does not fit at all. The only people who can report on this experience are people who have the particular form of disability under discussion and even then, in the case of acquired disability, the temporal factor must be carefully considered.

The whole rationale for QALYs within the quality of life context is invalid. So, too, are more recent formulations that rest on the same measurement process (e.g. utility adjusted life years; Richardson, 1991). Thus, the use of QALYs as a synonym for quality of life (e.g. Nord, 1991; Torrance, 1986) is totally inappropriate, as has also been argued by Romney, Brown & Fry (1994).

Conclusion

It has been argued that there is great danger in any conception of quality of life that is restricted to some minority group of the population. Inevitably, it seems, such conceptions are restricted in their scope and directed to measures of pathology or below-normal existence, rather than allowing for the determination of high life quality as judged on a norma-tive basis. To repeat, it is imperative that all definitions and models of life quality be referenced to the general population both in their conception and in their operational measurement.

DEFINITIONS VIA PERCEIVED DISCREPANCIES

The definitions so far discussed have focused on measures of satisfaction referenced to objective/subjective axes and discrete life domains. There are other approaches that take a quite different view and most commonly these are based on perceived discrepancies between what a person wants and what they actually have.

The oldest approach comes from the Environmental Protection Agency (1973) as cited by McCall (1976):

> The concept of quality of life has emerged in the last few years as an undefinable measure of society's determination and desire to improve

or at least not to permit a further degradation of its condition. Despite its current undefinability, it represents a yearning of people for something which they feel they have lost or are losing, or have been denied, and which to some extent they wish to regain or acquire.

(piii)

Despite its obvious limitations of restricted focus and rather nebulous wording, it does indicate that quality of life might be related to the fulfilment or non-fulfilment of wants or needs. Liu (1975) encapsulated this with the idea that 'quality of life expressed that set of "wants" which after having been supplied, when taken together, makes the individual happy or satisfied' (p1).

Numerous authors have taken up this theme, which can be considered under the banners of Relative Deprivation Theory or Discrepancy Theory. The general idea is that quality of life is the result of a match between an individual's wants or needs and their fulfilment (e.g. Brown, Bayer & MacFarlane, 1989; Karan, Lambour & Greenspan, 1990; Parmenter, 1988; Schalock, 1990). Some authors have provided various forms of elaboration regarding the precise nature of wants and needs. Quite commonly this is in the form of meeting expectations or aspirations (Calman, 1984; Hornquist, 1982; Milbrath, 1982) or life plans and goals (Cohen, 1982; Emerson, 1985; Milbrath, 1982). Others have related the needs to individual abilities (Bigelow *et al.*, 1982; Emerson, 1985; Goode, 1990) or to the needs created by normative societal expectations (Goode, 1990; Schalock, 1990).

MULTIPLE DISCREPANCY THEORY

The most comprehensive discrepancy model has been proposed by Michalos (1985) as Multiple Discrepancy Theory (MDT). He stated the basic hypothesis as:

Reported net satisfaction is a function of perceived discrepancies between what one has and wants, relevant others have, the best one has had in the past, expected to have three years ago, expects to have after five years, deserves and needs.

(p347)

The author presents an impressive empirical verification of the power of this formulation. Using undergraduates as subjects, he tested the ability of these seven discrepancy measures to predict global life satisfaction and found that they together explained 53% of the variance.

But what do these data really mean? What is the nature of the 'function' that links life satisfaction and MDT? Michalos (1985) cites and then dismisses the idea that satisfaction and self-want discrepancy variables might merely be two measures of the same thing. However, this idea deserves reconsideration, both in relation to the methodology used by MDT and as a more general conception.

In relation to the methodology a major problem is the degree of commonality between the questions that generate the dependent and independent variables for the MDT multiple regression analyses. Take the example of global measures. The dependent variable was generated on a seven-point 'delighted-terrible' scale (Andrews & Withey, 1976) in response to 'How do you feel about your life as a whole right now?'. Data for one of the independent variables were generated using the question 'Consider your life as a whole. Does it measure up to your general aspirations or what you want?'. This seven-point scale used three anchors: 'not at all', 'half as well as what you want' and 'matches or is better than what you want'.

These two questions are very similar to one another. It would certainly be surprising to find that the responses to them were not highly correlated.

At a more general level of conceptualization, MDT seems almost to be stating the obvious: that people who are dissatisfied with their lives see the quality of their lives as lying below (i.e. discrepant from) some reference point. Indeed, it is somewhat intuitive that satisfaction must be the outcome of a cognitive comparison process and that it must have a reference point. Then, as the result of such comparisons, a perceived negative discrepancy yields dissatisfaction. This broad notion has been formulated as Congruity Theory (Wilson, Rosenblood & Oliver, 1973) or Judgement Theory (Meadow *et al.*, 1992), and has been well articulated by Pavot & Diener (1993):

> Life satisfaction refers to a judgemental process, in which individuals assess the quality of their lives on the basis of their own unique set of criteria … A comparison of one's perceived life circumstances with a self-imposed standard or standards is presumably made, and to the degree that conditions match these standards, the person reports high life satisfaction. Therefore, life satisfaction is a conscious cognitive judgement of one's life in which the criteria for judgement are up to the person.
>
> (p164)

This is not the place to elaborate in detail on this conceptual framework, but three links to previously discussed processes can be mentioned. First, that there is likely to be a separate reference point for each type of cognitive comparison (e.g. for the judgement of satisfaction with each domain). Second, that such reference points might be expected to behave in accordance with the tenets of Adaptation Level Theory mentioned in the previous section. That is, they would vary over time and, at any instant, be a function of the weighted geometric mean of all relevant stimuli past and present. Third, the actual setting for each reference point would be a function of dispositional processes that act to constrain perceived discrepancies within some operational range of values (e.g. cognitive dissonance could be one such process), perceptions of external stimuli relevant to life quality and the cognitive, comparative process itself.

Are Multiple Discrepancy Theory and life satisfaction really the same?

What evidence does Michalos offer to defend satisfaction and discrepancy as separate processes? He tested his data according to the proposition that 'if two variables are measuring the same thing, then they ought to have similar relations to other theoretically relevant external variables ... in terms of direction, strength and consistency' (p388). He then generated 952 comparisons where both 'satisfaction' and a measure of 'self-want discrepancy' were correlated with some third variable. These 'third variables' included 12 putative life domains such as health, recreation and education, together with the five demographic variables of age, marital status, work status, educational level and course of study.

He then compared the extent to which satisfaction and self-want discrepancy correlated with these third variables and judged such correlations to be 'similar' if 'both had significant associations to the third variable in the set (whether the associations were positive or negative)' (p389). He then reported that 32% of the triples fulfilled the criterion of 'similar' and concluded that 'the satisfaction and self-want discrepancy variables are not merely two measures of the same thing' (p389).

This interpretation needs to be challenged. In the first place, the 'similarity' criterion requires that *both* satisfaction and discrepancy *significantly* relate to a third variable. Yet, non-significant relationships were certainly included in the 952 comparisons. In the second place, the comparisons are only valid if *both* satisfaction and discrepancy have some 'theoretical relevance' to the third variables. This criterion is violated in the case of the five demographic variables with the author's data (Exhibit 8: Michalos, 1985) indicating no significant relationships with satisfaction. This alone invalidates 304 of the 952 comparisons in terms of finding 'similarity'. A similar problem is evidenced from the data presented elsewhere (Exhibits 6 & 7; Michalos, 1985).

In summary, had Michalos used an appropriate basis for these comparisons, his discovered extent of 'similarity' would certainly have been higher than 32%. It is therefore concluded that this test of the alternative hypothesis is unconvincing. In addition, while Michalos found that 53% of global life satisfaction was explained by MDT, page 365 of his paper presents the results of a multiple regression where the same proportion of variance (53%) in global satisfaction was explained by the combination of satisfaction ratings on 12 life domains.

Several conclusions seem appropriate. First, while the extent to which self-want discrepancy and satisfaction co-vary remains open, there are very good reasons for believing that they are measuring much the same thing. Second, while it is of great theoretical interest to determine the relationship between discrepancy and satisfaction, the most robust measure in terms of estimating quality of life for people with or without disabilities is surely the most direct. Questions of satisfaction are the clearest measure of how people feel about their life quality.

Problems in operationalization

There are some major operational problems in the use of discrepancy theory to measure the quality of life of people with disabilities. The first concerns the interpretation of data. Presumably life quality is measured by practitioners with a view to mounting an intervention programme directed to those aspects of people's lives that are perceived to be in deficit. When the measurement unit is dissatisfaction the requirement for intervention is clear, but when measurement is in terms of discrepancy theory, it is not. When does a discrepancy get too large and require remediation? When it results in dissatisfaction, of course! This tautology reinforces the practical utility of measuring life quality directly through satisfaction.

The second issue relates to the rather intellectually demanding form of the questions asked in conjunction with the Michalos definition, referring to feelings at times different from the present, estimates of entitlement, etc. Because of this, the use of such scales with people who are cognitively impaired may pose considerable difficulties in terms of valid responding. It may therefore be considered appropriate to simplify the questions, making them refer to quite specific issues in the persons' lives. The danger, then, would be to equate the resultant responses with life quality, rather than as simple indicators of unmet need.

Finally, it should be noted that people's needs and expectations, and especially those of people in deprived circumstances, are very susceptible to change. According to classic theory on the hierarchy of needs (Maslow, 1943; Wicker et al., 1993), people organize their needs in a hierarchy of 'prepotency' from those required for basic survival to those of the highest 'self-actualizing' type. Accordingly, people will focus their attention on those needs, goals, etc. which are the lowest needs or goals not being met.

Consider, for example, the study by Hailstone (1989) which reported the elements considered to comprise a quality lifestyle as self-reported by people with intellectual disabilities. The list comprises: considering people first, rights and entitlements, dignity and respect, availability of

options, equality, opportunity, choice based on preference, empowerment, etc. While it is easy to see the reflected rhetoric of service
providers, the items are also recognizable as basic 'needs' that are a
consequence of the relative deprivation suffered by such people.
Consequently, in accordance with the theory of needs hierarchies, once
these needs are met a new set will emerge that reflect a further stage
towards self-actualization.

This, therefore, raises the operational question of what needs or expectations are going to be measured in order to deduce the magnitude of any
'discrepancy' that directly reflects quality of life. If only low-level needs
are used then, as they are fulfilled by changing circumstances or intervention programmes, new higher order needs will arise to take their place.

Conclusion

This has not been an exhaustive review of discrepancy theory and certainly additional evidence is available in support of multiple discrepancy
theory (e.g. Michalos, 1986). However, inconsistencies with the theory
have been found (e.g. Harwood & Rice, 1992) and theoretical complexities abound (e.g. Higgins *et al.*, 1986). While discrepancy theory is a
quite fascinating area for further study, it is certainly not recommended
as having practical utility in the measurement of life quality. The
simplest, most direct and most reliable measure of subjective quality of
life is to ask people to respond on a scale of satisfaction/dissatisfaction.

A COMPREHENSIVE QUALITY OF LIFE DEFINITION

> *Proposition 8*: Quality of life is defined as follows. Quality of life is both
> objective and subjective, each axis being the aggregate of seven
> domains: material well-being, health, productivity, intimacy, safety,
> community and emotional well-being. Objective domains comprise
> culturally relevant measures of objective well-being. Subjective
> domains comprise domain satisfaction weighted by their importance
> to the individual.

This highly operational definition is consistent with the Comprehensive
Quality of Life Scale (Cummins, 1993a, b, c; see later) that will be
described later in this chapter. It is also consistent with each of the quality
of life propositions that have been articulated. Specifically:

1. it incorporates both the objective and subjective axes of human existence;
2. the objective axis incorporates norm-referenced measures of well-being;
3. the subjective axis incorporates measures of perceived well-being
   based on satisfaction.

Proposition 4 suggested five domains as having very substantial support from the literature. These are material well-being, health, productivity, intimacy and emotional well-being. To this list has been added the domains of safety and community. The method for the selection of these seven domains has been described in detail elsewhere (Cummins *et al.*, 1994). The theoretical and empirical support for these additional two domains is as follows.

Evidence for a domain of safety

The domain of safety is intended to be inclusive of such constructs as security, personal control, privacy, independence, autonomy, competence, knowledge of rights and residential stability. In terms of quality of life, it is theoretically relevant to Antonovsky's (1987) Sense of Coherence, which refers to a disposition to look at life and its problems in a manner which makes coping easier by viewing the world as meaningful, comprehensible and manageable.

Of the 27 definitions located that attempt to identify quality of life domains, 22% identified a domain corresponding to safety. The terms used were: personal safety and justice (OECD, 1976), autonomy (Vitello, 1984), independence (Schalock *et al.*, 1989), stability (Borthwick-Duffy, 1990), a living environment that embraces security and autonomy (Stark & Goldsbury, 1990) and safety from harm and financial security (Halpern, 1993). It is interesting to note that, with the single exception of OECD, all of the other definitions pertained specifically to the life quality of people with an intellectual disability. This no doubt reflects the special concern that the safety domain has for the welfare of this particular group, but its influence is pervasive for the general population as well.

In terms of the objective axis, examples of the influences of the safety domain have been provided by Lehman (1983), who found a negative relationship between global well-being and having been a victim of crime, and Palmore & Luikart (1972) who found a positive relationship with residential stability. In terms of subjective quality of life, substantial correlations have been reported with feelings of safety (Headey, 1981; Lehman, 1983) and control over circumstances (Morris & Jones, 1989; Palmore & Luikart, 1972). Finally, using the domain of 'safety' within the Comprehensive Quality of Life Scale (ComQol), it has been found that in a sample of adults, adolescents and people with an intellectual disability (Cummins, 1993a, b, c), the domain-to-total objective axis correlations were .47, .29 and .16 respectively. For the satisfaction subscale, for adults, the domain-to-total correlation was .27 and for the importance subscale it was .45. Together these data provide reasonable empirical support for the inclusion of safety as a domain.

Evidence for a domain of community

The second new domain indicated by the definition is 'place in community'. This domain is intended to be inclusive of the constructs of (objective) social class, education, job status, community integration, community involvement and (subjective) a sense of self-esteem, self-concept and empowerment, in addition to feelings associated with the objective components. This 'community' domain reflects the influence of large-scale social structures and pressures on quality of life (Liem & Liem, 1978).

Perhaps the strongest traditional linkage of this domain with quality of life has been through its combination with material well-being to form the index Socio-Economic Status (SES). SES inevitably contributes significant variance to measures of life quality and the relative importance of the social component has been nicely demonstrated in a review by Adler *et al.* (1994). They found the literature supported the SES–good health link more strongly within, rather than between, countries. This suggests that the active ingredient may be more associated with relative position on a social hierarchy than absolute wealth *per se*.

The critical distinction between this domain and the other 'social' domain is that intimacy is provided by family and friends, with no implied status hierarchy, while place in community reflects hierarchical position within community life that implies no intimacy.

Of the 27 definitions mentioned earlier, 30% identified a domain corresponding to place in community. Most related to social relationships, activities or functioning (Felce & Perry, 1993; Hornquist, 1989; Schalock *et al.*, 1989; Schumaker *et al.*, 1993; Stark & Goldsbury, 1990; Wenger *et al.*, 1984), while Borthwick-Duffy (1990) referred to community involvement and Evans *et al.* (1985) to political activity and sporting activity.

The links of these community constructs to well-being are legion. Examples on the objective axis are education (Abbey & Andrews, 1985), job status (Makarczyk, 1962) and community involvement (Cutler, 1973). Of course, some researchers have also reported a lack of association, but the positive reports are clearly in the majority. In relation to the subjective axis, the relationship of self-esteem and self-concept to quality of life is almost by definition. Both Rosenberg (1965) and Coopersmith (1967) include 'self-worth' in their definitions of self-esteem, while self-concept is usually defined in ways that include 'a positive view of self' (e.g. Chene, 1991; Neugarten, Havighurst & Tobin, 1961). In empirical terms, almost all researchers find self-esteem, self-concept and feelings associated with the objective axis components to contribute substantial variance to subjective well-being.

Finally, in using the domain of community within ComQol, Cummins has reported that in a sample of adolescents and adults with and without an intellectual disability (Cummins, 1993a, b, c), the domain-to-total objective axis correlations were .63, .41 and .65 respectively. For the satisfaction subscale for non-disabled adults the domain-to-total correlation was .34 and for the importance subscale, it was .28. Together these data provide empirical support for the inclusion of community as a domain.

In conclusion, there is a strong theoretical and empirical rationale for each of the seven domains that has been proposed. Whether they are too numerous or too few is an empirical question to be answered through systematic determinations of the contribution each makes to the overall quality of life measurement. The definition of quality of life in terms of these seven domains, however, makes it clear that the requirement to accommodate Proposition 5 has been attempted. The seven domains are intended, in aggregate, to cover the spectrum of life quality.

THE MAINTAINED SEPARATION OF OBJECTIVE QUALITY OF LIFE AND SUBJECTIVE QUALITY OF LIFE

Proposition 6 states that the objective axis should reflect normative values, while the subjective axis should reflect the values of individual respondents. This has been achieved on the subjective axis through the use of satisfaction responses weighted by individual perception of domain importance.

In this construction, the two axes of quality of life are kept separate from one another and not combined to yield some overall measure. This differs from the suggestion of Felce & Perry (1993) that the importance of weightings should also be applied to the objective measurements.

This, if applied, would detract from the objective measures as primarily normative indicators of well-being. In their unweighted form the objective quality of life axis presents an estimation of how the individual is placed relative to societal norms of well-being. This provides information which can be viewed quite independently from subjective quality of life and yet is integral to the measurement of life quality. People adapt to quite gross deficits in their objective world, as has already been mentioned. Perhaps because of this, the correlation between objective and subjective variables has been generally found to be low and so both need to be measured and considered quite separately from one another.

Consider the reaction of the residents of Lawrence, Massachusetts, to the information that the *Places Rated Almanac* (Boyer & Savageau, 1981) had placed their town last of 277 metropolitan areas within the United States as a desirable place to live. Zautra (1983) describes their reaction:

> They told the media how much they valued sharing experiences with their family, friends, and neighbours in their community. Their attachment was both to people and also to the place itself. The physical setting, certain parks, city blocks, and other landmarks had meaning.
>
> (p84)

As Zautra points out, the basis for the objective rating of desirability and the subjective rating by inhabitants had been based on quite different criteria, yet both types of data are highly relevant to life quality. Only norm-referenced objective indicators can be used as reliable measures of people's actual circumstances of living.

The seventh proposition suggests that definitions of life quality should be broad enough to be equally applicable to all subgroups within the population. This requirement has been met through the parallel forms of the ComQol instrument (Cummins, 1993a, b, c).

CONCLUSION

In conclusion, the definition of life quality presented as Proposition 8 is consistent with all of the other propositions that have been deduced from this theoretical and empirical review. The matching of this total quality of life construct to a measurement instrument is the purpose of the Comprehensive Quality of Life Scale. This, together with other instruments that have been designed specifically for people with disabilities, is described in the appendix to this chapter.

RECOMMENDATIONS

- Several instruments are now available which allow people with cognitive impairments to record their subjective quality of life (see Appendix). It is recommended that such measurement be regarded as an essential, ethical requirement wherever issues of intervention, education or service delivery are under consideration.
- When quality of life for people with disabilities is defined in a way different from that of the general adult population, the implied standards tend to be lower. People with disabilities can be shown to have a life quality no different from that of the general population *provided that* they are not disadvantaged by discriminatory definitions or instrumentation. It is recommended that all definitions and instruments apply equally to people with and without disabilities.
- A large number of instruments to measure life quality have now been published. A copy of the author's *Directory of Instruments to Measure Quality of Life and Cognate Areas* is available on request and those that relate to intellectual disability are listed as an appendix to this chapter. It is recommended that anyone contemplating the development of a new scale be conversant with those that have already been produced.
- While research into discrepancy theory will undoubtedly continue to shed light on the theoretical construction of life quality, the use of perceived discrepancies should not be used to measure quality of life. It is

recommended that subjective quality of life be measured using the response mode of satisfaction/dissatisfaction.

APPENDIX – INSTRUMENTS

For research and teaching purposes, I have constructed an in-house document called the *Directory of Instruments to Measure Quality of Life and Cognate Areas* (Cummins, 1995b). As of the April 1995 edition, it contained 229 entries. Clearly only a fraction of these can be reviewed here and the ones that have been chosen are those that have direct utility for people with some form of cognitive impairment, be it through developmental disability, psychiatric impairment or adventitious brain damage. These will be presented in alphabetical listing of scale title.

ASSESSMENT OF RESIDENTS' SATISFACTION AND FAMILY PERCEPTIONS INDEX (BOWD, 1988)

Purpose: The instrument contains four parts: (a) Institutional/group home objective evaluation of normalization, (b) Family evaluation of their relative's accommodation, (c) Staff attitudes to normalization, (d) Residents' attitudes to their accommodation. **Scales**: (a) 29 items, (b) 18 items, (c) 40 items, (d) 19 items.

COMPREHENSIVE QUALITY OF LIFE SCALE (CUMMINS, 1993A, B, C)

Purpose: Three parallel versions of the Comprehensive Quality of Life Scale allow objective quality of life and subjective quality of life measurement for adolescents attending school, people with an intellectual or other form of cognitive disability and non-disabled adults. **Scale**: Objective quality of life (OQOL) is measured over the seven domains of material well-being, health, productivity, intimacy, safety, place in community and emotional well-being. Each domain is measured by the aggregate of three items. Subjective quality of life (SQOL) is measured over the same seven domains using satisfaction weighted by importance. The intellectual disability version contains a pretest to establish respondent competence in relation to the scale questions. **Psychometrics**: Cummins *et al.*, 1994, 1997; Ferris & Bramston, 1994.

CONSUMER SATISFACTION SURVEY (TEMPLE UNIVERSITY, 1988)

Purpose: To evaluate both consumer satisfaction and quality of life of people with a disability. **Scale**: Items are grouped into six areas: services received; satisfaction with services; independence/interdependence; community activities; productivity; need for supports, services and assistance. **Psychometrics**: Sands & Kozleski (1994).

LIFE EXPERIENCES CHECKLIST (VERSION 4) (AGER & EGLINTON, 1989; AGER *ET AL.*, 1989)

Purpose: Designed to assess a wide range of the life experiences of individuals who are intellectually disabled and receiving residential services. Its focus is on the quality of care practices within service settings and areas of human experience that are commonly judged as valuable by people in the general population. **Scale**: The checklist contains 50 items which are grouped into five sections reflecting different areas of experience: home, leisure, relationships, freedom and opportunities. Each section contains ten items. The LEC can be self-administered or an individual's response recorded on it by someone else.

PALS (ROSEN, SIMON & MCKINSEY, 1995)

Purpose: To measure perceived stress, affect, loneliness and satisfaction in people with intellectual disability.

LIFESTYLE SATISFACTION SCALE (HEAL & CHADSEY-RUSCH, 1985)

Purpose: Designed to be administered to people who are intellectually disabled. It measures manifest satisfaction of the individual with their lifespace, friends, community and opportunities. **Scale**: Requires 29 responses and includes an acquiescence scale. **Psychometrics**: Atkinson (1982).

The *Multifaceted Lifestyle Satisfaction Scale* (Harner & Heal, 1993) is derived from the Lifestyle Satisfaction Scale. **Scale**: It solicits responses from people with an intellectual disability relating to their happiness or satisfaction on seven subscales: community, friends and free time, job, recreation and leisure, services, interpersonal interactions, 'general' and an acquiescence subscale.

PERSONAL INTEGRATION INVENTORY (BERSANI & SALON, 1988)

Purpose: To record the extent to which the person is becoming integrated into the community. **Scale**: It is completed by another person, usually a staff member. It is basically a checklist with the occasional Likert scale.

QUALITY OF LIFE ASSESSMENT TOOL (JOHNSON & COCKS, 1989)

Purpose: Developed as an objective measure of quality of life for people with intellectual disability living in the community. **Scale**: It consists of a very large number of questions which can be completed by either carers or clients.

QUALITY OF LIFE CHECKLIST (MALM, MAY & DENCKER, 1981)

Purpose: Designed to provide information about which aspects of quality of life are particularly important to people with schizophrenia. **Scale**: Delivered as a semistructured interview containing 93 items. Contents include nine sections, seven of which resemble Comprehensive Quality of Life Scale. The ones which are additional are (a) Knowledge, education, leisure and recreation; (b) Communication and transport services. Most items are objective indices.

QUALITY OF LIFE INDEX FOR MENTAL HEALTH (BECKER, DIAMOND & SAINFORT, 1993)

Purpose: To measure quality of life for people with a psychiatric disorder. **Scale**: Contains nine domains with multiple questions within each. It utilizes importance and satisfaction, but the paper reports only on satisfaction. The items within domains are often taken from other instruments. It is intended to be completed by physician, family and patient and can be scored vicariously if the patient cannot complete it alone.

QUALITY OF LIFE INTERVIEW (LEHMAN, 1988)

Purpose: To assess the quality of life of people with severe mental illness. **Scale**: Delivered as a structured interview, it contains 143 items. Content includes leisure activities, employment, earnings, social interaction, perceived health, safety, religious activities. **Psychometrics**: Sullivan, Wells & Leake (1992); Fabian (1992); Lehman, Slaughter & Myers (1992); Lehman, Postrado & Rachuba (1993); Lehman, Rachuba & Postrado (1995).

Huxley & Warner (1992) describe the 'quality of life profile' which retains eight of Lehman's domains (health, social relations, law/safety, living situation, leisure, family, work and finances) and adds religion as a ninth. The domains are scored on a seven-point scale. It also includes a measure of positive and negative affect and self-esteem and a global quality of life measure using Cantrill's ten-step ladder.

QUALITY OF LIFE INTERVIEW SCALE (HOLCOMB *ET AL.*, 1993)

Purpose: To measure the objective quality of life of people with severe mental illness. **Scale**: Contains 87 items scored on a Likert scale and yields eight factors.

QUALITY OF LIFE INTERVIEW SCHEDULE (DEVELOPMENTAL CONSULTING PROGRAM, 1990)

Purpose: To measure quality of life in people who are disabled, including those who are non-verbal. **Scale**: Contains 12 domains, each rated on support, access, participation and contentment. It is completed by 'individuals who know him or her well'. **Psychometrics**: Ouellette-Kuntz (1990); Ouellette-Kuntz *et al.* (1994); Oullette-Kuntz & McCreary (1995).

QUALITY OF LIFE QUESTIONNAIRE (BIGELOW, GAREAU & YOUNG, 1991)

Purpose: To measure quality of life for people with an intellectual disability. **Scale**: The interviewer rating version contains 141 items, mainly objective, directed to people with psychiatric impairment. The respondent self-report version asks for subjective responses and appears to have little relationship to the other version. It contains ten domains. **Psychometrics**: Bigelow, McFarland & Olson (1991); Bigelow, Gareau & Young (1990); Bigelow & Young (1991); Bigelow *et al.* (1991).

QUALITY OF LIFE QUESTIONNAIRE (CRAGG & HARRISON, 1984, 1986) COMPASS: A MULTIPERSPECTIVE EVALUATION OF QUALITY IN HOME LIFE (CRAGG & LOOK, 1992)

Purpose: To measure quality of life according to the principles of normalization. **Scale**: Contains both subjective and objective measures, to questions of which 53 are completed by staff and residents, 17 by the questionnaire administrator, nine objective and eight subjective impressions. **Psychometrics**: Donegan & Potts (1988); Dagnan, Jones & Ruddick (1994).

REHABILITATION QUESTIONNAIRE: A PERSONAL GUIDE TO THE INDIVIDUAL'S QUALITY OF LIFE (BROWN & BAYER, 1992)

Purpose: To measure quality of life for people with an intellectual disability. **Scale**: Items are divided into 11 categories: home living, things you do, your health, your family and friends, you and your family, self-image, leisure time, employment, you and the law, the help you want, how you feel about life. A variety of response modes are employed including both closed and open-ended questions.

QUALITY OF LIFE SCALE (SCHALOCK & KEITH, 1993)

Purpose: To measure quality of life in people with an intellectual disability. **Scale**: 40 questions using three-point scales. The manual reports these items to load onto four factors: satisfaction, competence/productivity, empowerment/independence, social belonging/community integration. **Psychometrics**: Rapley & Lobley (1994); Rapley, Lobley & Bozatzis (1994); Schalock *et al.* (1994).

QUALITY OF LIFE SCALE (HEINRICHS, HANLON & CARPENTER, 1984)

Purpose: Designed for use with people with schizophrenia. **Scale**: Delivered as a semistructured interview by a trained clinician. Contains 21 items delivered over 45 minutes. Content includes commonplace activities, occupation, possessions, social relationships, sense of purpose, motivation and satisfaction. **Psychometrics**: Lehman, Postrado & Rachuba (1993).

RESIDENT LIFESTYLE INVENTORY (BELLAMY *ET AL.*, 1990)

Purpose: A quality of life instrument to be used for people with severe intellectual disability and completed by a carer. **Scale**: It measures 144 different leisure and personal management 'activities' performed during the last 30 days. It asks how many times each activity occurred, which activities were seen as preferred, the level of support necessary to participate and whether an activity typically occurred at home or in the community. **Psychometrics**: Kennedy *et al.* (1990).

RESIDENTIAL SATISFACTION INVENTORY (BURNETT, 1989)

Purpose: A self-report instrument designed for people with an intellectual disability, it assesses their level of satisfaction regarding their residential facility and its activities. **Scale**: 20 questions use a Yes/No response format. Four questions are devoted to each of four domains: physical environment, personal autonomy, organization, services. One item from each domain is oppositely worded to form a consistency scale.

SATISFACTION WITH LIFE DOMAINS SCALE (BAKER & INTAGLIATA, 1982)

Purpose: To evaluate the impact of a community support programme on quality of life of people with a chronic mental illness. **Scale**: It is a self-report scale, containing 18 'satisfaction' items administered by interview. Items concentrate on satisfaction with a wide variety of life areas. **Psychometrics**: Baker, Curbow & Wingard (1991); Baker *et al.* (1994).

STANDARD OF LIVING QUESTIONNAIRE (SKANTZE *ET AL.*, 1992)
QUALITY OF LIFE SELF-ASSESSMENT INVENTORY (QLS-100)

Purpose: A structured interview which yields an overall evaluation of standard of living for people with mental illness. **Scale**: Subscales measure: standard of housing, number of rooms per occupant, access to and use of community services (transport, telephone and home-help services), weekly activities, education, current employment and social network. It also provides information about social dependence (need to live with others), need for company to travel and need for help in handling money.

QLS-100 is a 100-item inventory organized into 11 domains, which ask people to indicate which they consider to be currently unsatisfactory. The domains are: housing (including household and self-care), environment (including community services), knowledge and education, contacts, dependence (including finances), inner experiences, mental health, physical health, leisure, work and religion.

REFERENCES

Abbey, A. and Andrews, F.M. (1985) Modeling the psychological determinants of life quality. *Social Indicators Research*, **16**, 1–34.

Abrams, M. (1973) Subjective social indicators. *Social Trends*, **4**, 35–50.

Adler, N.E., Boyce, T., Chesney, M.A. *et al.* (1994) Socioeconomic status and health: the challenge of the gradient. *American Psychologist*, **49**, 15–24.

Ager, A. and Eglinton, L. (1989) *Working Paper 4: Life Experiences of Clients of Services for People with Learning Difficulties: Summary of Findings From Studies Using the Life Experiences Checklist*, Mental Handicap Research Group, Department of Psychology, University of Leicester.

Ager, A., Annetts, S., Barlow, R. *et al.* (1989) *Working Paper 2 (revised): Life Experiences and Quality of Life in the General Population: A Study of Leicester and its Environs Using the Life Experiences Checklist*, Mental Handicap Research Group, Department of Psychology, University of Leicester.

Andrews, F.M. and Withey, S.B. (1976) *Social Indicators of Well-being: Americans' Perceptions of Life Quality*, Plenum Press, New York.

Antonovsky, A. (1987) *Unravelling the Mystery of Health*, Jossey-Bass, San Francisco.

Atkinson, T. (1982) The stability and validity of quality of life measures. *Social Indicators Research*, **10**, 113–32.

Baker, F. and Intagliata, J. (1982) Quality of life in the evaluation of community support systems. *Evaluation and Program Planning*, **5**, 69–79.

Baker, F., Curbow, B. and Wingard, J.R. (1991) Role retention and quality of life of bone marrow transplant survivors. *Social Science and Medicine*, **32**, 697–704.

Baker, F., Jodrey, D. and Intagliata, J. (1992) Social support and quality of life of community support clients. *Community Mental Health Journal*, **28**, 397–411.

Baker, F., Wingard, J.R., Curbow, B. *et al.* (1994) Quality of life of bone marrow transplant long-term survivors. *Bone Marrow Transplantation*, **13**, 589–96.

Barlow, J. and Kirby, N. (1991) Residential satisfaction of persons with an intellectual disability living in an institution or in the community. *Australia and New Zealand Journal of Developmental Disabilities*, **17**, 7–23.

Bech, P. (1993) *Rating Scales for Psychopathology. Health Status and Quality of Life: A Compendium on Documentation in Accordance with the DSM-m-R and WHO Systems*, Springer-Verlag, Berlin.

Becker, M., Diamond, R. and Sainfort, F. (1993) A new patient focused index for measuring quality of life in persons with severe and persistent mental illness. *Quality of Life Research*, **2**, 239–51.

Bellamy, G.T., Newton, J.S., Lebaron, N.M. and Horner, R.H. (1990) Quality of life and lifestyle outcomes: a challenge for residential programmes, in *Quality of Life: Perspectives and Issues*, (ed. R. Schalock), American Association on Mental Retardation, Washington DC.

Bersani, H. and Salon, R. (1988) *Personal Integration Inventory*, Research and Training Center on Community Integration, New York.

Bigelow, D.A. and Young, D.J. (1991) Effectiveness of a case management program. *Community Mental Health Journal*, **27**, 115–23.

Bigelow, D.A., Gareau, M.J. and Young, D.J. (1990) A quality of life interview. *Psychosocial Rehabilitation Journal*, **14**, 94–8.

Bigelow, D.A., Gareau, M.J. and Young, D.J. (1991) *Quality of Life Questionnaire. (a) Interviewer Rating Version: (b) Respondent Self-report Version*, Western Mental Health Research Center, Oregon.

Bigelow, D.A., McFarland, B.H. and Olson, M.M. (1991) Quality of life of community mental health program clients: validating a measure. *Community Mental Health Journal*, **27**, 43–55.

Bigelow, D.A., Brodsky, G., Stewart, L. and Olson, M. (1982) The concept and measurement of quality of life as a dependent variable in evaluation of mental health services, in *Innovative Approaches to Mental Health Evaluation*, (eds G.J. Stahler and W.R. Tash), Academic Press, New York.

Bigelow, D.A., McFarland, B.H., Gareau, M.J. and Young, D.J. (1991) Implementation and effectiveness of a bed reduction project. *Community Mental Health Journal*, **27**, 125–33.

Borthwick-Duffy, S.A. (1990) Quality of life of persons with severe or profound mental retardation, in *Quality of Life: Perspectives and Issues*, (ed. R. Schalock), American Association on Mental Retardation, Washington DC.

Borthwick-Duffy, S.A. (1992) Quality of life and quality of care in mental retardation, in *Mental Retardation in the Year 2000*, (ed. L. Rowitz), Springer-Verlag, New York.

Bowd, A.D. (1988) *Assessment of Residents' Satisfaction and Family Perceptions Index*, Lakehead University, Ontario.

Bowling, A., Farquhar, M. and Browne, P. (1991) Life satisfaction and associations with social network and support variables in three samples of elderly people. *International Journal of Geriatric Psychiatry*, **6**, 549–66.

Boyer, R. and Savageau, D. (1981) *Places Rated Almanac*, Rand McNally, Chicago.

Brickman, P. and Campbell, D.T. (1971) Hedonic relativism and planning the good society, in *Adaptation-level Theory: A Symposium*, (ed. M.H. Appley), Academic Press, New York.

Brickman, P., Coates, D. and Janoff-Bulman, R. (1978) Lottery winners and accident victims: is happiness relative? *Journal of Personality and Social Psychology*, **36**, 917–27.

Brown, R.I. and Bayer, M.B. (1992) *Rehabilitation Questionnaire and Manual: A Personal Guide to the Individual's Quality of Life*, Captus University Publications, Toronto.

Brown, R.I., Bayer, M.B. and MacFarlane, C. (1989) *Rehabilitation Programmes*, Lugus, Toronto.

Burnett, P.C. (1989) Assessing satisfaction in people with an intellectual disability: living in community-based residential facilities. *Australian Disability Review*, **1**, 14–19.

Butler, E.W. and Bjaanes, A.T. (1978) Activities and the use of time by retarded persons in community care facilities, in *Observing Behavior. Vol. 1. Theory and Applications in Mental Retardation*, (ed. C.P. Sackett), University Park Press, Baltimore.

Calman, K.C. (1984) Quality of life in cancer patients – an hypothesis. *Journal of Medical Ethics*, **10**, 124–7.

Campbell, A., Converse, P.E. and Rodgers, W.L. (1976) *The Quality of American Life*, Russell Sage Foundation, New York.

Chene, A. (1991) Self-esteem of the elderly and education. *Educational Gerontology*, **17**, 343–53.

Cohen, C. (1982) On the quality of life: some philosophical reflections. *Circulation*, **66**(Suppl. III), 29–33.

Coopersmith, S. (1967) *The Antecedents of Self-Esteem*, W. H. Freeman, San Francisco.

Cragg, R. and Harrison, J. (1984) *Living in a Supervised Home. A Questionnaire of Quality of Life*, West Midlands Campaign for People with Mental Handicap, Manchester.

Cragg, R. and Look, R. (1992) *Compass: A Multi-perspective Evaluation of Quality in Home Life*. Available from the authors at 302 Station Rd, Kings Heath, Birmingham B14 7TF, UK.

Cummins, R.A. (1993a) *The Comprehensive Quality of Life Scale – Adult, 4th edn (ComQol-A4)*, School of Psychology, Deakin University, Melbourne.

Cummins, R.A. (1993b) *The Comprehensive Quality of Life Scale – Adolescent, 4th edn (ComQol-AD4)*, School of Psychology, Deakin University, Melbourne.

Cummins, R.A. (1993c) *The Comprehensive Quality of Life Scale – Intellectual Disability, 4th edn (ComQol-ID4)*, School of Psychology, Deakin University, Melbourne.

Cummins, R.A. (1995a) On the trail of the gold standard for subjective well-being. *Social Indicators Research*, **35**, 179–200.

Cummins, R.A. (1995b) *Directory of Instruments to Measure Quality of Life and Cognate Areas*, April edn, School of Psychology, Deakin University, Melbourne.

Cummins, R.A., McCabe, M.P., Romeo, Y. and Gullone, E. (1994) The comprehensive quality of life scale: instrument development and psychometric evaluation on tertiary staff and students. *Educational and Psychological Measurement*, **54**, 372–82.

Cummins, R.A., McCabe, M.P., Romeo, Y., Reid, S. and Waters, L. (1997) An evaluation of the comprehensive quality of life scale – intellectual disability. International Journal of Disability, Development and Education, **44**, 7–20.

Cutler, S.J. (1973) Voluntary association, participation and life satisfaction: a cautionary research note. *Journal of Gerontology*, **28**, 96–100.

Dagnan, D., Jones, J. and Ruddick, L. (1994) The psychometric properties of a scale for assessing quality of life of people with learning disabilities in residential care. *British Journal of Development Disabilities*, **40**, 98–103.

Developmental Consulting Program (1990) *QUOLIS Kit for Interviewers: The Quality of Life Interview Schedule for Adults with Developmental Disabilities*, Available from 80 Queen St, Suite 301, Kingston, Ontario.

Donegan, C. and Potts, M. (1988) People with mental handicap living alone in the community: a pilot study of their quality of life. *British Journal of Mental Subnormality*, **34**, 10–22.

Dunst, C.J., Leet, H.E,. and Trivette, C.M. (1988) Family resources, personal well-being, and early intervention. *Journal of Special Education*, **22**, 108–16.

Emerson, E.B. (1985) Evaluating the impact of deinstitutionalization on the lives of mentally retarded people. *American Journal of Mental Deficiency*, **90**, 277–88.

Evans, D.R., Pellizzari, J.R., Culbert, B.J. and Metzen, M.E. (1993) Personality, marital and occupational factors associated with quality of life. *Journal of Clinical Psychology*, **49**, 477–84.

Fabian, E.S. (1992) Longitudinal outcomes in supported employment: a survival analysis. *Rehabilitation Psychology*, **37**, 23–35.

Feeny, D., Labelle, R. and Torrance, G.W. (1990) Integrating economic evaluations and quality of life assessments, in *Quality of Life Assessments in Clinical Trials*, (ed. B. Spilker), Raven Press, New York.

Fehring, R.J., Brennan, P.F. and Keller, M.L. (1987) Psychological and spiritual well-being in college students. *Research in Nursing and Health*, **10**, 391–8.

Felce, D. and Perry, J. (1993) *Quality of Life: A Contribution to its Definition and Measurement*, Mental Handicap in Wales Applied Research Unit, Cardiff.

Fernandez, R. M. and Kulik, J. C. (1981) A multilevel model of life satisfaction: effects of individual characteristics and neighborhood composition. *American Sociological Review*, **46**, 840–50.

Ferrans, C.E. (1990) Quality of life: conceptual issues. *Seminars in Oncology Nursing*, **6**, 248–54.

Ferrans, C.E. and Powers, M.J. (1985) Quality of life index: development and psychometric properties. *Advances in Nursing Science*, **8**, 15–24.

Ferris, C. and Bramston, P. (1994) Quality of life in the elderly: a contribution to its understanding. *Australian Journal on Ageing*, **13**, 120–3.

Flanagan, J.C. (1978) A research approach to improving our quality of life. *American Psychologist*, **33**, 138–47.

Flanagan, J.C. (1982) Measurement of quality of life: current state of the art. *Archives of Physical Medical Rehabilitation*, **63**, 56–9.

Goode, D.A. (1990) Measuring the quality of life of persons with disabilities: some issues and suggestions. *News and Notes*, **3**, 2–6.

Goodinson, S.M. and Singleton, J. (1989) Quality of life: a critical review of current concepts, measures and their clinical implications. *International Journal of Nursing Studies*, **26**, 327–41.

Guyatt, G.H., Townsend, M., Berman, L.B. and Pugsley, S.O. (1987) Quality of life in patients with chronic airflow limitation. *British Journal of Diseases of the Chest*, **81**, 45–54.

Hailstone, J. (1989) Quality lifestyles project. *Interaction*, **3**, 17–20.

Halpern, A.S. (1993) Quality of life as a conceptual framework for evaluating transition outcomes. *Exceptional Children*, **59**, 486–99.

Harner, C.J. and Heal, L.W. (1993) The Multifaceted Lifestyle Satisfaction Scale (MLSS): psychometric properties of an interview schedule for assessing personal satisfaction of adults with limited intelligence. *Research in Developmental Disabilities*, **14**, 221–36.

Harwood, M.K. and Rice, R.W. (1992) An examination of referent selection processes underlying job satisfaction. *Social Indicators Research*, **27**, 1–39.

Headey, B. (1981) The quality of life in Australia. *Social Indicators Research*, **2**, 155–81.

Headey, B. and Wearing, A. (1989) Personality, life events, and subjective well-being: toward a dynamic equilibrium model. *Journal of Personality and Social Psychology*, **57**, 731–9.

Headey, B., Holmstrom, E. and Wearing, A. (1984) Well-being and ill-being: different dimensions? *Social Indicators Research*, **14**, 115–39.

Heal, L.W. and Chadsey-Rusch, J. (1985) The Lifestyle Satisfaction Scale (LSS): assessing individuals' satisfaction with residence, community setting, and associated services. *Applied Research in Mental Retardation*, **6**, 475–90.

Heinrichs, D.W., Hanlon, T.E. and Carpenter, W.T. (1984) The Quality of Life Scale: an instrument for rating the schizophrenic deficit syndrome. *Schizophrenia Bulletin*, **10**, 388–98.

Helson, H. (1964) *Adaptation-level Theory*, Harper & Row, New York.

Higgins, E.T., Bond, R.N., Klein, R. and Strauman, T. (1986) Self-discrepancies and emotional vulnerability: how magnitude, accessibility and type of discrepancy influence affect. *Journal of Personality and Social Psychology*, **51**, 5–15.

Holcomb, W.R., Morgan, P., Adams, N.A., Ponder, H. and Farrel, M. (1993) Development of a structured interview scale for measuring quality of life of the severely mentally ill. *Journal of Clinical Psychology*, **49**, 830–40.

Hornquist, J.O. (1982) The concept of quality of life. *Scandinavian Journal of Social Medicine*, **10**, 57–61.

Hornquist, J.O. (1989) Quality of life: concept and assessment. *Scandinavian Journal of Social Medicine*, **18**, 69–79.

Huxley, P. and Warner, R. (1992) Case management, quality of life and satisfaction with services of long-term psychiatric patients. *Hospital and Community Psychiatry*, **43**, 799–802.

Johnson, R. and Cocks, H. (1989) *Quality of Life: An Assessment Strategy. Users Manual*, Challenge Foundation, Armidale.

Karan, O.C., Lambour, G. and Greenspan, S. (1990) Persons in transition, in *Quality of Life: Perspectives and Issues*, (ed. R. Schalock), American Association on Mental Retardation, Washington DC.

Kennedy, C.H., Homer, R.H., Newton, J.S. and Kanda, E. (1990) Measuring the activity patterns of adults with severe disabilities using the Resident Lifestyle Inventory. *Journal of the Association for Persons with Severe Handicaps*, **15**, 79–85.

Krupinski, J. (1980) Health and quality of life. *Social Science and Medicine*, **14A**, 203–11.

Lang, J.G., Munoz, R.F., Bernal, G. and Sorenson, J.L. (1982) Quality of life and psychological well-being in a bicultural Latino community. *Hispanic Journal of Behavioral Sciences*, **4**, 433–50.

Lehman, A.F. (1983) The effects of psychiatric symptoms on quality of life assessments among the chronic mentally ill. *Evaluation and Program Planning*, **6**, 143–51.

Lehman, A.F. (1988) A quality of life interview for the chronically mentally ill. *Evaluation and Program Planning*, **11**, 51–62.

Lehman, A.F., Slaughter, J.G. and Myers, C.P. (1992) Quality of life experiences of the chronically mentally ill: gender and stages of life effects. *Evaluation and Program Planning*, **15**, 7–12.

Lehman, A.F., Postrado, L.T. and Rachuba, L.T. (1993) Convergent validation of quality of life assessments for persons with severe mental illnesses. *Quality of Life Research*, **2**, 327–34.

Lehman, A.F., Rachuba, L.T. and Postrado, L.T. (1995) Demographic influences on quality of life among persons with chronic mental illness. *Evaluation and Program Planning* (in press).

Liem, R. and Liem, J. (1978) Social class and mental illness reconsidered: the role of economic stress and social support. *Journal of Health and Social Behavior*, **19**, 139–56.

Liu, B. (1975) Quality of life: concept, measure and results. *American Journal of Economics and Sociology*, **34**, 1–13.

Makarczyk, W. (1962) Factors affecting life satisfaction among people in Poland. *Polish Sociological Bulletin*, **1**, 105–16.

Malm, U., May, P.R.A. and Dencker, S.J. (1981) Evaluation of the quality of life of the schizophrenic outpatient: a checklist. *Schizophrenia Bulletin*, **7**, 34–42.

Maslow, A. (1943) A theory of human motivation. *Psychological Review*, **50**, 370–96.

McCall, S. (1976) Human needs and the quality of life, in *Values and the Quality of Life*, (eds W.R. Shea and J. King-Farlow), Science History Publications, New York.

Meadow, H.L., Mentzer, J.T., Rahtz, D.R. and Sirgy, M.J. (1992) A life satisfaction measure based on judgement theory. *Social Indicators Research*, **26**, 23–59.

Meyers, C.E. (1978) *Quality of Life in Severely and Profoundly Mentally Retarded People: Research Foundations for Improvement*, American Association on Mental Deficiency, Washington DC.

Michalos, A.C. (1985) Multiple Discrepancies Theory (MDT). *Social Indicators Research*, **16**, 347–413.

Michalos, A.C. (1986) An application of Multiple Discrepancies Theory (MDT) to seniors. *Social Indicators Research*, **18**, 349–73.

Milbrath, L.W. (1982) A conceptualization and research strategy for the study of ecological aspects of the quality of life. *Social Indicators Research*, **10**, 133–57.

Morris, P.L.P. and Jones, B. (1989) Life satisfaction across treatment methods for patients with end-stage renal failure. *Medical Journal of Australia*, **150**, 428–32.

Muthny, F.A., Koch, U. and Stump, S. (1990) Quality of life in oncology patients. *Psychotherapy and Psychosomatics*, **54**, 145–60.

Neugarten, B.L., Havighurst, R.J. and Tobin, S.S. (1961) The measurement of life satisfaction. *Journal of Gerontology*, **16**, 134–43.

Nirje, B. (1976) The normalisation principle, in *Changing Patterns in Residential Services for the Mentally Retarded*, (eds R.B. Kugel and A. Shearer), President's Committee on Mental Retardation, Washington DC.

Nord, E. (1991) *Methods for Establishing Quality Weights for Life Years. Working Paper No 8*, National Centre for Health Program Evaluation, Melbourne.

Organization for Economic Cooperation and Development (1976) *Measuring Social Well-being*, OECD, Paris.

Ouellette-Kuntz, H. (1990) A pilot study in the use of the Quality of Life Interview Schedule. *Social Indicators Research*, **23**, 283–98.

Ouellette-Kuntz, H. and McCreary, B.D (1995) Quality of life assessment for persons with severe developmental disabilities, in *Quality of Life in Health Promotion and Rehabilitation: Conceptual Approaches, Issues and Applications*, (eds R. Renwick, I. Brown and M. Nagler) (in press)

Ouellette-Kuntz, H., McCreary, B.D., Minnes, P. and Stanton, B. (1994) Evaluating quality of life: the development of the Quality of Life Interview Schedule (QUOLIS). *Journal on Developmental Disabilities*, **3**, 17–31.

Palmore, E. and Luikart, C. (1972) Health and social factors related to life satisfaction. *Journal of Health and Social Behavior*, **13**, 68–80.

Parmenter, T.R. (1988) *The Development of a Quality of Life Model as an Outcome Measure of Rehabilitation Programs for People with Developmental Disabilities*. Paper presented to Ninth Annual Conference of Young Adult Institute, Employment, Integration and Community Competence: The keys to quality of life and community coalescence. New York, April.

Pavot, W. and Diener, E. (1993) Review of the Satisfaction with Life Scale. *Psychological Assessment*, **5**, 164–72.

Rapley, M. and Lobley, J. (1995) *Factor Analysis of the Schalock and Keith (1994) Quality of Life Questionnaire: A Replication*, Mental Handicap Research, **8**, 194–202.

Rapley, M., Lobley, J. and Bozatzis, N. (1994) *Preliminary Validation of the Schalock & Keith (1994) Quality of Life Questionnaire with a British Population*, Department of Psychology, Lancaster University, Lancaster.

Revicki, D.A. and Kaplan, R.M. (1993) Relationship between psychometric and utility-based approaches to the measurement of health-related quality of life. *Quality of Life Research*, **2**, 477–87.

Richardson, J. (1991) What should we measure in health programme evaluation? in *Economics and Health: 1990*, (ed. C.S. Smith), Monash University, Melbourne.

Romney, D.M., Brown, R.I. and Fry, P.S. (1994) Improving the quality of life: prescriptions for change. *Social Indicators Research*, **33**, 237–72.

Rosen, M., Simon, E.W. and McKinsey, L. (1995) Subjective measure of quality of life. *Mental Retardation*, **33**, 31–4.

Rosenberg, M., (1965) *Society and the Adolescent Self-Image*, Princeton University Press, New Jersey.

Sands, D.J. and Kozleski, E.B. (1994) Quality of life differences between adults with and without disabilities. *Education and Training in Mental Retardation and Developmental Disabilities*, **29**, 90–101.

Schalock, R.L. (1990) Attempts to conceptualize and measure quality of life, in *Quality of Life: Perspectives and Issues*, (ed. R. Schalock), American Association on Mental Retardation, Washington DC.

Schalock, R.L. and Keith, K.D. (1993) *Quality of Life Questionnaire*, IDS Publishing Corporation, Ohio.

Schalock, R.L., Keith, K.D., Hoffman, K. and Karan, O.C. (1989) Quality of life: its measurement and use. *Mental Retardation*, **27**, 25–31.

Schalock, R.L., Lemanowicz, J.A., Conroy, J.W. and Feinstein, C.S. (1994) A multivariate investigative study of the correlates of quality of life. *Journal on Developmental Disabilities*, **3**, 59–73.

Schipper, H., Clinch, J. and Powell, V. (1990) Definitions and conceptual issues, in *Quality of Life Assessments in Clinical Trials*, (ed. B. Spilker), Raven Press, New York.

Schulz, R. and Decker, S. (1985) Long-term adjustment to physical disability: the role of social support, perceived control, and self-blame, *Journal of Personality and Social Psychology*, **48**, 1162–72.

Schumaker, J.F., Shea, J.D., Monfries, M.M. and Groth-Marnat, G. (1993) Loneliness and life satisfaction in Japan and Australia. *Journal of Psychology*, **127**, 65–71.

Shea, W.R. (1976) Introduction: the quest for a high quality of life, in *Values and the Quality of Life*, (eds W.R. Shea and J. King-Farlow), Science History Publications, New York.

Skantze, K., Malm, U., Dencker, S.J., May, P.R.A. and Corrigan, P. (1992) Comparison of quality of life with standard of living in schizophrenic outpatients. *British Journal of Psychiatry*, **161**, 797–801.

Spitzer, W.O. (1987) State of Science 1986: quality of life and functional status as target variables for research. *Journal of Chronic Diseases*, **40**, 465–71.

Spreitzer, E. and Snyder, E.E. (1974) Correlates of life satisfaction among the aged. *Journal of Gerontology*, **29**, 454–8.

Stark, J.A. and Goldsbury, T. (1990) Quality of life from childhood to adulthood, in *Quality of life: Perspectives and Issues*, (ed. R. Schalock), American Association on Mental Retardation, Washington DC.

Sullivan, G., Wells, K.B. and Leake, B. (1992) Clinical factors associated with better quality of life in a seriously mentally ill population. *Hospital and Community Psychiatry*, **43**, 794–8.

Taylor, S.E., Wood, J.V and Lichtman, R.R. (1983) It could be worse: selective evaluation as a response to victimization. *Journal of Social Issues*, **39**, 19–40.

Temple University (1988) *A National Survey of Consumers of Services for Individuals with Developmental Disabilities: Final Survey Instrument*, National Developmental Disabilities Planning Council, Washington DC.

Testa, M.A. and Nackley, J.F. (1994) Methods for quality of life studies. *Annual Review of Public Health*, **15**, 535–59.

Torrance, G.W. (1986) Measurement of health state utilities for economic appraisal: a review. *Journal of Health Economics*, **5**, 1–30.

Tversky, A. and Griffin, D. (1991) Endowment and contrast in judgements of well-being, in *Subjective Well-being; An Interdisciplinary Perspective*, (eds F. Strack, M. Argyle and N. Schwarz), Plenum Press, New York.

United States Department of Health, Education and Welfare (1969) *Toward a Social Report*, US Government Printing Office, Washington DC.

Vitello, S.J. (1984) Deinstitutionalization of mentally retarded persons in the United States: status and trends, in *Perspectives and Progress in Mental Retardation. Volume 1*, (ed. J.M. Berg), International Association for the Scientific Study of Mental Deficiency, New York.

Walker, S.R. (1992) Quality of life measurement: an overview. *Journal of the Royal Society of Health*, **112**, 265.

Watson, D. and Pennebaker, J.W. (1989) Health complaints, stress and distress: exploring the central role of negative affectivity. *Psychological Reviews*, **96**, 234–54.

Wenger, N.K., Mattson, M.E., Furberg, C.D. and Elinson, J. (1984) Assessment of quality of life in clinical trials of cardiovascular therapies. *American Journal of Cardiology*, **54**, 908–13.

Wicker, F.W., Brown, G., Wiehe, J.A., Hagen, A.S. and Reed, J.L. (1993) On reconsidering Maslow: an examination of the deprivation/domination proposition. *Journal of Research in Personality*, **27**, 118–33.

Wiklund, I., Lindvall, K. and Swedberg, K. (1986) Assessment of quality of life in clinical trials. *Acta Medica Scandinavica*, **220**, 1–3.

Wilson, A., Rosenblood, L.K. and Oliver, P.R. (1973) Congruity theory and linear models of attitude change. *Canadian Journal of Behavioral Science*, **5**, 399–409.

Wolfensberger, W. (1972) *The Principle of Normalization in Human Services*, National Institute on Mental Retardation, Toronto.

Wolfensberger, W. and Glenn, L. (1975) *Program Analysis of Service Systems (PASS): A Method for the Quantitative Evaluation of Human Services. Field Manual, 3rd edn*, National Institute on Mental Retardation, Toronto.

Wolfensberger, W. and Thomas, S. (1983) *Program Analysis of Service Systems' Implementation of Normalization Goals (PASSING): Normalization Criteria and Ratings Manual*, National Institute on Mental Retardation, Toronto.

Woodruff, S.I. and Conway, T.L. (1992) Impact of health and fitness-related behavior on quality of life. *Social Indicators Research*, **25**, 391–405.

Yetim, U. (1993) Life satisfaction: a study based on the organization of personal projects. *Social Indicators Research*, **29**, 277–89.

Zautra, A. (1983) Social resources and the quality of life. *American Journal of Community Psychology*, **11**(3), 275–90.

Zautra, A.J. and Goodhart, D. (1979) Quality of life indicators: a review of the literature. *Community Mental Health Review*, **4**, 1–10.

Developmental systems and narrative approaches to working with families of persons with disabilities   8

David Mitchell and John Winslade

INTRODUCTION

From the moment when parents are first informed that their child has a disability, a lifelong and life-wide process is set in motion. Those with responsibilities for planning, managing and evaluating services for persons with disabilities should recognize the powerful influences on this process. It is our intention in this chapter to look at these influences from two perspectives or sets of metaphors. One of these is drawn from an ecological or developmental systems model (Mitchell, 1984, 1985, 1986); the other derives from a narrative or social constructionist approach to making sense of what happens in family interactions (Pare, 1995). We shall draw from each of these perspectives in order to elaborate models for devising helping strategies.

In brief, a developmental systems model argues that the planning, management and evaluation of services for persons with disabilities and their families must be responsive to the changing developmental needs of the person with a disability. Such a system should be developed with reference to the evolving relational politics of their families and their social contexts at various stages of the person's life story. A narrative model argues that such services should take account of the social location of the person(s) affected by disability, particularly the influence of the discourses about disability that inform these social contexts.

DEVELOPMENTAL SYSTEMS PERSPECTIVE

A developmental systems perspective is built around two core assumptions. Firstly, it takes an ecological or systems perspective. Persons with disabilities do not live in a social vacuum. All have parents and most have siblings. And all exist in a society with its particular mix of subcultures and where disability is defined according to prevailing attitudes towards those who are different. This in turn reflects the value such people are attributed in the community (Johns, 1991; Oliver, 1990; Wolfensberger, 1983). Secondly, it is based on a developmental or life cycle perspective. The person with a disability, their family and social milieu change over time.

SYSTEMS PERSPECTIVE

The application of the study of cybernetics to a variety of systems, eventually including the study of the family as a 'system', provoked a series of shifts of thought. In order to acknowledge the advantages that these ideas offered to our thinking about the needs of families with a child with a disability, some of the principal assumptions of this theoretical orientation will be outlined. This will be followed by a discussion of the ecology of disability, using Bronfenbrenner's (1979) model of nested systems as a framework.

ASSUMPTIONS

Three core assumptions underpin the systems approach.

Wholeness

Although structurally a system is made up of a set of subsystems, these elements must comprise 'a whole' for the term 'system' to apply. A system can be thought of as a 'set of interrelated elements' (Ackoff & Emery, 1972). Thinking of families in this way led professionals to consider the interconnectedness of health, welfare and education systems. It also suggested considerations about disability which took the focus away from the individual diagnosed with a medically defined impairment and asked questions about the interactions within the family around the disability. This emphasis provides some interruption to the individualism promoted through an economic system that regards each person as a consumer or a labour unit, but which offers only very limited opportunities for full participation of people with disabilities. Shifting attention from the individual with the disability to the family might contribute to a reduction in the sense of isolation experienced by the person with the disability. A negative aspect of this emphasis is the danger of the family system becoming marked as different from other families.

Connectedness

Systems theory stresses the interactions between all the elements of a family system and draws attention to how these interactions add up to a pattern of communication that is greater than the sum of the actions of each of the individual persons in the system. Again, this idea has led to a less intense gaze on the individual with the disability and instead to a focus on how each family member is affected by any development that takes place in any other family member's life. It has also led to a recognition of the complexity of patterns of communication within families and to less reliance on a simplistic linear stimulus–response explanation of human behaviour.

Range of stability

According to Miller (1978) and Ramey, McPhee & Yates (1982), each variable within a system has a range of stability that is maintained in equilibrium (albeit constantly changing) by transactions within the system and between the system and its environment. This notion of equilibrium or steady state (Feiring & Lewis, 1978) in turn leads to the cybernetic principle that a successful system must have a mechanism for sensing perturbations and for regulating its behaviour to maintain a desired relationship between input and output (Griffiths, 1964; Pratt, 1982). In cybernetic terms, this requires a feedback loop of some kind that operates within its desired range of stability. Any variable that forces the system beyond this range constitutes a stressor which has to be dealt with, in case the system disintegrates. The presence in a family of a person with a disability can be characterized as a stressor in a family system. The extent to which a family system is able successfully to deal with the potential stressor of a disabled person depends on a variety of factors which will be dealt with later in this chapter. This homoeostatic principle has been criticized as the most dangerous aspect of the family systems way of thinking. It is socially conservative in nature. Change initiated by social movements is automatically framed as a stressor and the homoeostatic principle can be used to blind professionals to the operation of power within family relations. It can sometimes be seen as placing a value on stability ahead of justice or change (Hoffman, 1990; Pare, 1995).

THE ECOLOGY OF DISABILITY

From an ecological or systems perspective, a family of a person with a disability is seen as comprising an interpersonal system which, in turn, is embedded in other systems of varying degrees of remoteness from the family (Hayes, 1994; Hornby, 1994; Mitchell, 1986).

The basic theory of a systems approach as it applies to rehabilitation is that the behaviour of a disabled person cannot and therefore must not be considered in isolation from their social context. Or, as Bronfenbrenner (1979) has expressed it in relation to human development in general:

... the properties of the person and of the environment, the structures of the environmental settings, and the processes taking place within and between them must be viewed as interdependent and analyzed in systems terms.

(p41)

In meeting the needs of disabled persons and their families, consideration must be given to such factors as the transmission of information, the provision of support and the power relationships that exist in the interfaces between disabled persons, their families, human service agencies and the broader society. For example, the welfare of a person with a disability is very dependent upon their parents accepting a prolonged period of dependence, a relationship that is dramatically different from that which usually pertains between parent and offspring and one that is increasingly subject to scrutiny and challenge as disabled persons' rights to self-determination become accepted. A further example includes the continuous need of a family of a disabled person for information on a range of topics, including the child's developmental potential, the services available in the community and their legal entitlements. In turn, a family's capacity to cope with the problems presented by the disabled child will be influenced by the attitudes and beliefs of the community in which they live and of the broader society.

For a family with a disabled member, consideration must be given to the interactions that occur within and between the following four levels of social systems:

1. the *microsystem* of the family and its various subsystems;
2. the *mesosystem* with which the family members interact on a day-to-day basis (e.g. the extended family, specific health services, the school, the work setting);
3. the *exosystem* in which the mesosystem is embedded (e.g. the health system, the education system, voluntary agencies);
4. the *macrosystem*, made up of the broad values and beliefs that characterize the culture and subculture in which the family lives.

Figure 8.1 presents a diagrammatic summary of the main components of a total system which are of relevance to a family of a person with a disability, illustrated with reference to a nuclear family made up of a mother and father, a child with a disability and their sibling.

The microsystem

When viewed from a systems perspective, the family of a disabled person is seen as comprising a microsystem in which various activities, roles and reciprocal relationships are experienced between the disabled person

Microsystem

1   Mother–Father
2   Mother–Disabled Child
3   Mother–Non-disabled Child
4   Father–Disabled Child
5   Father–Non-disabled Child
6   Disabled Child–Non-disabled Child

Mesosystem

1   Medical and Health Workers
2   Extended Family
3   Friends/Neighbours
4   Work/Recreation Associates
5   Early Intervention Programmes
6   Other Parents
7   Parent Training Programmes
8   Local Community

Exosystem

1   Mass Media
2   Health
3   Voluntary Agencies
4   Social Welfare
5   Education

Macrosystem

1   Ethnic/cultural
2   Socioeconomic
3   Religious
4   Economic
5   Political

Fig. 8.1 The main systems of relevance to a family with a young child with a disability.

and their parents and siblings. In Western cultures, the family microsystem typically comprises three major subsystems (Minuchin, 1974):

1. the *spouse* subsystem (i.e. husband–wife interactions);
2. the *parental* subsystem (i.e. parent–child interactions);
3. the *sibling* subsystem (i.e. child–child interactions).

The number of reciprocal relationships (R) subsumed under these three
subsystems depends, of course, on the number of members in a family
(M), according to the following formula (Broderick & Smith, 1979):

$$R = \frac{M(M-1)}{2}$$

Thus, in a family comprising a mother, a father and two children, there
are six possible reciprocal relationships. Not only does the number of
relationships increase as family size increases but also, as Feiring & Lewis
(1978) have pointed out, indirect or *second-order* influences become possible. This point was taken up by Turnbull, Brotherson & Summers (1983)
when they argued that healthy family life involves a complex balancing

of individual and group interests in which equal importance should be accorded to the well-being of every family member. They illustrated how this balance can be disrupted when a mother works with a disabled child on a feeding programme during the family mealtime. While she is doing so, her availability for interactions with other members of the family are correspondingly reduced. As well, there may be consequential negative effects on future interactions involving the disabled child and others in the family because of resentment generated by the disabled child's taking so much of the mother's attention. To reiterate an earlier point: at the core of the systems approach is the notion of multiple interactions among elements, with the behaviour of any one element being influenced by the behaviours of other elements in the system (Simeonsson & Bailey, 1990).

The implication of this perspective for the planning and evaluation of services for persons with a disability is quite simply that intervention must at least take the dynamics of the family microsystem into account; better still, it should be directed at the total microsystem (Hornby, 1994; Marshak & Seligman, 1993). Research and services have recently shown an increased appreciation of the family ecology of disability, with an encouraging awareness of interactions between disabled persons, their parents and their siblings.

The mesosystem

Just as a person with a disability interacts with other members of their family microsystem, so too does the family interact with its wider social context, its mesosystem. This is made up of the extrafamilial (Minuchin, 1974) systems in which the family members, either collectively or individually, actively participate as they go about their daily lives. For a family with a disabled member, the mesosystem typically includes the extended kinship groups, friends and neighbours, work and recreation associates, other families with a member who is disabled, the local community and the host of statutory and voluntary agencies involved in delivering services to persons with a disability. These influences are bidirectional and can be either positive or negative.

Services for persons with a disability and their families must help them deal with these mesosystem elements. This process of negotiating what Rubin & Quinn-Curran (1983) refer to as a massive maze is by no means easy, particularly when the maze may lack the attributes of wholeness and connectedness. Helping parents to obtain information and support from the various mesosystem elements and to be able to make significant inputs into the mesosystem comprises a very legitimate goal for professionals working with disabled persons. Similarly, the task of acquainting the extended family and friends and associates of the family with the needs of disabled persons is one that should not be overlooked.

The exosystem

The mesosystem is, in turn, embedded in an exosystem. At this level, consideration is given to the various formal and informal organizations present in society which, through their procedures, regulations and value systems, have a bearing on a family with a disabled member. This impact is generally indirect and mediated by individuals or organizations at the mesosystem level. Included in the exosystem, then, are the health, employment, education, social welfare, recreation, voluntary societies and mass media systems.

The elements of the exosystem have a significant, albeit indirect, bearing upon the way a family perceives and interacts with its disabled member and on the ways in which systems at the mesosystem level interact with the family. The mass media, for example, can be quite powerful in creating or transmitting attitudes towards disabled persons.

Since the health system is one of the early elements of the exosystem to impinge on a family, it is important that attention be given to its collective ethos. The medical model, with its focus on disabilities and causation and on the physical care of disabled persons – often in institutional settings – has been antithetical to a developmental model in which the emphasis is on strengths through community care, socialization and education.

The education system is another exosystem element which has a major impact on the way in which a family perceives its disabled member. Like the health system, it is undergoing a series of rapid changes, with the emphasis shifting from a separate but equal model of services for children with disabilities to an inclusive model. Clearly, these philosophies, as they are manifested in the education provisions for students with special educational needs, will affect a family's expectations for and interactions with its disabled member.

On the basis of the systems approach presented in this chapter, it is suggested that it may be just as appropriate for professionals to bring about changes in the exosystem as it is to work with individual families. This may mean, for example, making conscious attempts to educate media representatives and to influence the various statutory and voluntary agencies into adopting more enlightened approaches towards persons with a disability and their families. In short, the best service may sometimes take the form of advocacy on behalf of those with disabilities. At the very least, it should take account of the impact of the exosystem on the families of disabled persons.

The macrosystem

And finally, there is the macrosystem, made up of the broad values, beliefs and ideologies that characterize a society. These influences may be broadly grouped under such headings as ethnic/cultural, socioeconomic, religious, economic and political – all of which have an indirect but significant impact on a family with a disabled person (Cocks, 1985; Johns, 1991). The ideologies of the systems at this level are frequently unexamined, mainly because they are taken for granted or are below the consciousness of the people. Also, because the prevailing ideologies underpin the power base of those exercising control over society, attempts to challenge them are frequently suppressed. In recent years normalization and inclusiveness have become the generally agreed approach used by consumers, clients, service providers, care givers and researchers.

How, then, does the macrosystem affect the family of a person with a disability? Factors such as ethnicity, religion and socioeconomic status – all of which spring from the macrosystem – seem to act as broad predictors of a family's reactions to disability. A society's prevailing political and economic ideologies are other macrosystem variables which have a major impact on persons with disabilities in such areas as the levels of financial assistance available for benefits, the recognition of human rights and employment opportunities. Here again, professionals must not only take prevailing ideologies into account in their work, but they must also accept some responsibility for bringing about changes where such ideologies are antithetical to the welfare of disabled persons and their families. The fact that these ideologies are deeply embedded in society and are the source of great sensitivity when they are raised should not be a deterrent. In the last analysis, a political stand is taken whether one seeks to bring about structural change in society or goes along with the prevailing ideology. There is no middle ground.

ADAPTING TO PERSONS WITH DISABILITIES

Earlier in this section, reference was made to the range of stability possessed by a system and how the family microsystem must evolve coping strategies or face the threat of disintegration. While it is possible to detect broad trends from the literature on families of persons with a disability, it is abundantly clear that particular individuals and particular families have unique reactions to disability (Challela, 1981). Just as some seem to benefit from their association with a person with a disability in the family, some seem to have their development put at risk. Thus, some marriages seem to be strengthened, while others are placed in jeopardy (Brotherson *et al.*, 1986; Featherstone, 1981; Gallagher & Bristol, 1989; Howard, 1978; Lamb, 1983; McConachie, 1982; Meyer, 1986; Price-Bonham & Addison, 1978; Wikler, 1981). Similarly, while some siblings appear to derive benefits from having a brother or sister with a disability, others do not and may even be psychologically harmed by the experience (Hayes, 1994; Parfit, 1975; Seligman, 1983; Simeonsson & McHale, 1981; Skrtic *et al.*, 1983).

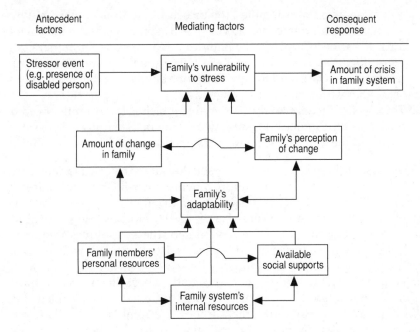

Antecedent factors	Mediating factors	Consequent response

Fig. 8.2 Factors that influence a family's response to disability.

Further, as Hewett (1970) and Mittler & Mittler (1982) caution, we should beware of drawing too sharp a distinction between families of disabled and non-disabled persons; they have more in common with each other than is often recognized.

A useful framework for conceptualizing the factors that influence a family's response to disability, based on the writings of Hill (1949), Burr (1973), McCubbin et al. (1980), and Turnbull, Brotherson & Summers (1983), is presented in Figure 8.2.

From this model, it can be seen that the extent to which the presence of a disabled person in a family creates stresses is dependent upon many interacting conditions. At the broadest level, three factors determine a family's vulnerability to stress.

1. Consideration should be given to the amount of change imposed on a family by the presence of a disabled person. For some families, a person with a disability will require quite dramatic changes in earning power and lifestyle, while for others only minor adjustments might be required.
2. A family's perception of the seriousness of the changes required in its functioning will influence its responses to its disabled member. Socioeconomic status has long been associated with a family's perceptions of disability, Farber (1962), for example, noting that for high

socioeconomic status families, the presence of a disabled person typically represents a tragic disparity between aspirations and reality, while for low socioeconomic status families it requires a less traumatic role reorganization. According to Reiss (1981), people with the same culture or social class tend to agree with one another on the magnitude of stress that various life events engender.

3. There is family adaptability, a variable which is in turn influenced by three sets of resources. The first two reside in the family microsystem itself and the third in the family's interactions with its mesosystem.

The first of these comprise the personal resources of each family, particularly their educational accomplishments, their health and their self-esteem. The second set is made up of the family system's internal resources. As various writers (Hayes, 1994; Hornby, 1994; Turnbull, Brotherson & Summers, 1983) have noted, these resources frequently reflect the membership and style characteristics of families. The size of the family, for example, can influence the way in which it adapts to a disabled member. Thus, there is evidence to the effect that a larger number of children in a family can reduce the negative effects of a disabled child (Trevino, 1979). Clearly, too, the number of parents in a family can be important in determining parental availability for working on programmes. Research suggests that single-parent families are more likely than two-parent families to institutionalize their disabled child (German & Maisto, 1982). There is evidence, too, that mothers are placed under more stress by the presence of a disabled child in the family than are fathers (Wilkin, 1979; Wing, 1975) – although fathers seem to have more difficulty in accepting disability, particularly if it occurs in a son (Hornby, 1994) – but that marital satisfaction helps alleviate this stress (Friedrich, 1979). Religious commitment also influences the family system's internal resources. In Turnbull, Brotherson & Summers' (1983) study, for example, religious commitment was mentioned with unanticipated frequency as being the source of important coping strategies for parents. Family adaptability is also conditioned by a third set of resources, namely the amount and quality of the informal and formal social supports available to it from the mesosystem level of the community (Friedrich & Friedrich, 1981; Howard, 1978; Parke & Lewis, 1981; Suelzle & Keenan, 1981).

DEVELOPMENTAL PERSPECTIVE

Just as human service professionals should think of disabled persons as living in social contexts, so too should they think of disabled persons and their contexts as changing over time. The second assumption of the developmental systems approach, then, is that families typically develop through a life cycle. Although this life cycle approach to family analysis has a long history in family sociology (Alpert, 1981; Nock, 1982), it has only recently been applied systematically to families of disabled persons (Mitchell, 1985; Rubin & Quinn-Curran, 1983; Skrtic et al., 1983; Suelzle & Keenan, 1981; Turnbull, Brotherson & Summers, 1983; Turnbull, Summers & Brotherson, 1986; Wikler, Wasow & Hatfield, 1981).

From the life cycle perspective, families are considered to pass through a series of stages related to the development of the person with a disability, each of which is characterized by a set of *developmental tasks* (Havighurst, 1972). These tasks result from interactions within the microsystem of the family, as well as from interactions between the family and the social systems in which it is embedded. While many of these tasks are common to all families as they assist in the development of their members, others are quite specific to the families of a person with a disability. It is argued that these tasks have to be at least partially mastered if families are to reach a satisfactory equilibrium in adapting to the stresses associated with the presence of a disabled person (O'Hara, Chaiklin & Mosher, 1980; Seligman, 1979; Simeonsson & Simeonsson, 1981; Suelzle & Keenan, 1981). As a corollary, human service agencies should offer assistance that is appropriate not only to the changing developmental needs of disabled persons as they grow older, but also to the changing needs of the family over its life cycle.

Changes in the life cycle are bounded by what Wikler (1981) terms *transition points*. These occur when there is a major discrepancy between expected (or idealized) achievement and actual performance and/or when there are major changes in service delivery systems. An example of the former is when parents are first informed that their child is disabled or at risk – a point at which many parents feel a sense of grief for the death of their hoped-for child. The latter type of transition occurs, for example, when a child commences school or when they finish school and enter into an occupation or some form of sheltered employment. Using these criteria, it is possible to identify four broad stages in the life cycle of a family with a disabled member when the initial diagnosis is made at or near birth:

1. initial diagnosis;
2. infancy and toddlerhood;
3. childhood and early adolescence;
4. late adolescence and adulthood.

For the purposes of this chapter, the fourth stage only will be discussed below.

A DEVELOPMENTAL SYSTEMS PERSPECTIVE

The systems and life cycle perspectives described above come together to make up the developmental systems approach. In planning and evaluating services for persons with disability, each perspective is necessary; one without the other is insufficient for it will lead to inappropriately narrow programmes.

This section will examine the range of developmental tasks that confront the family microsystem of late adolescents or adults with disabilities as they and their families interact with their surrounding mesosystem, exosystem and macrosystem.

Developmental tasks during late adolescence and adulthood

During this stage, the family microsystem typically undergoes major structural changes as the non-disabled siblings leave home and as the person with a disability takes on increasing independence, even to the extent of pursuing a life outside their family origin. And, of course, the parents eventually die. Major changes take place, too, in the type of agencies at the mesosystem level with which the disabled person and their family interact. The school system no longer plays a dominant role and is replaced with work and/or long-term residential settings, typically operated in Western societies by non-government agencies.

Several developmental tasks confront the families of disabled persons during their late adolescence and adulthood; these must be taken into account in the planning and administration of services.

Adapting to the disabled person's needs for dependence/independence

This task involves accepting that while the person with a disability has a right to enjoy maximum independence, some will continue to have dependency needs which might have to be met by their families. The latter needs require an emotional adjustment to the chronicity of the disabling condition (Turnbull, Brotherson & Summers, 1983) and may sometimes involve assuming a full-time care role (Mittler & Mittler, 1982), a role that greatly inhibits parents from moving on to the next stage of personal development that parents of non-disabled children can normally aspire to (Rubin & Quinn-Curran, 1983). The other end of the continuum – accepting that the person with a disability may wish to live outside the family home – can be equally demanding for parents to adjust to. Whatever the balance of dependence or independence that is appropriate to the particular family, Mittler & Mittler (1982) feel that teaching social independence and community living skills constitutes one of the most important and distinctive roles of parents and families during this stage.

There is limited information on how those with an intellectual disability define themselves and their preferences in respect to accommodation, care giving and care receiving and work expectations. While there has been extensive research on care givers during the early stages of children's lives, little emphasis has been placed on the phenomenon of 'letting go' and on how to assist older parents to achieve a life cycle family development typical for their culture and in keeping with their aspirations (Grbich & Sykes, 1990; Griffith & Unger, 1994).

Intergenerational care giving and care receiving has been comprehensively researched internationally and the results indicate the need to recognize the complexity of the transactions that occur. Some areas which are pertinent to the present discussion include the effect of marital history and early family relationships which influence intergenerational support (Kramer, 1993; Mauldon, 1992; Webster & Herzog, 1995; Whitbeck, Hoyt & Huck, 1994); the duration of care giving and the influence of life activities (Hoyert & Seltzer, 1992); reciprocity of relationships (Walker, Pratt & Oppy, 1992); the impact of workplace support on work and family role strain (Warren & Johnson, 1995); and interpersonal conflict, emotional and personal strain (Baine *et al.*, 1993; Sheehan & Nuttall, 1988; Suitor & Pillemer, 1993). Strategies of transactions have been recorded which indicate that empowerment of both the care giver and the person with a disability can be achieved which improves both parties' quality of life (Pratt, Wright & Schmoll, 1987).

Before enumerating the developmental tasks appropriate to maturing young adults, reference must be made to certain demographic factors which have been highlighted in research on intergenerational care giving. Of particular importance is the issue of gender, as more sisters of persons with disabilities are likely to be involved in care giving relationships than are brothers (Lee *et al.*, 1993). This situation reflects the impact of gender role expectations on this support process in most Western countries (Barbee *et al.*, 1993; Sonntag, 1993; Spitze *et al.*, 1994). Socioeconomic and ethnic influences are important determinants in the acceptance of long-term intergenerational care-giving roles (Speare & Avery, 1993). Geographical proximity, marital and parent status and the number of children born to parents also influence the assistance which can be expected in a crisis (Connidis, 1994).

Understanding and accepting the sexuality of a person with a disability and their possible wish for close and enduring relationships outside the family

This task may even include families coming to accept the notion that the person with a disability may wish to marry and have children. This in turn draws attention to the role of the person with a disability as a parent (Feldman *et al.*, 1985; Llewellyn, 1990; Tymchuk, Andron & Rahbar, 1988).

A good deal of work has been done in recent years to help people with disabilities understand their rights and options in the field of human relationships (Johnson, 1984), but rather less has been done to help parents and non-disabled siblings to develop philosophies and strategies to assist the disabled person to obtain fulfilment in this area.

Becoming familiar with and helping the person with a disability to pursue their legal rights

As a result of the very recent emergence of concern among human service professionals and legal experts for the rights of people with disabilities, the broader community is becoming increasingly attuned to the notion that people with disabilities should enjoy the same or broadly similar rights as non-disabled persons (Herr, 1980). This awareness has been heightened by the growth of self-advocacy movements in most Western countries. As noted earlier, many parents who have been accustomed to thinking of their disabled offspring as eternal children with circumscribed rights will experience difficulty in accepting the modern view of disabled persons having rights, especially when such rights are exercised in a way which they perceive to be in conflict with their own interests or those of their disabled family member.

Ensuring satisfactory future provisions for the person with a disability

Of particular concern is what happens to the person with a disability after the incapacitation or death of the parents (Seligman, 1979, 1983). This involves consideration of social as well as economic support for the disabled person, issues that have been covered in some detail in various guardianship proposals that have been advanced (McLaughlin, 1979; New Zealand Institute of Mental Retardation, 1982). Planning for the future affects siblings as well as parents and for the former is all too frequently surrounded with doubts and ambiguities that can be a major source of anxiety (Skrtic et al., 1983). To help them cope with this task, families need clear information from relevant human service agencies, as well as opportunities to discuss the issues with well-informed professionals (Mittler & Mittler, 1982).

Helping the person with a disability gain access to and fulfilment in work and recreational settings

The notion of disabled persons, particularly those who are intellectually disabled, being considered capable of developing work and recreational skills is relatively new even for sheltered settings, let alone for integrated settings within the community at large (Brown, Bayer & MacFarlane, 1989). As well as demanding well-designed and competently staffed rehabilitation services, meeting the vocational and leisure needs of disabled persons requires a major adjustment on the part of the broader community

(Beck-Ford & Brown, 1984; Day & Marlett, 1984). This frequently requires, in turn, a high degree of advocacy on behalf of such persons and their families. Issues to be addressed if people with disabilities are to compete successfully in the job market include other employees' attitudes, social expectations and the availability of suitable work (Bigby, 1992; Dempsey, 1991; Grant, 1989; Gray & Neale, 1991; Jiranek & Kirby, 1990; Tse, 1994).

In the case of the non-disabled siblings, additional developmental tasks occur during this stage, including:

Coming to terms with feelings upon leaving their family of origin

In some cases, siblings can have strong feelings of guilt when they leave their parents with the prime responsibility for caring for the disabled person. In others, there is a sense of relief at being able to pursue their own lives, while in others close relationships are maintained with their sibling who is disabled. Counselling opportunities for siblings should be provided by service agencies to help them come to terms with their feelings towards the person with a disability and their parents. On the whole, however, there is evidence that only a small majority of adult siblings felt that having an intellectually disabled sibling affected commitments in career, marriage and family (Cleveland & Miller, 1977).

Coping with any anxieties regarding capacity to be a parent

Siblings of a person with a disability can identify with them to the extent that they lack confidence to marry and have children of their own (Simeonsson & McHale, 1981). In order to counteract any misplaced fears in this area, as Parfit (1975) has noted, non-disabled adolescents need information on the genetic implications of their sibling's disability for their own potential offspring.

THE NARRATIVE PERSPECTIVE

INTRODUCING THE NARRATIVE METAPHOR

At this point we would like to add to the systems approach a new perspective which has been emerging in the field of family therapy and which offers some fresh challenges to our thinking about the developmental paths of people with disabilities. David Pare (1995) has described this new perspective as a shift away from metaphors borrowed from biology or cybernetics (systems, homoeostasis, feedback, etc.) and towards metaphors borrowed from literary theory (text, story, account, counterplot, etc.). This shift has several important consequences. One is that the view of families as systems can be subsumed by a view of families as 'interpretive communities, or storying cultures' (Pare, 1995, p2). The emphasis in professional consultation can be much more explicitly focused on the interpretive task of making meaning from events within the family rather than on explaining how the world 'really' is. Therefore the professional interest in matters of development might be upon the stories that are operating on developmental processes rather than just on the 'realities' of developmental tasks.

The idea of stories or narratives that guide the direction of life and give meaning to events along the way provides a way of understanding the coherence and consistency that we experience in our lives (Bruner, 1986, 1987). We can think of ourselves as characters in a story participating in its dialogues and acting in ways that produce the twists and turns of its plot. Development can be thought of as the unfolding of a story over time. This perspective allows us the flexibility that comes with the possibility of different stories or narrative traditions. Rather than the assumption that our lives are bound and determined by the realities of our environment, we can start to think about how we are caught up in narratives but also that there are other stories that can be lived. In fact, often conflicting narratives intersect in the problematic events of our lives.

While systems thinking widened the purview of service provision from a narrow focus on the individual, the interest in stories has again widened the focus beyond the functioning of systems. The stories that operate on and through the systems become the subjects of our attention. Stories are not just told *about* developments in family life. Rather, the stories that are to be found in circulation are seen as *constitutive* of the developments in the family (White, 1992). Stories exert influence and often have profound effects. Therefore we might expect that the developmental issues encountered in a family of a child with a disability will be influenced by discourses circulating in the language communities around the family, rather than just by the communication within a family system.

The idea of living according to stories begs the question of the authorship of these stories. The liberal viewpoint that we are the author of our own stories is too difficult to sustain in the face of chance events and in the face of, for example, the understanding of the shaping effects of cultural and gender differences on the social conditions of people's lives. The social constructionist answer is that the stories that shape our lives are given to us in the discourses that surround us in the language communities in which we live (Fairclough, 1992; Gergen, 1985; Harre, 1986). But since we are also participants in these language communities we are also part of the ongoing production of the dialogues in which these discourses are evolving. Through our creative use of language we are always contributing to the authorship of the stories that position us.

This concept of culturally produced narratives which lend coherence to experience can be useful in explaining how systems interact together around and within families. Fulcher (1992) has described the various levels of systems at work in relation to disability as operating in a range of 'arenas'. She suggests that we might profitably investigate the discourses that give shape to interactions in *all* of these arenas and argues that each of the levels of system share some organizing ideas in common which provide a coherence to social systems in general. These organizing ideas or discourses can be given voice as statements of meaning that often lie unspoken just beneath the surface of the language used in relation to disability.

DISABILITY DISCOURSES

Fulcher (1992) goes on to identify some dominant themes which give shape to the lives of people with disabilities and their families. She calls these discourses the medical discourse, the charity discourse and the lay discourse and adds the idea of a newer rights discourse. Each of these discourses coheres around a web of language usages which circumscribe the relations between people within any level of system. And it is within these language usages that 'policy' about service provision for people with disabilities is developed.

Her argument is that the politics of disability is not primarily about centralized decision-making processes, say through influential government committees, but about contests over ways of speaking in daily conversations that take place in every kind of arena. She shows how the policies implemented in special education are produced at all levels of political activity and that the parent–teacher interview, for example, may be subject to the same linguistic influences, or discourses, as the government committee that makes funding decisions. This perspective means that, when we are talking about service provision, we are never just talking about a politically neutral activity. We are talking about arenas in which policy is being made, in which political contests are taking place or in which power relations are being manifested. Moreover, if language is central to the shaping of our consciousness then it is possible to conceive of every conversation as a site in which power relations are being shaped.

Let us now examine the four themes which Fulcher identified as operating in the ways of speaking that give shape to the lives of people with disabilities.

Medical discourse

In this discourse, disability is thought of primarily as an individual physiological deficit that belongs to the person who is physically impaired. The person with a disability is invited within this discourse to think of themselves as a deficient human being. Medical opinion is given weight ahead of the views of the person with the disability or their family members when decisions are being made about their life. Such decisions become formulated as technical problems rather than as social or political issues. The person in the wheelchair is seen as having a mobility problem rather than as living in a society which is often not organized for the full participation of people in wheelchairs in social interaction. Once problem issues are defined in technical terms by diagnostic and assessment procedures under the control of medical personnel, it follows that they are resolvable only through the application of objective expert knowledge. In this way power becomes professionalized and depoliticized. Professionals of a variety of disciplines enter into the medical discourse when they adopt medical metaphors and use words like 'diagnosis' and 'treatment', which leads to 'knowing' what is 'in the best interests' of their clients better than they do themselves.

Charity discourse

This way of speaking is related to and supportive of the medical discourse but it operates in slightly different social circles, such as through corporations which provide welfare assistance to people with disabilities. Notions of 'pity' and 'tragedy' are associated with disability to mobilize a spirit of generosity among people who do not have disabilities. The social conscience of citizens is thus appealed to in order to provide services designed to benefit people with disabilities. In this kind of thinking the person with the disability is positioned as an object of pity with an expectation that they should be grateful for what is being done for them, even if it is simply what most people might expect to be able to provide for themselves or their family members. Claiming anything as their right or not showing the requisite amount of saintly patience easily provokes anger towards people with disabilities within this discourse because it does not fit with the position of being the recipient of charity. Employers who offer openings to people with disabilities may convey a message of expectation that the recipients should gratefully accept what they have been offered, even if the work is demeaning to the intelligence and capabilities of the person. In the social relation between benefactor and welfare recipient there is a built-in power differential. Those with disabilities are never considered the equals of their benefactors in this discourse.

Lay discourse

What Fulcher calls the lay discourse has many echoes of the medical and charity discourses but it also features other responses to disability such as fear, prejudice, misplaced patronage or resentment. It becomes manifest when people demonstrate ways of speaking or social practices that are objectifying or demeaning of people with disabilities. Examples of practices that feature in this discourse include speaking to a person with a disability as if they are unable to comprehend things like other people; speaking to other family members about the person with the disability as if they were not in the room; labelling people with disabilities and viewing them as disabled first and persons second; excusing people with disabilities from requirements to be responsible; telling jokes that make fun of people with disabilities.

Rights discourse

Finally, Fulcher identifies the rights discourse as standing in contradiction to the other three discourses. This is the way of speaking that stands upon traditions of political protest and advocates for the rights of people with disabilities as a minority group. It emphasizes liberal concerns for self-reliance, independence and consumer wants, using strategies of confrontation and demand and challenging the conventional notions of privilege evident in the other three discourses. People with disabilities have often adopted this way of speaking in recent years in preference to the positions offered to them in the other discourses.

Of course, these discourses must circulate in contexts where there are other discourses also at work to produce the ways of speaking that are manifest in our social practices and institutions. The discourse of the market is a powerful economic discourse at present, but there are also discourses that produce relations between genders, sexual orientations, religions, races and classes.

All this leads us to consider how the lives of persons with disabilities are laid down in stories about what it is like to be disabled or to have a member of your family with a disability. From a narrative perspective, such stories are culturally scripted and persons are invited by these stories to take up positions within them, to be the 'long-suffering patient' or 'patient care giver' of the medical discourse, to be the 'grateful beneficiary' of the charity discourse, to accept the positions of 'second-rate citizen' or 'poor, burdened, grieving parent' of the lay discourse (Winslade, 1994). In this way a family 'system' is created. Other social systems can be thought of in the same way, including the pervasive systems of social privilege organized around gender, class or culture. The emphasis is on the organizing principle of discourse rather than on structure – hence the use of the term 'poststructuralism'. From this viewpoint, the influence of the epistemologies that shape our thinking about disability need to be understood as provisional stories rather than as a kind of truth which corresponds simply with ontological reality (Pare, 1995). So the stories or discourses that circulate in professional circles are seen as having real effects in the lives of people with disabilities.

POWER RELATIONS

The narrative metaphor makes relations of privilege and power much more noticeable. Issues of race, gender and class do not fit well with biological metaphors and therefore have often been overlooked from the systemic perspective (Pare, 1995). But the narrative perspective promotes an explicit attention to the politics of the family as well as to the politics of relations between professionals and their clients. It requires professionals to eschew neutrality and to examine the possible marginalizing effects of the ideologies and practices of their work. This is important for the families of children with disabilities for two reasons. It raises questions about how the politics of gender, race, class and age might become implicated in the 'realities' of experience and development within a family system. And it opens the way for a family to consider how ablebodied privilege and the politics of disability might shape the relations within their family and the family's relations with the world around it.

Central to the idea of discourse as developed by Foucault (1980) are the sets of power relations constituted within a discourse. Particular discourses or stories offer people patterns of relation. For example, the medical discourse produces a relation between medical practitioner and patient. It also legitimates authority within such a relation. When people enter such a relation, they take up the positions offered in the discourse. In this way relations of power and authority are created at the local level. This poststructuralist analysis of power does not emphasize the centralized, top-down, structural power that has been dominant in most political analyses and which influences most thinking about systems theory. Instead, power is thought of as capillary and produced from the bottom up through the stories and ways of speaking that circulate through communities.

The poststructuralist analysis of power relations has an important corollary, though. Power is considered always to be unstable, always needing to reproduce itself, always subject to the changes brought about through shifts in discourse or social movements. The disability movement is an example of a social movement which gives people with disabilities opportunity to take a different stance towards the social positions offered to them by the discourses of disability. It is notable for challenges to the linguistic practices that embody discursive assumptions about disability and these challenges afford openings for persons affected by disability to re-situate their identities and relationships and developmental needs within different stories that may be more of their own choosing, less defined by others. Because these kinds of challenges are possible and do take place, even dominant and accepted realities or knowledges, produced within social systems at any level, can be regarded as provisional. Stories can be revised. And the existence of alternative knowledges, often forgotten or overlooked or disregarded, can be assumed and searched out in order to increase the range of options available for people to choose from in the definition of their developmental paths. As new ways of speaking are taken on board, new relations are forged.

This is an important point for the provision of services for the families of people with disabilities because it suggests where we should direct our attention when problems and stresses arise in the family. That is, we might look to amplify and support or seek sustenance for the development of the stories of protest against dominant 'truths' about disability (and their inhibiting effects on normal development). And we might do this in collaboration with the family by seeking to bring to full expression family members' experiences that run contrary to the dominant discourses about disability. We might work with the emerging narratives of competence and rich possibility, rather than with those of discouragement and constraint, always building the sense of coherence of the new story through connecting it to otherwise unnoticed aspects of lived experience.

QUALITY OF LIFE

Bach (1994) has suggested an approach to the problems of defining quality of life that starts from a narrative perspective. In a search for a vantage point for research into matters of quality of life for people with intellectual disabilities, he rejects a liberal perspective based on simple measures of client satisfaction, as well as approaches that stress objective standards of functional 'normality' or an ecological fit between the person and their environment. Rather, he proposes a 'social well-being' approach in which quality lies in the extent of the presence in a person's life of a set of conditions for developing and realizing life plans or life projects. In the process of formulating and realizing life plans or projects, people inevitably draw from available narratives in the scripting of their sense of self and their social relations. How the narratives are put together becomes central to a social well-being approach to quality of life issues. Bach argues that this is an ethical (rather than a technical) matter in which principles of social justice are paramount and that communities have a responsibility to ensure that room is created to allow people with disabilities to participate in the scripting of the narratives from which they will draw in the development of their lives.

Personal agency

From this perspective it would be unthinkable to develop ideas of quality of life for persons with disability and their families without including them in the process of defining the meaning of this concept. Otherwise, there is grave danger of professional colonization taking place. Indeed, it may be useful to include the concepts of 'voice' and 'personal agency' as central ideas in any definition of quality of life. In other words, the struggle for quality of life may be thought of primarily as the struggle to establish agency in one's own life, in the face of powerful discourses which are marginalizing in their effects. Agency can be thought of as having the authority to be an actor rather than to just be acted upon (Davies, 1991). Unless the discourses setting up the relative authority to act are inclusive of people with disabilities and their family members as actors, then a satisfying quality of life is unlikely to be achieved.

Voice

The concept of 'voice' is related. It implies not just the ability to speak but to speak in one's own authority rather than only in words given by someone else's definition (Sampson, 1993). This authority to have a say in the decisions of one's life is granted within the relations set up by a discourse. Stories about disability are often marginalizing or exclusive of the voice of the person with the disability. Such stories have real effects in constituting the relational politics of lives affected by disability, so much so that the possibilities of authoring one's own decisions in life are severely constrained or disqualified. On the other hand, having a voice in the definition of the social conditions of one's own life opens possibilities for a quality of life that offers much greater opportunity for achieving life projects of one's own choosing.

Implications for service provision

Therefore services that were dedicated to enhancing quality of life for persons with disabilities would need to ensure that they were responsive to a person's own voice in the design and delivery of service provisions. They would also need to pay critical attention to the implicit narratives conveyed in information being transmitted by professionals to people with disabilities and their families. The content of any information may be assumed to contain epistemological assumptions which shape people's lives through offering them positions within power relations. These power relations might be those that pertain within the family, between the family and human service agencies and in relation to the wider society. For example, information about the 'realities' of job opportunities for persons with disabilities is not socially neutral information, but is constructed through the discourses about work and disability that exist within a particular community. If vocational counselling services provide this information in language that suggests it is simply factual data or essential truth about life for people with disabilities, then they may be colluding with an oppressive social discourse that is limiting of the life plans possible for these people.

Similarly, support services for families need to be critically examined. For example, the welfare of a person with a disability might be assumed within some ways of speaking to require their parents to accept a prolonged period of dependence, in contrast with some dramatically different assumptions for families not affected by disability. From a narrative perspective these assumptions themselves need to be considered as part of the social construction of disability in a particular historical and social context, rather than as essential truths about the nature of disability and its effects on family life. Once this position is taken seriously, we can contemplate the possibility of different kinds of developmental patterns rather than trying to build services which lock people into accepting the inevitability of what the 'realities' of disability prescribe, no matter how empirically supported they might appear.

The nature of relations between professionals and people with disabilities and their families also needs to be subject to ethical scrutiny. We might acknowledge the regular need of a family with a disabled child for information on a range of topics, including the range of services in the community, their legal entitlements and feedback about their child's developmental progress. Such information can always be given from a professional expert position which positions the parents and children with disabilities as subject to the superior truth of the professional discourse, be it medical or educational or otherwise. Or such quests for information can be developed into dialogues by a service dedicated to the production of a sense of agency amongst the people affected by the disability.

These dialogues can recognize that quality of life depends on having a sense of ownership and authorship of your own developmental direction (in consultation with professional experts when necessary). Professionals working towards this end need to develop a relational stance of genuine and respectful curiosity about the knowledge that those most closely involved with the disability through its presence in their family have to offer. Parents know a lot about the particular developmental trajectories of their children. Children with disabilities know a lot about how they want to progress in their lives and how adults can support them. Service providers need to learn to speak in ways that validate the voicing of this knowledge rather than subsuming it beneath professional knowledge even when they are confronted with a request for professional opinion. Families affected by disability need to be treated ethically as owners of the knowledge about their own experience even when it might be contributing to the accumulated knowledge of professional persons. A narrative family therapist like David Epston often speaks of his professional role as one in which he is seeking to consult (rather than the other way around) the families who come to see him about the expertise they have (but may have forgotten that they knew or may not be trusting in deference to the authority of professional knowledges) for dealing with the developmental challenges they are facing (Epston, 1989). These are ways in which professional providers of services to families affected by disability can make room for the kind of agency that makes for a subjective sense of 'quality of life' which is not just grounded in a subjectivity dominated by the prevailing discourses of disability.

EXTERNALIZING CONVERSATIONS

The narrative approach to working with families also offers a rhetorical method which helps to delineate the relations between persons and discourses. It is known as the practice of developing externalizing conversations (Tomm, 1989; White, 1992; White & Epston, 1989). This way of speaking involves a language shift which avoids any suggestion of attaching personal blame or personal deficits to people when discussing a problem issue. White has captured the spirit of this approach in the aphorism: 'The person is not the problem. The problem is the problem' (White, 1992).

For the developmental issues of people with disabilities, White's approach suggests a way of speaking about disability that avoids any invitation to the person or their family members to make disability a central feature of their identity or relationships. Instead, the disability can be talked about as an external object separate from the persons in the family. It might even be personified at times and spoken about as if it were another family member. In this way people can be addressed as persons in their own right rather than as disabilities first and foremost. Social practices which are objectifying of people or marginalizing attitudes towards people with disabilities can be turned on their heads by this approach. They become the objects instead of the people. Discourses about disability can thus be acknowledged and space opened for people to contradict the positions offered to them in the dominant story. Let us examine some examples of this way of speaking.

Internalizing ways of speaking such as these would be avoided:

- How are you coping with your disability? with having a disabled child?
- Have you been feeling guilty about your parenting because your daughter has been making slow progress?
- Are you feeling jealous of the attention your brother receives because of his disability?
- I want to affirm your right to express your sexuality.

Instead, externalizing ways of speaking in which a linguistic separation is maintained between the person and the problem are preferred:

- How is disability affecting your life at the moment? your family's life at the moment?
- Does disability have a history of inviting you to feel guilty about your parenting? What has it suggested to you as a way of making sense of Debbie's slow progress? Is this fair on you?
- Do you think disability has been making a difference to the way Mum's and Dad's attention is shared out in the family?
- Can you tell me some of the ways in which you have been standing up to the idea that disability and sexual relationships don't go together?

This way of speaking produces its greatest emancipatory force when it is applied to the discourses which are most active in shaping the internalized notions of self and family and disability. For example, the discourses that encourage people with disabilities to see themselves as deficient human beings or less worthy citizens than the able-bodied are ripe for externalizing. For an extensive discussion of this kind of language use, readers are referred to the writings of White & Epston (1989, 1992).

CONCLUSION

In this chapter, we argued that the planning, management and evaluation of services for disabled persons should be based on a developmental systems approach. From the systems perspective, each family should be viewed as comprising a unique microsystem with complex reciprocal relationships existing among the family members. Families, in turn, are embedded in a range of social systems, some of which impinge very directly on a disabled person and their parents and siblings, while some have more indirect influences. Moreover, families and social systems are scripted by stories or discourses which give shape to people's experiences of them. The developmental approach leads us to look at the changing patterns and needs of families over the life cycle of the disabled person. From this perspective, the following specific principles should form the basis of service planning.

1. The uniqueness of each family microsystem and its interactions with its social environment should be recognized.
2. Since siblings play an important role in families, their contributions should be recognized and their needs met.
3. Given that family structures and needs change over the life cycle of the disabled person, these should be regularly re-evaluated.
4. Agencies concerned with the health, education and welfare of disabled persons should be integrated into a whole human service system, centred on the principle of working in partnership with families.

5. Dealing with the broader community's perceptions of disability and acting as an advocate of disabled persons is as much the responsibility of professionals as working with a disabled individual.
6. Successful integration of disabled persons requires that they and the community be helped to adapt to each other. For the former, this means teaching them social skills and for the latter there should be widespread education on the characteristics and needs of disabled persons. For both, there must be opportunities to make contact.

From a narrative perspective, the following principles arise:

7. Consideration is given to the meaning of concepts like independence or care giving for a particular family. Service provision for families affected by disability might explore the effects of the stories about dependence and independence on each of the family members in order to work towards a quality of life for the family based on their preferences rather than on the assumptions of established professional knowledge.
8. Professionals might engage a family in deconstructive conversations about the lay discourses that might be at work in the assumptions about sexuality and disability. In so doing, the way might be opened up for some ways of speaking and acting that contradict the dominant discourses in this area of life.
9. The practice of externalizing conversations might be of advantage. The idea of the 'eternal child' might be externalized and spoken about as an object rather than as an internal representation of anyone's thought. Then the effects of this idea might be traced on the lives of the parents and the person with the disability in a way that positions them together as separate from this discursive idea. Once this separation is achieved, the possibility opens up for the development of a new relation built more around the kind of agency that the person with the disability is seeking through their insistence on their rights.
10. Planning would be most effective if people with disabilities and their families have been supported by professionals to develop a voice and a sense of agency in their lives over a period of time.
11. The addressing of these issues might often entail establishing exceptions to the dominant stories about disability and work which are influenced heavily by medical and charity discourses. Such exceptions might take the form of innovative practices, the establishment of new rights for people with disabilities or personal victories in securing recognition for a person's vocational potential. But they might also be small shifts in people's understandings of themselves, of each other and of disability that break away from the understandings most common in the discourses of disability. As such small shifts begin to cohere together, shifts in discourse take place.

12. The kind of counselling assistance that might be undertaken in a narrative way might aim to widen the language community in which people with disabilities are accorded voice and agency in their lives.
13. A professional with a narrative understanding might engender a discussion with people about these anxieties in an externalizing kind of way that removed the personal guilt about thinking such thoughts. The discourses that might be exerting an influence on the persons might be explored and the possibility of taking personal decisions based on a preferred stand in relation to these discourses canvassed.

Acknowledgement

The authors wish to acknowledge the assistance of Vivien Webb Hendy with parts of this chapter.

REFERENCES

Ackoff, R. and Emery, F.E. (1972) *On Purposeful Systems*, Tavistock Publications, London.

Alpert, J.L. (1981) Theoretical perspectives on the family life cycle. *Counseling Psychologist*, **9**, 25–33.

Bach, M. (1994) Quality of life: a social wellbeing approach, in *Disability is Not Measles: New Research Paradigms in Disability Research*, (eds M. Rioux and M. Bach), Roeher Institute, North York, Ontario.

Baine, D., McDonald, L., Wilgosh, L. and Mellon, S. (1993) Stress experienced by families of older adolescents or young adults with severe disability. *Australia and New Zealand Journal of Developmental Disabilities*, **18**, 177–88.

Barbee, A., Winstead, B., Gulley, R., Yankeelov, P. and Druen, P. (1993) Effects of gender role expectations on the social support process. *Journal of Social Issues*, **49**, 175–90.

Beck-Ford, V. and Brown, R.I. (1984) *Leisure Training and Rehabilitation: A Program Manual*, Charles C. Thomas, Springfield, IL.

Bigby, C. (1992) Access and linkage: two critical issues for older people with an intellectual disability in utilising day activity and leisure services. *Australia and New Zealand Journal of Developmental Disabilities*, **18**, 95–109.

Broderick, D. and Smith, J. (1979) The general systems approach to the family, in *Contemporary Theories about the Family, Vol. II*, (eds W.R. Burr *et al.*), The Free Press, New York.

Bronfenbrenner, U. (1979) *The Ecology of Human Development*, Harvard University Press, Cambridge, MA.

Brotherson, M.J., Turnbull, A.P., Summers, J.A. and Turnbull, H.R. (1986) Fathers of disabled children, in *The Developing Father*, (eds B.E. Robinson and R.L. Barrett), Guilford, New York.

Brown, R.I., Bayer, M.B. and MacFarlane, C. (1989) *Rehabilitation Programmes: Performance and Quality of Life of Adults with Developmental Handicaps*, Lugus, Toronto.

Bruner, J. (1986) *Actual Minds, Possible Worlds*, Harvard University Press, Cambridge, MA.

Bruner, J. (1987) Life as narrative. *Social Research*, **54**, 12–32.

Burr, W.R. (1973) *Theory Construction and the Sociology of the Family*, John Wiley and Sons, New York.

Challela, M.L. (1981) Helping parents cope with a profoundly mentally retarded child, in *Coping with Crisis and Handicap*, (ed. A. Milunsky), Plenum Press, New York.

Cleveland, D.W. and Miller, N. (1977) Attitudes and life commitments of older siblings of mentally retarded adults: an exploratory study. *Mental Retardation*, **15**, 38–41.

Cocks, E. (1985) Roadblocks to appropriate services for persons with intellectual disability in Australia. *Australia and New Zealand Journal of Developmental Disabilities*, **11**, 75–82.

Connidis, I. (1994) Sibling support in older age. *Journal of Gerontology: Social Sciences*, **49**, 309–17.

Davies, B. (1991) The concept of agency: a feminist poststructuralist analysis. *Postmodern Critical Theorising*, **30**, 42–53.

Day, H. and Marlett, N. (1984) Vocational rehabilitation and employment, in *Dialogue on Disability: A Canadian Perspective*, (eds N.J. Marlett, R. Gall and A. Wight-Felske), University of Calgary Press, Calgary.

Dempsey, I. (1991) Parental roles in the post-school adjustment of their son or daughter with a disability. *Australia and New Zealand Journal of Developmental Disabilities*, **17**, 313–20.

Epston, D. (1989) *Collected Papers*, Dulwich Centre Publications, Adelaide.

Fairclough, N. (1992) *Discourse and Social Change*, Polity Press, Cambridge, MA.

Farber, B. (1962) Effects of a severely mentally retarded child on the family, in *Readings on the Exceptional Child*, (eds E.P. Trapp and P. Himmelstein), Appleton-Century-Crofts, New York.

Featherstone, H. (1981) *A Difference in the Family*, Penguin, Harmondsworth.

Feiring, C. and Lewis, M. (1978) The child as a member of the family system. *Behavioural Science*, **23**, 225–33.

Feldman, M., Case, L., Towns, F. and Betel, J. (1985) Parent education project 1: development and nurturance of children of mentally retarded parents. *American Journal of Mental Deficiency*, **90**, 253–8.

Foucault, M. (1980) *Power/Knowledge: Selected Interviews and Other Writings*, Pantheon Books, New York.

Friedrich, W.N. (1979) Predictors of the coping behaviour of mothers of handicapped children. *Journal of Consulting and Clinical Psychology*, **47**, 1140–1.

Friedrich, W.N. and Friedrich, W.L. (1981) Psychological assets of parents of handicapped and nonhandicapped children. *American Journal of Mental Deficiency*, **85**, 551–3.

Fulcher, G. (1992) *Disabling Policies? A Comparative Approach to Education Policy and Disability*, Falmer, London.

Gallagher, J.J. and Bristol, M. (1989) Families of young handicapped children, in *Handbook of Special Education: Research and Practice, Volume 3: Low Incidence Conditions*, (eds M.C. Wang, M.C. Reynolds and H.J. Walberg), Pergamon Press, Oxford.

Gergen, K. (1985) The social constructionist movement in modern psychology. *American Psychologist*, **40**, 266–75.

German, M.L. and Maisto, A.A. (1982) The relationship of a perceived family support system to the institutional placement of mentally retarded children. *Education and Training of the Mentally Retarded*, **17**, 17–23.

Grant, G. (1989) Letting go: decision-making among family carers of people with a mental handicap. *Australia and New Zealand Journal of Developmental Disabilities*, **15**, 189–200.

Gray, A. and Neale, J. (1991) *Survey of Employment and Training Experiences of People with Disabilities*, Department of Labour, Wellington, New Zealand.

Grbich, C. and Sykes, S. (1990) A study of persons with severe intellectual disabilities: gender, the home environment, schooling and outcomes. *Australia and New Zealand Journal of Developmental Disabilities*, **16**, 259–73.

Griffiths, D. (1964) The nature and meaning of theory, in *Behavioral Science and Educational Administration*, (ed. D.E. Griffiths), National Society for the Study of Education, University of Chicago Press, Chicago.

Griffiths, D. and Unger, D. (1994) Views about planning for the future among parents and siblings of adults with mental retardation. *Family Relations*, **43**, 221–7.

Harre, R. (1986) The step to social constructionism, In *Children of Social Worlds*, (eds M. Richards and P. Light), Polity Press, Cambridge, MA.

Havighurst, R.J. (1972) *Developmental Tasks and Education*, 3rd edn, David McKay, New York.

Hayes, A. (1994) Families and disabilities, in *Educating Children with Special Needs*, 2nd edn, (eds A. Ashman and J. Elkins), Prentice-Hall, New York.

Herr, S.S. (1980) Rights of disabled persons: international principles and American experiences. *Columbia Human Rights Law Review*, **12**, 1–55.

Hewett, S. (1970) *The Family and the Handicapped Child*, Allen & Unwin, London.

Hill, R. (1949) *Families Under Stress*, Harper & Row, New York.

Hoffman, L. (1990) Constructing realities: an art of lenses. *Family Process*, **29**, 1–12.

Hornby, G. (1994) *Counselling in Child Disability: Skills for Working with Parents*, Chapman & Hall, London.

Howard, J. (1978) The influence of children's developmental dysfunctions in marital quality and family interaction, in *Child Influences on Marital and Family Interaction*, (eds R.M. Lerner and G.B. Spanier), Academic Press, New York.

Hoyert, D. and Seltzer, M. (1992) Factors related to the wellbeing and life activities of family caregivers. *Family Relations*, **41**, 74–81.

Jiranek, D. and Kirby, N. (1990) The job satisfaction and/or psychological wellbeing of young adults with an intellectual disability and nondisabled young adults in either sheltered employment, competitive employment or unemployment. *Australia and New Zealand Journal of Developmental Disabilities*, **16**, 133–48.

Johns, K. (1991) *Employment and Training Policies for People with Disabilities: A Literature Review*, Department of Labour, Wellington, New Zealand.

Johnson, P.R. (1984) Interpersonal relationships: self esteem, sexual intimacy and life-long learning, in *Integrated Programmes for Handicapped Adolescents and Adults*, (ed. R.I. Brown), Croom Helm, London.

Kramer, B. (1993) Marital history and the prior relationship as predictors of positive and negative outcomes among wife caregivers. *Family Relations*, **42**, 367–75.

Lamb, M.E. (1983) Fathers of exceptional children, in *The Family with a Handicapped Child*, (ed. M. Seligman), Grune & Stratton, New York.

Lee, G., Dwyer, J. and Coward, R. (1993) Gender differences in parental care: demographic factors and same-gender preferences. *Journal of Gerontology: Social Sciences*, **48**, 9–16.

Llewellyn, G. (1990) People with intellectual disability as parents: perspectives from the professional literature. *Australia and New Zealand Journal of Developmental Disabilities*, **16**, 369–80.

Marshak, L.E. and Seligman, M. (1993) *Counselling Persons With Physical Disabilities*, PRO-ED, Austin, TX.

Mauldon, J. (1992) Children's risks of experiencing divorce and remarriage: do disabled children destabilize marriages? *Population Studies*, **46**, 349–62.

McConachie, H. (1982) Fathers of mentally handicapped children, in *Psychological Aspects of Fatherhood*, (eds N. Beail and J. McGuire), Junction, London.

McCubbin, H.I., Joy, C.B., Cauble, A.E. *et al.* (1980) Family stress and coping: a decade review. *Journal of Marriage and the Family*, **42**, 855–71.

McLaughlin, P. (1979) *Guardianship of the Person*, National Institute on Mental Retardation, Downsview, Ontario.

Meyer, D.J. (1986) Fathers of handicapped children, in *Families of Handicapped Children*, (eds R.R. Fewell and P.F. Vadasy), PRO-ED, Austin, TX.

Miller, J.G. (1978) *Living Systems*, McGraw-Hill, New York.

Minuchin, S. (1974) *Families and Family Therapy*, Harvard University Press, Cambridge, MA.

Mitchell, D.R. (1984) *The Family as Partner – The Parents and Siblings*. Paper presented at the Third Pacific Regional Conference of the International League of Societies for the Mentally Handicapped, Wellington, New Zealand.

Mitchell, D.R. (1985) Guidance needs and counselling of parents of mentally retarded persons, in *Mental Retardation: Research and Services in New Zealand*, (eds N.N. Singh and K.M. Wilton), Whitcoulls, Christchurch.

Mitchell, D.R. (1986) A developmental systems approach to planning and evaluating services for persons with handicaps, in *Rehabilitation Education, Volume 2*, (ed. R.I. Brown), Croom Helm, Beckenham, Kent.

Mittler, P. and Mittler, H. (1982) *Partnership with Parents*, National Council for Special Education, Stratford-upon-Avon.

New Zealand Institute of Mental Retardation (1982) *Guardianship for Mentally Retarded Adults: Submissions to the Minister of Justice*, New Zealand Institute of Mental Retardation, Wellington.

Nock, S.L. (1982) The life cycle approach to family analysis, in *Handbook of Developmental Psychology*, (ed. B. Wolman), Prentice-Hall, Englewood Cliffs, NJ.

O'Hara, D.M., Chaiklin, H. and Mosher, B.S. (1980) A family life cycle plan for delivering services to the developmentally handicapped. *Child Welfare*, **59**, 80–90.

Oliver, M. (1990) *The Politics of Disablement*, Macmillan Education, London.

Pare, D. (1995) Of families and other cultures: the shifting paradigm of family therapy. *Family Process*, **34**, 1–19.

Parfit, J. (1975) Siblings of handicapped children. *Special Education: Forward Trends*, **2**, 19–21.

Parke, R.D. and Lewis, N.G. (1981) The family in context: a multilevel interactional analysis of child abuse, in *Parent-Child Interaction: Theory, Research and Prospects*, (ed. R.W. Henderson), Academic Press, New York.

Pratt, C., Wright, S. and Schmoll, V. (1987) Burden, coping and health status: a comparison of family caregivers to community dwelling and institutionalized Alzheimer's patients. *Journal of Gerontological Social Work*, **10**, 99–112.

Pratt, D. (1982) A cybernetic model for curriculum development. *Instructional Science*, **11**, 1–12.

Price-Bonham, S. and Addison, S. (1978) Families and mentally retarded children: emphasis on the father. *Family Coordinator*, **27**, 221–30.

Ramey, C.T., McPhee, D., and Yates, K.D. (1982) Preventing developmental retardation: a general systems model, in *Facilitating Infant and Early Childhood Development*, (eds L. Bond and J. Jaffe), University Press of New England, Hanover, NH.

Reiss, D. (1981) *The Family's Construction of Reality*, Harvard University Press, Cambridge, MA.

Rubin, S. and Quinn-Curran, N. (1983) Lost, then found: parents' journey through the community service maze, in *The Family with a Handicapped Child: Understanding and Treatment*, (ed. M. Seligman), Grune & Stratton, New York.

Sampson, E. (1993) Identity politics. *American Psychologist*, **49**, 412–16.

Seligman, M. (1979) *Strategies for Helping Parents of Exceptional Children*, Free Press, New York.

Seligman, M. (1983) *The Family with a Handicapped Child: Understanding and Treatment*, Grune & Stratton, New York.

Sheehan, N. and Nuttall, P. (1988) Conflict, emotion, and personal strain among family caregivers. *Family Relations*, **37**, 92–8.

Simeonsson, R.J. and Bailey, D.B. (1990) Family dimensions in early intervention, in *Handbook of Early Childhood Intervention*, (eds S.J. Meisels and J.P. Shonkoff), Cambridge University Press, Cambridge.

Simeonsson, R.J. and McHale, S. (1981) Review, research on handicapped children: sibling relationships. *Child Care, Health and Development*, **7**, 153–72.

Simeonsson, R.J. and Simeonsson, N.E. (1981) Parenting handicapped children: psychological aspects, in *Understanding and Working with Parents of Children with Special Needs*, (ed. J.L. Paul), Holt, Rinehart & Winston, New York.

Skrtic, T.M., Summers, J.A., Brotherson, M.J., and Turnbull, A.P. (1983) Severely handicapped children and their brothers and sisters, in *Young Severely Handicapped Children and their Families: Research in Review*, (ed. J. Blacher), Academic Press, New York.

Sonntag, E.J. (1993) *Caregiving and Activism: The Experience of Women with Daughters and Sons with Intellectual Disability*. Master of Social Sciences degree thesis, University of Waikato, Hamilton, New Zealand.

Speare, A. and Avery, R. (1993) Who helps whom in older parent-child families. *Journal of Gerontology: Social Sciences*, **48**, 64–73.

Spitze, G., Logan, J., Joseph, G. and Lee, E. (1994) Middle generation roles and the well-being of men and women. *Journal of Gerontology: Social Sciences*, **49**, 107–16.

Suelzle, M. and Keenan, V. (1981) Changes in family support networks over the life cycle of mentally retarded persons. *American Journal of Mental Deficiency*, **86**, 267–74.

Suitor, J. and Pillemer, K. (1993) Support and interpersonal stress in the social networks of married daughters caring for parents with dementia. *Journal of Gerontology: Social Sciences*, **48**, 1–8.

Tomm, K. (1989) Externalizing the problem and internalizing personal agency. *Journal of Strategic and Systemic Therapies*, **8**, 54–9.

Trevino, F. (1979) Siblings of handicapped children: identifying those at risk. *Journal of Contemporary Social Work*, **60**, 488–92.

Tse, J. (1994) Employers' expectations and evaluation of the job performance of employees with intellectual disability. *Australia and New Zealand Journal of Developmental Disabilities*, **19**, 139–47.

Turnbull, A.P., Brotherson, M.J. and Summers, J.A. (1983) The impact of deinstitu-tionalization on families: a family systems approach, in *Living and Learning in the Least Restrictive Environment*, (ed. R.H. Bruininks), Brookes, Baltimore.

Turnbull, A.P., Summers, J.A. and Brotherson, M.J. (1986) Family life cycle: theoretical and empirical implications and future directions for families with mentally retarded members, in *Families of Handicapped Persons: Research, Programs, and Policy Issues*, (eds J.J. Gallagher and P.M. Vietze), Brookes, Baltimore.

Tymchuk, A., Andron, L. and Rahbar, B. (1988) Effective decision-making/problem-solving training with mothers who have mental retardation. *American Journal of Mental Retardation*, **92**, 510–16.

Walker, A., Pratt, C. and Oppy, N. (1992) Perceived reciprocity in family care-giving. *Family Relations*, **41**, 82–5.

Warren, J. and Johnson, P. (1995) The impact of workplace support on work-family role strain. *Family Relations*, **44**, 163–9.

Webster, P. and Herzog, R. (1995) Effects of parental divorce and memories of family problems on relationships between adult children and their parents. *Journal of Gerontology: Social Sciences*, **50**, 24–34.

Whitbeck, L., Hoyt, D. and Huck, S. (1994) Early family relationships, inter-generational solidarity, and support provided to parents by their adult chil-dren. *Journal of Gerontology: Social Sciences*, **49**, 85–94.

White, M. (1992) *Recent Developments in Narrative Therapy*. Paper presented at the 50th Anniversary Conference of AAMFT, Miami Beach, Florida, October 1992, recorded on video by D. Sollee, *Learning Edge Series*, AAMFT, Washington, DC.

White, M. and Epston, D. (1989) *Literate Means to Therapeutic Ends*, Dulwich Centre Publications, Adelaide.

White, M. and Epston, D. (1992) *Experience, Contradiction, Narrative and Imagination*, Dulwich Centre Publications, Adelaide.

Wikler, L. (1981) Chronic stresses of families of mentally retarded children. *Family Relations*, **30**, 281–8.

Wikler, L., Wasow, M. and Hatfield, E. (1981) Chronic sorrow revisited: parent vs professional depiction of the adjustment of parents of mentally retarded chil-dren. *American Journal of Orthopsychiatry*, **51**, 63–70.

Wilkin, D. (1979) *Caring for the Mentally Handicapped Child*, Croom Helm, London.

Wing, L. (1975) Problems experienced by parents of children with severe mental retardation, in *Right from the Start*, (eds B. Spain and G. Wigley), National Society for Mentally Handicapped Children, London.

Winslade, J. (1994) The social construction of disability: some implications for counselling. *New Zealand Journal of Counselling*, **16**, 44–54.

Wolfensberger, W. (1983) Social role valorization: a proposed new term for the principle of normalization. *Mental Retardation*, **21**, 234–9.

Quality of life – issues for children with handicaps

9

Vianne Timmons and Roy I Brown

INTRODUCTION

The study of quality of life for people with disabilities is a fairly recent phenomenon. The term emerged in the late 1950s and early 1960s in relation to global concerns such as environmental pollution and the deterioration of urban living (Szalai, 1980). The phrase 'quality of life' also came to have relevance in connection with dying patients whose lives were being sustained with respirators, intravenous feeding and other medical interventions (Wortis, 1984). Researchers such as Goode (1988), Parmenter (1988) and Brown (1988) have examined quality of life in relation to people with disabilities. Their investigations have moved the focus of quality of life to a more person-centred concept incorporating life experiences, knowledge and opinions of people with the disabilities and their families.

In 1988, Goode organized a work group of consumers aged 13–21, along with professionals and advocates, to discuss issues around quality of life. Goode concluded from these discussions that it is important to discover the extent to which children are involved in the decision-making process. If empowerment and decision making are goals for adults with disabilities then it is vital that attention be paid to this issue in programmes for children with disabilities, for it seems likely that many of the issues pertaining to quality of life are developmental and cover the lifespan. Furthermore, the development of self-concept, control and problem-solving abilities in relation to choice are important skills which need to be encouraged amongst young children. But there are some major questions which arise, not least why so few studies on quality of life have been carried out with children.

AGE AND QUALITY OF LIFE

Apart from the development of models of quality of life relating to children, there are a number of key questions which should be raised. How early should we start looking at issues of quality of life – infancy, school-aged children or later? Different age groups may require very distinct approaches and research methods. Investigating the quality of life of a five-year-old is likely to be very different from looking at the quality of life of a teenager and quality of life issues for an older adult may have different accents and priorities.

Overall there is very little research available on quality of life and children of any age. In the last five years some researchers have focused on teenagers (Halpern, 1993; Timmons, 1993). Information on younger children has to be extracted from research which focuses on specific areas of children's lives, such as education and leisure, but has not been carried out specifically in the area of quality of life. An overview of the literature on research of children with special needs has demonstrated that various components of children's lives have received scrutiny and although they relate to quality of life, a holistic approach incorporating children's perspectives has not for the most part guided thinking in the field. This may seem extraordinary when books and articles are written on the quality of education. It seems alarming to us that the development of quality in education, parenting or society can be pursued without consulting with those whom it most affects. Yet, this frequently happens in health and health-related areas where the professionals believe they know best or perceive person involvement as non-scientific (see Romney, Brown & Fry, 1994). Indeed, we are arguing that one of the virtues of conceptualization around quality of life is its ability to enable us to view behaviour and conditions from other people's perspectives.

However, due to the paucity of research in the area of children and quality of life, it is difficult to establish a baseline, let alone a comparison on quality of life. For each age group, relevant and, often, different issues need to be identified and measurement procedures selected. For example, Moss (1994) identified quality of life issues and factors which related specifically to older people with intellectual disability. Goode (1988) identified a taxonomy of quality of life issues for children which included home, education, leisure and personal areas. He felt that these components fitted together to provide a holistic view of quality of life of children with mental handicaps. This chapter explores the quality of life of children in relation to the literature and to practice. To some extent it leans on research from older age groups but an attempt is made to identify with children's issues. In the next decade quality of life research involving children will be critical, for it will not only identify key issues, but possibly challenge some of the different views of children and their families. Already research into family perceptions of quality of life is underway (MacKenzie, 1997; Rasmussen, 1993). Such studies not only identify some of the stresses facing families with children who have disabilities, but also underline positive features which arise from individual adaptation or outlook.

MEASUREMENT

Measurement of quality of life is a focus of discussion for researchers. Schalock (1990) stated that we are just beginning to understand the concept of quality of life and we must continue in our efforts to measure it. There are three types of orientation around quality of life measurement which stand out in the literature: objective measures, subjective measures and the person–environment interaction. All types of measurement provide valuable information that should be viewed together. 'Objective data about such phenomena as unemployment, hospitalization and crime rates would be lifeless unless some implications about their human meaning could be drawn' (Rodgers & Converse, 1975). In the area of disabilities, the role of subjective indicators is vital because it reflects personal concerns as perceived by the individual.

The measurement of quality of life in children has some unique challenges. First, quality of life is about value and, if we argue for the observation and measurement of children and their perceptions, they (the children) must be seen as valued. As indicated elsewhere, the issue is not whether such values correlate with extrinsic measures or parents' or teachers' perceptions, but whether each child's perceptions or children's perceptions collectively have value in the overall research. How such information should be weighted needs further debate. Further, when we look at children we do not have an accurate yardstick on quality of life of children without special needs to give us comparison data. There are no norms with which to compare. Despite the concerns about normative measurement, the lack of such data is seen as a major omission, as noted in Cummins' chapter in this volume and in Evans (1994).

There has been some research which has looked at the area of measurement of quality of life of children. Brown (1992) obtained information on quality of life of adolescents with disabilities through interviews, observations, diaries and checklists. Timmons (1993) utilized extensive interviews based on a questionnaire which modelled that developed by Brown & Bayer (1992) for adolescents and adults. Timmons, when investigating quality of life, found acceptable reliability between the parental information and the teenager information. In addition, there was satisfactory reliability on repeat questions during the interviews. Brown, Bayer & MacFarlane (1988) also found consistency between the responses of adolescents and adults with disabilities and their sponsors in their quality of life study. Such agreement, though not a requirement for accuracy, lends support to the argument that teenagers' views bear some positive relationship to events as perceived by others. However, perceptions which are incorrect in other people's terms have an important message and are therefore relevant to measure. Brown, Bayer & Brown (1994) noted how the views of parents and their adolescent/adult children became closer as rehabilitation took place. In other words, the objective correctness of views may be less important than harmonious interactions between persons. But some, particularly young children and language-disabled children, may be unable to provide oral information. In these circumstances, other forms of observation are essential. It has been argued (Brown, Bayer & Brown, 1992) that the inclusion of the perceptions of professionals and relations is also relevant, but that the individual's perceptions must be the central measurement considered in looking at quality of life, because the decisions are about them and it is their behaviour which is the focus of observation and intervention.

CHOICE AND DECISION MAKING

Mittler (1984) stated that an essential component of quality of life is the opportunity for individuals to make choices between perceived alternatives. He felt that the failure to canvass opinions of people with special needs condones the exclusion of people with disabilities from taking an active role in decisions which affect their lives. Schloss, Alper & Jayne (1994) found that the majority of special education graduates remained underemployed or unemployed for reasons associated with lack of decision-making skills. In their review of the literature they found that normalization and quality of life are closely associated with choice and decision making.

If one of society's goals is to empower people with disabilities and foster choice, then we need to begin with children. The lack of opportunity for choice of teenagers with special needs can be illustrated by the following example. Timmons (1993) asked 47 teenagers with special needs questions regarding their quality of life. These questions were framed around decision making. The answers were compared to responses from teenagers of approximately the same age and sex who lived in the same geographical areas but were not disabled. They were asked questions such as, 'Who decides your bedtime?'. Only 21% of the teenagers with special needs decided themselves, compared to 72% of teenagers without special needs. At an in-service training session given to residential staff from three communities, Timmons posed the same question. Not one adult with special needs decided their own bedtime. When this was explored further, the workers were not able to identify one area where the people they lived with exercised choice. Yet, there have been studies which documented that people with profound and multiple disabilities can learn to make choices (Dattilo & Rusch, 1985). The response made by the residential staff illustrates the lack of emphasis on empowerment which actually exists in the lives of people with disabilities. Persons with severe disabilities can often make choices. For example, Timmons (1993) interviewed a client with an IQ of 30 who was able to express clear needs and desires and had an ability to make choices and participate in decision making regarding her life.

Choice and decision making are viewed as vital aspects of quality of life. They enhance human dignity and can provide people with more effective environments for learning and adapting. Schloss, Alper & Jayne (1994), for example, state that the application of quality of life models can encourage skills required and valued by employers. Halpern's (1993) study on transition from school to work supports the need for quality of life models through the late adolescent stage of development. Children must be encouraged to develop choice and decision-making skills. Consistent with the holistic views of quality of life, these opportunities must exist throughout every aspect of children's lives and should be incorporated into their education, community, home living, social and leisure activities.

On occasions, developing these skills may result in exposing a child to risk; a reason given by some teachers and parents for denying choice. Many choices have risk associated with them: for example, cycling to school or exploring a neighbourhood. If a child is protected from such experiences, how do they learn? Many risks may be minimal. We generally allow non-disabled children to decide what to wear – it is a way to begin the development of personal tastes and interests. Brown, Bayer & Brown (1994) stated that 'Choice is the right of the client and, unless it is likely to cause physical harm to the individual or to others, should automatically be accepted' (p47). We are not suggesting exposure to grave dangers and, of course, children should be protected from harm. But as Brown & Hughson (1993) point out, total protection (and removal of choice) can lead to psychological deprivation and, in its broadest sense, abuse. Persons who cannot learn how to choose are constantly in danger from their environment.

The issue of abuse is, however, a major and growing area. We recognize that children, particularly young children, are vulnerable to physical and sexual abuse and that this is much more common amongst children who are disabled (Sobsey & Doe, 1991). We therefore need to develop structures and experiences which, while ensuring experience is rich, normal and provides choices, recognize the potential for abuse and the need for protection. It is obvious from the above examples that children often suffer from unintentional deprivation and abuse, as well as being subject to the rigours of pathological abuse. It is in this context that the rights of the child come to the fore, for children with disabilities have only recently started to gain rights. Indeed, one of the probable reasons for the lack of quality of life studies amongst children with disabilities is the paucity of personal pressure groups and consequent lack of awareness by professionals, parents and the public of the role played by environmental stimulation in the context of choice. The work of Barnes (1991) clearly highlights some of these challenges.

EDUCATION

At what level can children make choices? Can children make effective choices about the schools they attend or the activities in which they wish to be involved? Do integrated settings improve a child's quality of life? School has been highlighted as a major life setting for children in the area of quality of life (Goode, 1988). The principle of inclusion has been heralded as a way to improve quality of life of children with various disabilities. For example, Borthwick-Duffy (1990) noted that integrated educational placements can decrease transportation time, provide closer proximity to special school activities, expose children to non-handicapped peers along with more normal standards of behaviour and increase the variety of experiences and stimulation. These are the obvious benefits. However, not all professional models portray such inclusion. Gartner & Lipsky (1987) stated that 'the medical model that undergirds special education inextricably leads to the belief that persons with a handicap … are not capable of making choices or decisions' (p394).

Timmons (1993) asked teenagers with special needs about their preferences. She compared their responses with teenagers in regular education and then analysed the patterns which emerged. Teenagers who attended regular classes had more choices available to them at school. They not only selected schools which offered programmes suited to their learning needs, they also had a wide choice of courses within their schools. Students in special education settings not only had fewer options regarding where to attend school, they had limited choice in course or class selection. Only half of the students in special education stated they were attending the school of their choice, compared with approximately 80% of teenagers in regular education. The students in special education, who expressed dissatisfaction, stated that their preferred school was their neighbourhood high school. Teachers may claim that such views came from their parents. In some cases this may be correct, but all views are engendered, at least in part, by our environmental experiences. The point is whether we believe the views we state. If we do, they are likely to influence our behaviour profoundly. As Andrews (1974) stated, people take actions based on their views, not on objective data.

If we explore further these students' activities and preferences in their school lives we see other patterns emerging. When teenagers with special needs were asked how they travelled to and from school, 94% took the school bus, compared to 55% of the students in regular education. When asked what they did on their way to school, 60% of the students in special education said they did nothing, compared to 17% of the students in regular education. Sixty-two percent of the regular education students indicated they talked to their friends, compared with 23% of the students in special education.

Teenagers spend a considerable amount of time socializing. This helps formulate their identities and develop their interests and enhances their communication skills. When teenagers are bused to schools outside their neighbourhoods, this has an obvious and subtle impact on developing behaviour. Borthwick-Duffy (1990) noted that inclusion may decrease transportation time for students with special needs. This decrease in time can actually affect the child in a variety of ways. Brown, as early as 1968, identified the effects of busing through the deterioration of motor behaviour, fatigue, increased aggressiveness and in a few instances, epileptic seizures.

Students with special needs in this study had significantly lower verbal abilities compared with visual-spatial abilities. They would probably benefit from greater opportunities for language stimulation such as conversations with peers who have no disabilities. There are many additional reasons; exclusion in separate classes and mixing primarily with other disabled persons are likely to lead to less stimulation. Separation from neighbourhood schools lessens personal contact with the local community.

However, the non-inclusion practice cannot simply be laid at education's door. The family and local community members also have their part to play. Here quality of life underlines the importance of the environment in increasing handicap, while administration and management react to what they believe is the disability. Why the discrepancy? The children may have been placed in special facilities because of poor verbal skills but as noted above, this can compound the disability. In the Brown & Timmons (1994) study, many of the children wished to select, more appropriately, the environment which gave the greater verbal stimulation.

Indeed, quality of life evaluation underscores the fact that all aspects of life are interactive and the education of the future must ensure social, community and family aspects of learning are fully taken into account. This, we argue, cannot be carried out by professionals alone devising and applying curricula, but by equal and valued opportunities for design and application by all parties. Schooling, in this model, cannot be seen as separate from home, parents, friends or community. This is why issues of inclusion are not simply school issues, they are about received and per-ceived quality of life. They not only require teachers to consider and accept inclusion, but require parents to modify family behaviours at home. Inclusion within a quality of life model requires joint, consultative and agreed intervention in all events. Many teachers are still wary of inclusion, but many parents have not recognized that, to work, inclusion means inclusion practices at home (e.g. asking a child what they want to do, who they want to have time with, the games and home activities in which they would like to be included). These may all seem obvious, but parents within the study quoted above were often surprised when a qual-ity of life questionnaire brought out such concerns. However, once enlightened, most parents took immediate action.

What do teenagers talk about on the way to school? They review what they did the night before, they discuss the upcoming school day, they make plans for their social time and they talk about themselves and others. These conversations have impact beyond language development; they affect leisure activities, social relationships, choice and decision making and the formulation of interests and ideas. In other words, language inter-action is a means of developing an individual's social structure.

The opportunity for language interaction can affect a number of areas in a teenager's life which then impacts on the individual's quality of life. Indeed, the examples we have given all relate to the richness of quality of life and to the breadth of choices for the individual. One can argue that it is the diversity of environmental stimuli which enables the individual to develop an internal social structure, which then can result in a repertoire from which appropriate and varied choices can be made. For example, Stainback *et al.* (1994) stated that 'to develop a positive self-identity, young people need opportunities to exercise and express choices about friendships and group affiliations'. These opportunities can be realized in a variety of ways but one characteristic is critical: we must be cautious that the decisions which are made about a person's life do not limit opportunities to make such choices. Decisions such as where a child attends school have to be viewed in a broader context than just where a programme is offered. It is also important to take into account the choices parents make about inclusive practices within the home and local com-munity. Do they take account of their child's comments and behaviours? Do they consult with the child? Data from our own studies suggest that parents often make decisions based on assumptions rather than checking with the child. Indeed, it is frequently the lack of consultation and choice over minor items which leads to a sense of disempowerment over the larger issues.

More than half of the students interviewed in special education said that they would like to be involved in school clubs. When asked about involve-ment in school clubs, only 11% of the teenagers in special education said they belonged to such clubs compared to 55% of the students in regular education. There are many possible explanations for this, although one obvious reason is that club events are scheduled after school and these children often have to catch a bus to their distant home. There are a number of obvious benefits to belonging to such clubs – enhanced opportunities for communication, friendships, development of leisure interests and skills and the gaining of leadership and decision-making abilities. McGill (1987) noted that many friendships are either started or strengthened during leisure time and that leisure plays a vital role in expanding personal networks. Again, these opportunities are likely to affect personal planning skills and self-image.

Social interaction is an ongoing concern of parents of children with special needs (see Guralnick, Connor & Hammond, 1995). These authors also found that mothers of children in integrated settings reported that their children played more effectively and were 'more social'. This seems to be one of the effects of inclusion and is also found in the behaviour of preschool children within inclusive settings (Butler Dunn, 1991).

Schools should provide more than academic preparation. To fulfil a more comprehensive role, schooling has to viewed in a holistic manner by educators and parents, which is also consistent with quality of life models described elsewhere in this book. Even non-structured time should be examined in terms of its relevance to quality of experience. Timmons (1993) found that 23% of the students with special needs interviewed spent their lunch hours alone. They operated as an isolated entity in their schools. Their story is one of loneliness in a school filled with teenagers. Stantrock (1993) stated that involvement in group activities satisfies adolescents' personal needs, rewards them, provides information, raises self-esteem and gives them identity. These are powerful outcomes which are not being realized by some teenagers with special needs. In other words, inclusion is not simply 'being there'; it relates to the quality of experience. But even when activities become included, other issues remain. A child who is now included in about 80% of the school day goes to sports practice at weekends in a joint school/parent-run activity. He is seven years old and is never selected for team events. Although the event is said to be fun rather than competitive, the youngster's poor attention is cited as a reason for exclusion. Inclusiveness means the involvement of other parents in supporting the inclusion of children with disabilities, to ensure social handicap is not added to disability. The quality of life model requires a societal change relating to individual teacher and parental (all parents, not just the parents of the child with a disability) perception and responsibility.

Another area to consider when viewing education beyond the classroom is the preparation of students for employment. Twenty-six percent of the teenagers in the special education study expressed a desire to go on to college or universities. This is currently not a possibility in many areas, although some colleges do provide programmes for adults with intellectual disabilities and colleges and universities are gradually becoming more accessible to persons with other disabilities. The education of students with special needs must move beyond the K-12 classroom and look at lifelong learning. A successful attempt at this in Alberta, Canada, has been described by Westwood (personal communication, 1996).

Halpern (1993), noting that transition from adolescence into adulthood can be difficult for any young person, stressed the importance of dealing with transition issues while a teenager is still in high school. If students wish to receive tertiary education, then they need to explore this education. Halpern's questionnaire on quality of life issues is a tool that may be used in this context.

The recurring theme is that education cannot be viewed as simply classroom instruction. If quality of life issues are addressed by educators, the approach has to go beyond classroom walls and involve both community and family. Again, the need for close collaboration between the various interested parties is stressed.

LEISURE

Leisure, hobbies and recreation have been identified as other major life settings critical for children's quality of life (Stark & Goldsbury, 1990). Leisure activities have the potential to give richness and break the monotony of the lives of children with disabilities but we see them as much more integral to well-being and development. According to McGill (1987), leisure involves skills which are developed throughout childhood. Indeed, it is often during leisure time that children learn to choose, share and collaborate.

Timmons (1993) found that teenagers with special needs appeared to be involved in fewer leisure activities than their peers in the regular classroom. The activities in which they did participate were apparently less frequently taken up than their peers in regular classrooms. Firth & Rapley (1990) also observed that people with disabilities largely participate in solitary and passive activities. They concluded that it was lack of opportunity rather than capability that restricted the involvement of people with disabilities, yet lack of opportunity necessarily leads to decreased capability. The first requirement is appropriate environments for experiencing stimulation with and opportunities for learning.

Personal choice is a vital component in obtaining a repertoire of leisure activities. People with disabilities have preferences, but their choices are typically limited by minimal exposure to recreational activities (Schloss, Smith & Kiehl, 1986). When Brown, Bayer & MacFarlane (1988) studied leisure in relation to the quality of life of adults, they found that the activities engaged in were primarily observational and solitary. If we want adults to enjoy full lives with a variety of leisure activities then we need to foster participatory leisure and recreation in children of all ages. Exclusion restricts such development.

Schalock (1990), in discussing quality of life, indicated that people with disabilities should have the same opportunities as people without disabilities. But Timmons (1993) found that some teenagers with special needs did not experience even basic and routine activities. For example, she found there were teenagers with special needs who had never attended a movie, yet physically they were able to do so. Such activities as seeing a movie involve many skills – partnering, money exchange, purchasing food, accessing transportation, etc. When leisure activities are limited, so are opportunities to develop these skills. Of course, there are secondary gains, other than learning from the event itself. However, it is often these secondary gains which are overlooked when parents or teachers decide against an event on the grounds that it is not suitable for the child with a disability. Activities should not simply be considered for their obvious characteristics, but also for their side effects on learning and experience. If an activity is denied, other natural experiences must be made available so that compensation can occur.

Brown (1990) stressed that activities which promote planning and thinking are important for people with disabilities. Children should not only be exposed to a variety of leisure activities but also participate in the planning of these activities. When Timmons asked teenagers how they chose their leisure activities, a number said their parents decided for them. None of their non-handicapped peers stated that their parents made these decisions. As Brown mentioned, it is vital that opportunities are created where children can take an active role in decision making. Leisure planning can provide this framework. McConkey (1985), for example, illustrated how play can aid learning through choice, empowerment and the fostering of autonomous decision making.

As Janicki (1990) stated, physical well-being is fundamental to a person's quality of life. Brown, Bayer & MacFarlane (1988) found that, on average, adolescents and adults with disabilities had very little physical exercise and poor leisure skill development. Stark & Goldsbury (1990) noted that over the last decade the number of teenagers with medical problems has been on the increase. But the skills and habits involving exercise and physical well-being need to be established in childhood. We are suggesting that physical and mental well-being are important to and part of effective quality of life. Such developments need to be established in childhood, but the bulk of the quality of life literature is concerned with adults, when some of the determinants of quality of life have already been cast. The messages arising from quality of life studies are that life experience needs to be seen holistically and across the lifespan. Therefore the focus of research and practice needs to be changed to accent childhood and disabilities.

FRIENDSHIPS

McGill (1987) found that leisure activities build and strengthen friendships and expand personal networks. Friendships and relationships overlap with leisure activities. Quality of life is not simply holistic; it requires integration. Activities link together, promoting gain. When environments become artificial or isolating, they promote a breakdown in this integrated activity network.

Parents of children with special needs see friendships as critical to the happiness and well-being of their children (Stainback & Stainback, 1987). Goode (1990) also pointed out that quality of life is highly responsive to the social relationships of the individual with disabilities. But social relationships may not always be positive. For example, Lawrence *et al.* (1992) quote parents who recognize that inclusive education can result in teasing and bullying of a child with a disability. Yet this is understood by some parents as an unpleasant but necessary experience in learning how to deal with life. In other words, developing improved quality of life may involve some stress – 'no pain, no gain!'. It is essential that quality of life is not seen as a static concept but one where improved quality of life results from healthy interactions and experience. It is also not simply a measure of happiness. The more aware and knowledgeable people become, the more dissatisfaction they may experience with their environment. This is one of the factors which appears to promote further change. Teachers and parents need to be sensitive mediators of change, allowing experience but protecting their children from long-term harm.

Stantrock (1993) stated that adolescent friendship served six functions: companionship, stimulation, physical support, ego support, social comparison and intimacy, and affection. Discussions concerning quality of life of children need to pay attention to the multifaceted function of friendships and their importance. In this context the review by Denholm (1992) is important; as he pointed out, children with disabilities wish to realize the same goals as children without disabilities. The top ten sources of greatest enjoyment for adolescents in order of stated interest are, according to Bibby & Posterski (Denholm, 1992): friendship, music, mother, girl/boyfriend, stereo, father, dating, television, sports and reading. This may be obvious, but actual activities carried out amongst adolescents with developmental disabilities are different, with television clearly the most extensive time absorber.

There are many obstacles to developing and increasing the child and community relationships of children with special needs. The challenges may be geographical, opportunity, access and attitudinal. Seward (1987), in a description of the integration experiences of a 15-year-old girl, stated that 'Everybody entering adolescence needs friends who are dealing with the same fears and apprehensions'. Timmons (1993) asked teenagers with special needs whether there were people who would turn to them if they needed help. The responses were very limited compared to teenagers without disabilities. But the issue is somewhat wider than this, because friendship includes the notion of reciprocity or mutuality. Historically children and adults with disabilities have been seen as receivers (G. Allan Roeher Institute, 1990). When children can provide support for others their value and self-esteem is increased. Sharing and giving can also provide an inner sense of achievement and positive self-image and teenagers utilize their social network for these and many other reasons.

Timmons found that even when teenagers with disabilities had friends, the quality of the relationship seemed to be different. Teenagers with special needs went out with their friends less often, were involved in fewer activities and often did not have a best friend with whom they did everything. Children with special needs require opportunities to form relationships and then opportunities to strengthen and add depth to relationships. If children are bused out of neighbourhoods for schooling and participate less in leisure activities in the community, then these opportunities will be fewer. Such children will find it more difficult to form relationships.

Firth & Rapley (1990) have provided a practical list of issues and discussion topics for workshops on friendship. This is an example where choice may have to be supported by structured learning. However, the solution to the 'friendship challenge' has not been resolved. Brown, Bayer and Brown (1992) note that the resolution often comes about through opportunities in the community when self-image has developed to a level that allows the individual to share directed and spontaneous behaviour. Information and skilled behaviour are part of the repertoire and activities such as drama can enable the processes to be developed through modelling (see Chapter 13).

Relationships with members of the opposite sex have been recognized as lacking in the lives of many adults with disabilities (Firth & Rapley, 1990). Experience and relationships with the opposite sex often begin during the teenage years as dating becomes one of the ways to experiment with relationships. If people do not have the experience of dating during their teenage years it may very well impact on their lifetime relationships. Goode (1990) found that love, acceptance and sexuality were factors considered important in the lives of adults with mental handicaps. Teenagers should be encouraged to participate in activities which will provide opportunities to meet members of the opposite sex. Through the experience of dating they may develop ideas about what they value in members of the opposite sex and become more discriminating about their choice of partners. This is an area that should be explored in more depth and also given more attention by practitioners and researchers. Again, the lifespan nature of friendship is critical in the development of intimacy and the gaining of normalcy. The issue of partnership and marriage amongst persons with disabilities is now receiving attention. The opportunity for developing relationships starts not with the person with disability but with their parents.

Brown (1995) cites the story of a mother who had a baby with Down syndrome accompanying the author on an interview with a married couple. The wife had Down syndrome. After the interview, the mother said, 'Through that interview, I have recognized that my son has a future'. The need for families to appreciate the potential longevity and normalcy of prospective experience is an important step to providing appropriate choices and opportunities.

CONCLUSIONS

Quality of life has largely been employed as a concept based on research with adults. The literature, until recently, has essentially ignored children. Indeed, one can argue that quality of life has been first employed with those who are most empowered. Children are not amongst this group, largely having things done to and for them by an adult community. Children with disabilities are even less empowered and, therefore are likely to have poorer quality of life. Quality of life, then, can be seen as an empowering concept, helping us to recognize the holistic nature of needs and allowing us to pursue developments which incorporate the child's perspective. In this context it is also important to recognize that the definition and conceptualization of quality of life must be clear. In our view not only is quality of life a concept involving the lifespan, but it is holistic and integrates diverse aspects of the child's life. It critically involves personal perceptions and choices. As an applied concept, it does not imply that 'everything goes' but highlights choices within a structured context. Personal choices and needs are recognized, but are mediated through environmental change and counselling. There is dignity in recognizing children's choices in attempting to meet their personal needs. However, it is also recognized that some needs cannot be met either in the present or over time. This also allows for decision making and problem solving with the child as a partner, which forms part of the developmental cycle.

Research suggests that children with disabilities experience a lower quality of life than their non-handicapped peers. They are socialized differently, have fewer experiences and opportunities, have generally fewer choices and are not as involved in decision making as their non-handicapped peers. Quality of life of children needs to be viewed holistically. We cannot look at one component in isolation. School cannot be viewed separately from community or home. Nor can we look at quality of life as a static entity. It is a fluid concept with different foci at different age levels. It is a developmental process, as are its components of choice and decision making.

Quality of life cannot be connected to any one item or situation. It presents itself in different forms over many domains. It is a complex concept requiring attention to the connectiveness of experiences. We have illustrated this through the example of busing students to a school outside their neighbourhood.

Children need to experiment with choice and therefore be allowed to take risks. The role this plays in development is of considerable relevance. Risk taking is limited in the lives of many children with special needs. In some of the research quoted teenagers are the source of enquiry yet, by this age, many restrictions have been imposed, thereby limiting opportunities for improved quality of life. Quality of life must be seen as a lifelong concept relating to parents' attitudes to disability and their views about the potential lifestyle of their children when they grow to adulthood.

There has to be a concerted effort to allow situations to happen where children can exert choice in their lives. This means that parents and care givers need to encourage assertiveness. Unfortunately, in the education of children with special needs, we frequently value and encourage submissiveness. If we allow children more control over their lives this requires us to 'let go'. We can no longer simply exert our preferences and choices over their lives. We may not like the clothes they choose or disapprove of the games they play. To recognize their growing and different values requires a significant switch in our thinking. This does not mean accepting all of children's choices, nor does it imply a *laissez-faire* environment. It argues for recognition of children's choices, providing environments for experimentation, reducing seclusion and promoting inclusion, while promoting guidelines and structure within which choices can be mediated.

As teenagers grow so they begin to pull away from their families and make greater decisions for themselves. Teenagers with special needs may not be able to initiate this separation themselves. Peer pressure has a great influence on teenagers. If teenagers with special needs do not develop normal relationships with others they may be deprived of opportunities to develop this aspect of their lives. The next decade should involve a drive to explore quality of life for children and their families.

REFERENCES

Andrews, F.M. (1974) Social indicators of perceived life quality. *Social Indicators Research*, **1**, 279–99.

Barnes, C. (1991) *Disabled People in Britain and Discrimination: A Case for Anti-discrimination Legislation*, Hurst, London and University of Calgary, Calgary.

Borthwick-Duffy, S. (1990) Quality of life of persons with severe or profound retardation, in *Quality of life: Perspectives and Issues*, (ed. R.L. Schalock), American Association on Mental Retardation, Washington DC.

Brown, I. (1992) *Quality of Life Project – Phase I*, The Centre for Health Promotion, University of Toronto.

Brown, R.I. (1988) *Quality of Life for Handicapped People*, Croom Helm, London.

Brown, R.I. (1990) Quality of life, in *Special Education across Canada: Issues and Concerns for the '90s*, (eds M. Csapo and L. Goguen), Centre for Human Development and Research, Vancouver, BC.

Brown, R.I. (1995) Social life, dating and marriage, in *Down Syndrome: Living and Learning in the Community*, (eds L. Nadel & D. Rosenthall), Wiley-Liss, New York.

Brown, R.I. and Bayer, M. (1992) *Rehabilitation Questionnaire and Manual*, Captus, Toronto.

Brown, R.I. and Hughson, E.A. (1993) *Behavioural and Social Rehabilitation and Training*, 2nd edn, Chapman & Hall, London.

Brown, R.I. and Timmons, V. (1994) Quality of life: adults and adolescents with disabilities. *Exceptionality Education*, **4**, 1–11.

Brown, R.I., Bayer, M.B. and MacFarlane, C. (1988) Quality of life amongst handicapped adults, in *Quality of Life for Handicapped People*, (ed. Roy I. Brown), Croom Helm, London.

Brown, R.I., Bayer, M.B. and Brown, P.M. (1992) *Empowerment and Developmental Handicaps*, Captus, Toronto.

Brown, R.I., Bayer, M.B. and Brown, P.M. (1994) A quality of life model: new challenges arising from a six year study, in *Quality of Life for Persons with Disabilities*, (ed. D. Goode), Brookline Books, Cambridge, MA.

Butler Dunn, L. (1991) *The Effects of Toy and Group Composition on the Social Play of Young Children With and Without Handicaps*. Unpublished PhD Thesis, University of Calgary.

Dattilo, J. and Rusch, F. (1985) Effects of choice on leisure participation for persons with severe handicaps. *Journal of the Association for the Severely Handicapped*, **10**, 194–9.

Denholm, C. (1992) *Developmental Needs of Adolescents: Application to Adolescents with Down Syndrome in Building our Future*. 1992 National Conference, Proceedings of the Canadian Down Syndrome Society, pp125–133.

Evans, D.R. (1994) Enhancing quality of life in the population at large, in *Improving the Quality of Life in Normal and Disabled Populations*, (eds D.M. Romney, R.I. Brown and P. Fry), Kluwer Academic Publishers, New York.

Firth, H. and Rapley, M. (1990) *From Acquaintance to Friendship: Issues for People with Learning Disabilities*, British Institute of Mental Handicap Publications, Kidderminster.

G. Allan Roeher Institute (1990) *Making Friends*, The G. Allan Roeher Institute, Toronto, Ontario.

Gartner, A. and Lipsky, D. (1987) Beyond special education: toward one quality system for all students. *Harvard Educational Review*, **57**, 367–95.

Goode, D.A. (1988) *Quality of Life for Persons with Disabilities: A Review and Synthesis of the Literature*, Mental Retardation Institute, New York.

Goode, D.A. (1990) Thinking about and discussing quality of life, in *Quality of Life: Perspectives and Issues*, (ed. R.L. Schalock), American Association on Mental Retardation, Washington DC.

Guralnick, M., Connor, R. and Hammond, M. (1995) Parent perspectives of peer relationships and friendships in integrated and segregated programs. *American Journal of Mental Retardation*, **99**, 457–76.

Halpern, A.S. (1993) Quality of life as a conceptual framework for evaluating transition outcomes. *Exceptional Children*, **59**, 486–98.

Janicki, M. (1990) Growing old with dignity: on quality of life for older persons with a lifelong disability, in *Quality of Life: Perspectives and Issues*, (ed. R.L. Schalock), American Association on Mental Retardation, Washington DC.

Lawrence, P., Brown, R.I., Mills, J. and Estay, I. (1992) *Adults with Down Syndrome*, Captus, Toronto.

Lichty, J. and Johnson, P. (1992) Client intervention: another team's experience, in *Empowerment and Developmental Handicaps*, (eds R. Brown, M. Bayer and P. Brown), Captus, Toronto.

MacKenzie, S. (1997) The study of the life experience of parents of children with disabilities: a rationale for using quality of life as a framework, in *Studies in Quality of Life* (ed. R.I. Brown) (in preparation).

McConkey, R. (1985) Changing beliefs about play and handicapped children. *Early Child Development and Care*, **19**, 79–94.

McGill, J. (1987) Our leisure identity. *Entourage*, **2**, 23–5.

Mittler, P. (1984) Quality of life and services for people with disabilities. *Bulletin of the British Psychological Society*, **37**, 218–25.

Moss, S. (1994) Quality of life and aging, in *Quality of Life for Persons with Disabilities*, (ed. D. Goode), Brookline Books, Cambridge, MA.

Parmenter, T. (1988) An analysis of the dimensions of quality of life for people with physical disabilities, in *Quality of Life for Handicapped People*, (ed. R.I. Brown), Croom Helm, London.

Rasmussen, L. (1993) *Quality of Life for Parents of a Child with a Developmental Disability*. Unpublished Masters thesis, University of Calgary.

Rodgers, W. and Converse, P. (1975) Measures of the perceived overall quality of life. *Social Indicators Research*, **2**, 127–52.

Romney, D.M., Brown, R.I. and Fry, P.S. (1994) Improving the quality of life: prescriptions for change, in *Improving the Quality of Life in Normal and Disabled Populations*, (eds D. M. Romney, R. I. Brown and P. Fry), Kluwer Academic Publishers, New York.

Schalock, R. (1990) Attempts to conceptualize and measure quality of life, in *Quality of Life: Perspectives and Issues*, (ed. R.L. Schalock), American Association on Mental Retardation, Washington DC.

Schloss, P., Smith, M. and Kiehl, W. (1986) Rec Club: a community centered approach to recreational development for adults with mild to moderate retardation. *Education and Training of the Mentally Retarded*, **21**, 282–8.

Schloss, P., Alper, S. and Jayne, D. (1994) Self-determination for persons with disabilities: choice, risk, and dignity. *Exceptional Children*, **6**, 215–25.

Seward, K. (1987) That's what friends are for. *Entourage*, **2**, 26–31.

Sobsey, D. and Doe, T. (1991) Patterns of sexual abuse and assault. *Sexuality and Disability*, **9**, 243–50.

Stainback, W. and Stainback, S. (1987) Facilitating friendships. *Education and Training in Mental Retardation*, **20**(1), 18–25.

Stainback, S., Stainback, W., East, K. and Sapon-Shevin, M. (1994) A commentary on inclusion and the development of a positive self-identity by people with disabilities. *Exceptional Children*, **60**, 486–91.

Stantrock, J.W. (1993) *Adolescence*, 5th edn, Brown & Benchmark, Wisconsin.

Stark, J. and Goldsbury, T. (1990) Quality of life from childhood to adulthood, in *Quality of Life: Perspectives and Issues*, (ed. R.L. Schalock), American Association on Mental Retardation, Washington DC.

Szalai, R. (1980) The meaning of comparative research on the quality of life, in *The Quality of Life*, (ed. A. Szalai), Sage, London.

Timmons, V. (1993) *Quality of Life of Teenagers with Special Needs*. Unpublished doctoral thesis, University of Calgary.

Wortis, J. (1984) Introduction: Quality of life, in *Mental Retardation and Developmental Disabilities*, Vol. 13, (ed. J. Wortis), Plenum Press, New York.

An ecological perspective on the quality of life of people with intellectual disabilities as they age

10

James Hogg and Loretto Lambe

INTRODUCTION

THE DEMOGRAPHICS OF AGEING AND IMPLICATIONS FOR THE FUTURE
LIVES OF OLDER PEOPLE

Throughout Europe and the developed world, the life expectancy of men
and women has increased throughout the 20th century (Thane, 1989). The
social and medical factors leading to this improvement in longevity have
similarly dramatically increased the lifespan of people with intellectual
disabilities (mental retardation). Increased longevity among people with
intellectual disabilities is reported throughout European countries. This is
illustrated in studies from Austria, Germany and Switzerland (Wieland,
1987), Denmark (Dupont, Vaeth & Videbech, 1987), France (Reboul *et al.*,
n.d.), The Netherlands (Maaskant, 1993), Ireland (Mulcahy & Reynolds,
1984) and the United Kingdom (Hogg, Moss & Cooke, 1988), as well as in
the United States (Seltzer, 1992). Though people with profound and
multiple intellectual disabilities (Eyman, Call & White, 1989), and to a
lesser extent those with Down syndrome (Eyman, Call & White, 1991),
have a lower than average life expectancy, half of those with intellectual
disabilities can be expected to live for as long as the wider population.

This changed state of affairs has had a dramatic impact on the challenges
faced by policymakers, front-line service providers and family members.
Policymakers are now planning services that reflect the philosophy of normalization with its emphasis on an ordinary and productive life in the
community and the right of people with intellectual disabilities to make
choices about the way in which they live. In many countries this has
resulted in a programme of closure of long-stay hospitals or institutions,
with the residents returning to the community to enjoy day, residential and
leisure services (Emerson & Hatton, 1994).

Front-line staff providing these services have, in turn, had to consider what form of provision best meets the needs of those people with intellectual disabilities living in the community as they age. As with younger people with intellectual disabilities, however, the application of normalization principles has dictated a move towards community-based services and participation in the life of the community. Many parents, too, have maintained their daughters and sons in the community, engaging in the caring role in the family home. They now anticipate, however, that their daughter or son may outlive them, for the first time in history. For such parents, the burden of care may increase as they themselves age and become less able to cope. This has implications not only for the caring role as such, but for future planning for their son or daughter 'after they have gone'. Similar issues are raised for relatives who care, principally sisters or sisters-in-law.

An increasing community presence has also drawn attention to another issue pervasive in the field of intellectual disability, that of the quality of life of the individual and their carer. In the context of the present study of ageing and intellectual disability, Goode's (1988) ecological perspective guided the research, mapping as it does onto a similar position articulated in the wider field of elderly studies by Cantor & Little (1985). This theoretical position was utilized by Hogg, Moss & Cooke (1988) to organize an extensive review of the field of ageing and intellectual disability, as well as in a population study of this group (Hogg & Moss, 1994), while Moss (1994) has further explored the applicability of ecologically based quality of life concepts to older people with intellectual disabilities. In brief, the life of the older person is conceptualized with respect to their relation to family, neighbours, friends and service provision, as well as informal community supports and ultimately the wider administrative, political and philosophical context in which all these elements operate. Elements of all these relations are represented throughout this chapter.

A CASE STUDY OF ECOLOGICAL DETERMINANTS OF QUALITY OF LIFE FOR OLDER PEOPLE WITH INTELLECTUAL DISABILITY

The present study was undertaken in the Grampian Region of Scotland at the request of the principal agencies, both statutory and voluntary (i.e. not for profit). It was framed from the outset from the ecological perspective noted above, in that all elements of Cantor's model were to be explored and integrated, and was informed by Goode's (1988) conceptualization of quality of life. A report which more fully represents the comments of respondents with and without intellectual disabilities and illustrates their lives through case studies is also available (Lambe & Hogg, 1995).

RESEARCH STRATEGY

POLICY ISSUES IN GRAMPIAN REGION

Regional policy with respect to people with intellectual disabilities on the one hand and elderly people on the other is covered in a wide range of documents. These have been analysed from the viewpoint of the present study to establish what explicit policies are in effect for older people with intellectual disabilities in the region complemented by interviews with senior administrators.

SELECTION OF PARTICIPANTS

The methodology suggested therefore entailed selective interviews with service users (older people with and without intellectual disabilities), their families and professional carers and relevant service managers. Forty-two older people in all were interviewed. Thirty-two had intellectual disabilities. Ten older people without intellectual disabilities who had experience of integrated provision were also interviewed. The families and professional carers of the 32 people with intellectual disabilities were interviewed, as were management and staff of day services.

The qualitative nature of this study, involving as it does an intensive analysis of a variety of themes related to the lives of individuals, precluded conventional statistical sampling of the population of older people with intellectual disabilities in Grampian Region. For that reason an approach entailing theoretical sampling was adopted (Glaser & Strauss, 1967). This involves the careful selection of cases in such a way that key dimensions of difference are represented. As interviews proceed, so new hypotheses emerge and the sample may be progressively expanded. Overall, individuals were selected on the basis of:

1. place of residence (long-stay hospital, group house, independent living, family home, generic elderly service);
2. geographical location (urban, rural, coastal);
3. age/health status of individual;
4. age/health status of carers;
5. day service;
6. competence of individual.

Interviews were also conducted with two small groups of older people with experience of participating in an integrated setting for older people with intellectual disabilities, seven in a day service and three in a private nursing home.

The final breakdown of the sample of people with intellectual disabilities is shown in Table 10.1. Of the 13 people living at home, five had a single carer, the mother, while three lived with both parents though the mother

Table 10.1 Residential and geographical location of interviewees with intellectual disabilities

| Location | Place of residence | | | | |
	Family	Independent	Group house	Hospital/ hostel	Elderly generic
Urban	8	2	2	7	–
Rural	3	–	3	–	2
Coastal	2	*1	2	6/1	–
TOTALS	13	3	7	7	2

* Very sheltered housing but travels independently.
Ten elderly people without intellectual disabilities were also interviewed in generic day and residential services for elderly people. In addition, variations in the other dimensions (3–6 above) were built in to ensure adequate contrasts between the likely needs of the interviewees and their carers.

was the primary carer. In four families the sister was the primary carer and in one the sister-in-law.

The three people in the independent group were all female, two living without any in-home support and one in very sheltered accommodation. Six lived in small group houses and one in a larger group house of 10 residents. Of these seven, four had moved from long-stay hospitals, one had moved on the death of a parent and two had moved prior to parents becoming unable to cope, i.e. a planned relocation. Six people still lived in the principal long-stay hospital: five males and one female. One person lived in a hostel (20+ residents). Of the two people who lived in a nursing home for elderly people, one had moved from the hospital and one from the family home following the death of a parent.

Table 10.2 Characteristics of individuals and family carers

Person	Age	Carer(s)	Age
Anne Grassick	44	Mother	74
Moira Curry	45	Mother (+ Father)	75 (76)
Colin Law	45	Mother	71
Madge Fraser	70	Sister	57
Edith Erskine	47	Mother	81
Sophie Balmain	58	Sister	63
Hattie Napier	62	Sister	64
Chae MacFarlane	56	Sister	59
Alice Spence	42	Mother	81
Fergus Thompson	54	Sister-in-law	57
Cynthia McHoul (step sister/brother)	37	Mother (+ Father)	84 (76)
Hamish Gillies (step brother/sister)	54	Mother (+ Step Father)	84 (76)
George Glass	44	Mother	80

Table 10.3 Characteristics of people living in residential settings

Person	Age	Residential provision
Independent living		
Victoria Reid	51	–
Ellen Muir	65	–
Else Queen	59	–
Group houses		
Jimmie Simpson	60	Partnership
Ernest Urquhart	57	Partnership
Chrisie Beattie	61	Ark
Colin Eldrum	56	Partnership
Scott Taylor	54	Partnership
Sarah Sinclair	38	Cornerstone
Marget Strachan	47	Cornerstone
Hostel		
Christopher Knapp	62	–
Hospital		
Alec Mutch	84	–
Dod Guthrie	75	–
Alec Fraser	63	–
Ralph Stirton	63	–
Maggie Jean	61	–
Norrie Yuille	69	–
Generic elderly, nursing home		
Lizzie Annandale	79	–
Jessie Moultrie	70	–

The characteristics of the people living with family members appear in Table 10.2 and those in other forms of residential setting in Table 10.3. All names are pseudonyms. Of the 32 individuals interviewed, 15 were male and 17 were female. Seven people had Down syndrome and three were wheelchair users.

INTERVIEW AND ASSESSMENT INSTRUMENTS

Interviews from the diverse sources noted were subsequently collated for each individual with intellectual disabilities on an interview summary document which provided the basis for analysis of the key topics.

Interviews with policymakers

Interviews with policymakers were adapted to the particular agency and responsibilities of the person. They all dealt, however, with the following areas:

- development of community care provision from the agency's viewpoint;
- the service objectives for older people with intellectual disabilities;
- service models through which to realize these objectives;
- other specific issues related to this group, including integration with generic services for elderly people.

Interviews with managers of facilities

Interviews with the managers of residential or day services in which the older interviewees with intellectual disabilities were based were again tailored to the types of facility and service. Principally, however, the nature of provision for older people was discussed and any specific policies within the facility were considered. Deficits in service provision for this group and staff training needs were considered.

Interviews with individuals with intellectual disabilities, their carers and keyworkers

Three separate questionnaires were developed for interviews with older people with intellectual disabilities, their carers and keyworkers. The responses to the questions were linked to specific codes but for the present purposes the results are generally treated qualitatively in line with the original proposal. Where respondents introduced topics not directly addressed in the questionnaires, these were nevertheless discussed and recorded.

Each questionnaire explored the following issues:

1. Interview with older person with intellectual disability. The experience of ageing and expectations for the future – particularly with respect to residential change. In addition, the *Rehabilitation Questionnaire: A Personal Guide to the Individual's Quality of Life* (Brown & Bayer, 1992) was used to explore issues to do with satisfaction, where the person lived, activities engaged in, feelings about health, social and family relationships, self-image, use of leisure time, management of money, employment, help and support needed. Where the person was unable to respond to the Quality of Life Questionnaire, information was collected from the keyworker.
2. Interview with keyworker. Here basic information was collected, e.g. past history, age and other demographic information, as well as questions specifically on ageing, future plans and requirements, integration of intellectual disability services with generic elderly services and staff needs.
3. Interview with carers. A detailed review of the person's past history was taken, together with a full account of the person's present service

provision. Where the carer was a family member the impact of caring on the family was discussed, as were the consequences of ageing for the person with intellectual disability and family members. Issues related to coping and future provision were considered from the viewpoints of continued caring, financial considerations and legal matters. The issue of leaving the family home was central to this discussion and knowledge of residential options was discussed. Factors that enable the carer to continue this role were explored.

POLICY AND PLANNING IN GRAMPIAN REGION

Recent legislation, notably the National Health Service and Community Care Act 1990 which was implemented in April 1993, has led to the statement of detailed plans to realize community care policy (Grampian Regional Council & Grampian Health Board, 1992, 1993, 1994). These documents expressed commitment to an overall objective of enabling individuals, wherever feasible and sensible and taking full account of their wishes and those of their carers, to remain in their own homes or local community for as long as they wished to do so. The concomitant of this objective was the relocation to their place of origin of individuals resident in institutions. No explicit differentiation of older people with intellectual disabilities from their younger peers, nor from older people generally, is made in this documentation. Indeed, older people with intellectual disabilities are viewed as 'older people first'.

In contrast, ENABLE (Scottish Society for the Mentally Handicapped), the principal intellectual disability voluntary agency in Scotland, has taken a policy decision to consider the needs of older people with intellectual disability, taking note:

> ... of the lack of appropriate facilities for older people with intellectual disabilities. When one reaches about 50 years of age it is quite normal for our needs to vary from those of a person in their early 20s. On the whole services have not developed to take this factor into consideration.
>
> (ENABLE, 1993, p2)

It should be added that the view expressed represents the perception and needs of a substantial segment of ENABLE's older membership, i.e. parents and other relatives who typically are concerned about the present and future life of their relative with intellectual disabilities. In general, voluntary organizations concerned with the general ageing population make little reference to those with intellectual disabilities and have no formal policy towards this group.

A wide variety of statutory and voluntary agencies provide and purchase services for people with intellectual disabilities in Grampian Region. The principal providers of services are Grampian Regional

Council Social Work Department and Grampian Healthcare (NHS) Trust, Moray Healthcare (NHS) Trust and the voluntary sector. The principal purchasers are Grampian Health Board and Grampian Regional Council. A wide range of residential services is offered by residential care providers. There is also a strong voluntary sector input with respect to both older people generally and people with intellectual disabilities.

SERVICE PROVISION

A wide range of residential provision was found in the region including home (family) based accommodation, independent living with various degrees of support, service-run community accommodation in group houses, hostels, etc. for people with intellectual disabilities, use of general elderly accommodation and the persistence of long-stay hospitals, due, however, for closure under the community care policy. Day service provision was also wide ranging and included day centre-based facilities, employment opportunities, education activities and leisure. With respect to health services, the Joint Community Care Plan emphasizes that people with intellectual disabilities should be able to access the full range of primary care and other general health services, with these complemented by Community Intellectual Disability Nurses and Clinical Psychologists, though the need for specialist therapeutic services has also been addressed.

RESEARCH FINDINGS

The research findings are organized around six principal themes, which will be summarized and followed by an overall comment on their bearing on quality of life issues.

THE PERSON WITH INTELLECTUAL DISABILITIES AS REFLECTED IN THEIR OWN ASPIRATIONS AND THOSE OF CARERS AND STAFF

The perspective of the participants with intellectual disabilities was explored through use of the Quality of Life Rehabilitation Questionnaire. The degree to which individuals were able to reflect on their own lives varied considerably. Those who were able to do so, while only very rarely commenting on the nature and consequences of their disability, typically presented a positive self-image. For several, their Scottish identity was highly significant, even to the extent of resenting staff members who were incomers.

Except for some of those living in the long-stay hospital, none indicated that they would wish to live elsewhere. This applied equally to those living at home with relatives and those in non-family community houses. However, three of the six hospital residents expressed deep dissatisfaction with their continued containment in hospital and were intent on returning to their original neighbourhoods. Similarly, expressed satisfaction with day service provision and, where applicable, employment was high. One woman who had recently been made redundant reported that she missed work, found herself unoccupied and was becoming deskilled through lack of opportunity.

In line with Third Age expectations, several respondents reported that they continued to make progress in a variety of skills, a view confirmed by care staff. Nevertheless, some invoked age as a reason for not continuing formal learning, particularly in the area of literacy. The two principal skill deficits they reported were in the areas of budgeting and telephone use, a situation which clearly inhibited their autonomy and ability to function independently in the community.

The persistent finding that friendship networks were restricted to other people with intellectual disabilities or family was confirmed in this study. This limited friendship network is, in the main, a reflection of the wider situation in which the person leads their life. Virtually all those involved in the study lived in specialized settings or with their family and attended specialized day services. For those living in integrated residential settings or independently or attending a generic elderly day service, such provision had come late in life and did not appear to have had a significant impact on the formation of friendships with people without intellectual disabilities.

The experience of ageing was investigated through use of the White Top Research Unit Ageing Questionnaire. This explores a variety of themes related to ageing including self-perceptions of ageing and what it meant for their future life. Individuals' ability to describe the ageing process in themselves and others varied markedly. Some showed good awareness of cognitive and physical changes in themselves and others, as well as the consequences of such changes for their present and future lives. Others could express little that was meaningful, a situation particularly noticeable in three of the long-stay hospital residents. This lack of understanding argues for a more constructive approach that would assist people to appreciate the changes that occur over the lifespan and the ways in which they relate to the individual. The experience of ageing is a fundamental one for most people, nearly as significant as birth or death and as legitimate a target for education as the more obvious skill-based activities.

The experience of bereavement and the response to it also showed similar variation. Some were aware of past losses and visibly moved by this, while others had little to say about those they had lost and their consequent feelings. Again, one must raise the question of how far the opportunity to come to terms with the experience of bereavement and death might have conditioned the apparent loss of response. Following the interview one woman raised with her carer-sister, for the first time, her wish to be buried rather than cremated.

None of the individuals had independent advocates. Among staff there was confusion as to the nature of independent advocacy, with many regarding themselves as the person's advocate. In addition, aspects of the advocate's role, such as befriending, were emphasized without much consideration being given to the advocate as the person's representative. If priorities had to be set, then clearly hospital residents have the greatest need, particularly where there is a keen and strongly felt wish to leave the hospital and where staff, sometimes in agreement with quite peripheral relatives, oppose such a move. Nevertheless, the development of participation by some individuals with intellectual disabilities in the running of the principal voluntary organization in Scotland, ENABLE, was well advanced.

Positive and negative views were expressed regarding life satisfaction and the influence of the family, community and service provision. The wider influences of available provision from the statutory, private and voluntary agencies, themselves conditioned by legislation and resource availability, as well as the wider service philosophy, also clearly have a bearing on the overall situation in which the person finds themselves (e.g. expressed satisfaction with the move from hospital to community, as was typically the case). However, a fuller understanding of the person's value system, history and cognitive and affective status would be necessary to determine the person–environment interaction in detail. This situation with respect to the individual is elaborated in the following consideration of the various environments in which they live.

THE FAMILY SITUATION

As will be anticipated from the composition of the sample, there was a continuum of contact between the individual and relatives. This ranged from limited involvement, in the case of some people in residential settings, to full-time, long-term caring. This section deals principally with the 13 families with whom individuals are at present living. We will also note two families whose daughters left the family as a planned move a few years ago, but with whom parents maintain close contact. Finally, we will comment on the role of relatives in the lives of individuals living in both community and institutional settings.

If a single word can capture carers' views of their role it is 'acceptance', regardless of the consequences of engaging in such long-term caring. The interviews confirmed Grant's (1986) characterization of the quality of care that families can provide with its emphasis on reliability and the personal nature of many caring activities. A wide range of positive aspects of caring from the point of view of family carers was also reported, related to the person and social advantages including friendship, company and love, as well as help in the home. However, a strong ethical motivation was also present, with caring having been adopted as the only acceptable course. Problems were acknowledged, including restriction of the family's social life, as well as increased expenses attendant on heating, laundry, etc.

Other family members were reported as feeling positive about the individual with intellectual disabilities. Contact, however, was generally very restricted and did not make a direct contribution to day-to-day caring activities. Indeed, with few exceptions the wider informal care network was limited with respect to other family members, friends and neighbours. In only a small number of families was a member not involved in the primary care role regularly in contact. In some instances strong anta-gonisms within families emerged, notably to siblings who were perceived not to have made a suitable contribution. Even where a father, brother or brother-in-law was also in the family home, his role tended to be broadly one of support rather than direct instrumental involvement. Nor was the primary role of women as carers changed in any significant way by the absence of a husband through divorce, the spouse's retirement or his death.

As may be inferred from the acceptance of the caring situation, continuation of the role came down firmly to the direct support required by the primary carer or indirect support resulting from relief from caring, if they were to continue with their accepted role as both they and the individual with intellectual disabilities aged. The principal form of direct support was domiciliary provision in the home, though in reality this was rarely received. In one instance it was anticipated that such support would in future be welcome in order to assist in dealing with a daughter's personal care needs. More typically, indirect support resulting from the relative receiving respite care and/or a reliable day service was seen as the main requirement for continued care.

A reliable day service was considered crucial to continued caring. Typically, such services were highly valued by carers, though not neces-sarily without some criticism of their operation. That alleged 'retirement' policies might jeopardize this element of support was a concern to some carers, engendered by the general confusion over the issues of retirement among day service staff. With the growing emphasis on dispersed day provision, i.e. the person not necessarily attending a day centre five days a week, it is important to emphasize that reliable provision, whatever the location, is guaranteed in the interest of carers as well as service users. If the move to dispersed services results in inconsistent provision with the person remaining at or returning home, there can be little doubt that pressure on older and elderly carers will result and their ability to cope be diminished.

All carers interviewed were aware that the fact that they and their relatives were ageing had significant implications for future care. Obviously, their actual ages and present health had a strong bearing on how acutely they saw the future as presenting a problem. In some extreme instances the process of ageing was clear and an immediate source of concern.

Few relatives had taken, or been given assistance to take, any steps to planning the future, either adopting a fatalistic attitude or putting off a decision indefinitely. Against a background of long-term commitment within the immediate family, planning was seen almost as a contravention of the principles that have guided that commitment. And yet behind this view could be discerned a major anxiety regarding the future. In response to the question, 'What would you like to see done?', several carers suggested that information on what could be done was the starting point. It is significant that a number of carers commented on the value of the research interview in raising and beginning to explore issues of future planning of residential provision.

Lack of future planning, so clear with respect to future residential provision, was also evident with regard to general legal and financial planning, issues relevant to families generally but with special relevance to families caring for an individual with intellectual disabilities. In only one instance out of the 13 where the person with intellectual disabilities lived in a family home had a will specifically making provision for that person been made. Discussion during the interview tended to raise awareness of this as an issue which should be addressed. An important point made by one respondent was that to make a will making provision for the individual implies that one will die first, i.e. an admission of one's own mortality but also of their daughter's or son's disabilities. It is also an acknowledgment that brings one face to face with the fact that the present arrangement will change radically and that no steps have been taken to prepare for this.

The lack of future planning described above is in no way confined to parents in Grampian Region. A wide range of studies have confirmed this picture, including work by Cooke (1987), Prosser (1994) and Richardson & Ritchie (1986, 1990).

If the relative was to move from the family home, what was demanded from such provision? Carers usually referred to typical facilities such as independent living with staff back-up or group houses or hostels – generally a situation with which they were familiar, rather than a well-grounded picture of the options that might be developed through a personalized residential programme. In terms of the social aspects of the residents, a homely atmosphere with a private room ('home from home'), together with friendly and compatible co-residents (all female, with respect to one daughter), and in one instance a 'no smoking' house, were the principal demands. Staff with a commitment to and knowledge of people with intellectual disabilities were viewed as crucial to good quality provision. The word 'vocation' was mentioned by some carers. Personal care was what carers believed they effectively provided and acceptable care standards by staff were invariably a theme in all discussions.

A placement in a setting for generic elderly people was deemed worth considering by a majority of carers, but at the right age. Principal objections were the lack of stimulation from older residents and the fear that specialist input from staff with a vocation to work with people with intellectual disabilities would be lacking.

Two families had enabled their adult daughters to move to a small group house well before the parents' own old age. This was achieved through the creation of a parents' self-help group co-ordinating both local voluntary and statutory provision acceptable to them and their daughters at a time at which they themselves could monitor and influence provision. The demand by carers that they should have a continued role in their children's lives also signals that in making provision they have not abrogated their life-long commitment.

Finally, we will comment on family carers' attitudes to the overall service context. Few had a clear view of their rights and entitlements and those of the person cared for. Who was responsible for a given service was often not known. Issues related to recent developments in community care were a closed book and few had heard of Care Managers or Care Management, let alone come into contact with those responsible for implementing this policy.

The family, particularly the family actively engaged in care, is the bridge between the individual and the wider service context. The impact of that service context on their care role is both direct, i.e. providing support in the home, and indirect, i.e. provision of day service to the person or the availability of respite permitting continuation of caring. However, carers typically have only the most limited knowledge of the principles underpinning services and their own and their relative's rights in this situation. Although the ecological model entails two-way processes between all the nests, that between family carers and the nests surrounding them seems particularly tenuous. This is important given the emphasis explicitly placed in national legislation and local community care plans on consultation with carers and the development of needs-led services.

RESIDENTIAL NEEDS OF INDIVIDUALS

We noted above five broad classes of residential provision: the family, independent living, managed community residences, provision for generic elderly people and hospitals. In this section we will focus on the views of residents and staff with respect to the last four of these areas.

With respect to the two women living independently as tenants of council flats, there were a number of common features. Both greatly valued their own homes and their independence. Both, however, were dependent upon a measure of support from sisters. Despite the emphasis placed on independence, neither had a rich social life or access to extensive day provision. For one, the Age Concern day service for generic elderly people, offering one day each week, had been a major breakthrough and may provide a platform for fuller community involvement. The other, too, was relatively isolated, even within a community where she had lived for many years. There was little statutory sector input, voluntary organizations making what limited provision there was. On the other hand, neither woman was subject to the abuse and exploitation found in Flynn's (1988) study in a Manchester inner city area and certainly neither was looking for a fundamental change in her living circumstances.

From one perspective such people stand on the threshold of an ideal situation with respect to community integration and participation. The sensitive facilitation of such involvement requires a co-ordinated effort that we would suggest can best be achieved through a professional worker responding to individual aspirations and building on present achievements, rather than a radical attempt to 'place' either woman in some centralized service. The enhancement of leisure opportunities, participation in voluntary work or employment would expand both women's horizons. The possibility of combining further education appropriate to meeting domestic demands would enhance independence, particularly in the areas of cooking and budgeting.

Six people in group houses were interviewed, including the two noted above who had moved with support from their parents. The ability range covered in the study embraced a man with profound intellectual disabilities, multiple impairments and medical difficulties through to able individuals with a high degree of independence.

The four group houses catered for from four to 11 people. All were in residential areas with little to differentiate them from their neighbours. The environment in each was essentially domestic and all were well furnished. Residents had individual rooms (with the exception of two men who chose to share) and their own possessions. All had 24-hour staffing. Three residents of group houses interviewed had come from their family home, one of whom had moved on the death of his mother. Three residents of long-stay hospitals had successfully returned to the community, one man after 49 years in two institutions. They and keyworkers reported on benefits in social behaviour and the learning of new skills. In all cases there was a strong preference for life in the group house as compared to life in the hospital.

Satisfaction with life in group houses was high, with involvement in domestic life and a good range of hobbies. Family contact was maintained by a majority of those living in group houses. Friends tended, however, to be from within the house or day service or in some cases a person with intellectual disabilities living elsewhere. Visitors appeared to be few.

Day services varied markedly for residents of group houses. Basically they received part or full-time day centre provision though a small number spent part of the week in employment or voluntary work, e.g. in a charity shop.

Changes in health status, actual and anticipated, were a concern for staff. This was particularly so where declining health would create difficulties in mobility or carrying out basic care activities. Where such expectations existed, moving to alternative accommodation was not ruled out, though clearly this would have a significant impact on the social composition of the residents and the life of the person. It is just such situations that critics of group houses are talking about when they urge more flexible responses to residential provision.

Earlier research has shown that, even without a stated policy of integrating older people with intellectual disabilities, a significant proportion do find their way into residential accommodation for older people (Hogg & Moss, 1994). Many of these are not known to those in intellectual disability services. Two types of accommodation where they did live were identified in this study, i.e. a conventional nursing home and very sheltered accommodation. Two women with profound learning and physical disabilities lived in the former, a more able woman with mild intellectual disabilities but serious medical problems in the latter.

Within differing frames of reference and the ethos of these residences, the three women have already successfully integrated and benefitted from the respective regimes which cater for their very contrasting ability levels. It would be difficult to envisage a more appropriate environment for the resident of the very sheltered housing facility, either with respect to its physical quality or the degree of independence it permits. With respect to the co-residents of the nursing home, judgement on their placement depends ultimately on how one would envisage an ideal service for two women in their 70s. Again, the quality of their environment, though typical of congregate care settings, is of a very high order, apparently enjoyed by other older people who were also interviewed. Well-qualified nursing staff are on hand to meet their complex needs. It was reported that they had both progressed in communication since arriving. A small-scale residence for people with intellectual disabilities, with clearly programmed aims, might offer a higher level of stimulation and give their lives a clearer direction. However, the issue may well be one of scale rather than a specialized setting *per se*, i.e. life in a small, integrated setting could offer the benefits of both specialized intellectual disability input and contact with peers of their own age.

For all three women, acceptance into their integrated settings was not an issue. Residents of the very sheltered accommodation did not see their co-resident as in any way problematical. Three women interviewed in the nursing home, ages 78, 79 and 91 years, discussed the mix of residents within the house and expressed more concern about the residents with dementia than those with intellectual disabilities.

The relative success of these placements provides confirmation of the attitudes reflected in the interviews with the individuals themselves and their family carers to integration into residences for generic older people, particularly 'old folks' homes', described above. Similarly, the opinions of staff in group houses and hospitals tended to concur with this view, where it was judged that the person would benefit from integration and the ensuing social stimulation and that such placements would not be stigmatizing. Reservations that were expressed related to fears that the person would be patronized and not treated as adult and this might occur in both day and residential services. However, even against this positive background, the need for specialist intellectual disability input was urged by most of those interviewed.

On the basis of the above findings, we would suggest that integrated living within the wider population of older and elderly people can be a positive experience. This judgement is not neutral with respect to the kind of model that provides the most adequate provision and sheltered and very sheltered settings in urban areas particularly offer ready access to the community and its facilities. Nor does such a view imply that a specialist intellectual disability input, either through staff from the intellectual disability field or training of non-specialist staff, is not called for. A blending of expertise would offer positive advantages. A proactive exploration of such opportunities developed through contact between those administering services for people with intellectual disabilities and those whose concern is with provision for elderly people is recommended.

We have described above Grampian Healthcare (NHS) Trust's policy with respect to closure of the principal hospital. The six individuals interviewed were selected as representing a range of views on hospital life and relocation and were of varying levels of intellectual disability. It is important to note here that, though the selection intentionally represents individuals keen to leave the hospital and those who prefer to stay, the even split in no way reflects the overall pattern of aspirations with respect to relocation to the community or the typical outcome of such relocation. It was reported that of over 300 people who have been relocated to date, only seven have chosen to return.

Here we consider these residents' views on life in the hospital and their aspirations for the future. Two, a woman of 61 years who had spent 32 years in the hospital and a man of 84 resident there for 23 years, had both returned to the hospital following unsuccessful placements in the community. In both instances it was clear that significant misjudgements had been made with respect to the transition and the experience in the community setting. While the woman, however, was still intent on leaving the hospital, the man felt that his friendships in the hospital were sufficient to keep him there.

In addition to faulty preparation, a second barrier emerged which was the influence of relatives on the process of relocation. Typically, relatives did not wish relocation to the community, despite their very limited contact with the resident and the fact that it would impinge little on them. Interviews with relatives typically revealed a lack of understanding of what was entailed in community living, coupled with a high level of satisfaction with hospital provision. Staff, often implicitly hostile to the move to the community, gave undue weight to relatives' views that bolstered their own opposition to relocation. Against this opposition must be set the intensity with which three of the residents wished to return to the community.

Two points need to be made with respect to the very diverse residential settings in which people in this Region find themselves. First, the policies stated by statutory sector agencies bear only a partial relation to the reality. It is clear that only in certain instances are older people with intellectual disabilities treated as 'older people first'. Even where they are, as with placement in a nursing home, the objective of community participation is hardly facilitated. However, in one instance involving sheltered accommodation, both of these aims were successful realized, with consequent high life satisfaction on the part of the individual concerned.

DAY-TIME ACTIVITIES AND LEISURE

A broad pattern of day provision may be found in Grampian Region for older people with intellectual disabilities. Nevertheless, the principal emphasis remains on centre-based services and specific developments for older people sometimes reinforce this model by segregating them further within such centres. Questioning regarding centre-based services by service providers was, however, prevalent, with a move towards a more varied pattern of community-based provision mooted.

Ten of the 13 people living at home received some form of day service, while one person was in full-time sheltered employment and two people received no formal day service. Five of the seven people living in group houses attended a day centre for part of the week, while the remaining two people were in part-time non-sheltered employment.

The availability and activities offered in conventional day services were typically highly valued by the service users and their carers, particularly other family members. However, there were a substantial number of critical comments regarding the activities on offer and the lack of a proper curriculum. One mother referred to the irrelevance of projects about other countries which appear to be modelled on primary school activities. Why, she asked, was there not more emphasis on basic training? Another mother was highly critical of centre staff for having failed to identify significant age-related decline in her daughter, leading to the loss of well-established skills, and even more critical of their lack of response to this decline when it was noted.

The middle and later years were viewed by staff and service users alike as having great potential for development. Several professionals reported positive progress in service users for whom they were responsible. The wider literature on ageing has emphasized the potential for growth in the Third Age in the wider population (Laslett, 1989). It is clear that the individuals with whom this chapter is concerned, their carers and service providers also view middle age and the later years as an opportunity for growth and that services should play an enabling role in meeting this aim.

We have noted in passing the detrimental effect of loss of a job on one woman living independently in the community. Of those studied here, only four people were in any form of employment, three part time and one full time in sheltered employment. Two were involved in broadly horticultural work, both indicating that this was a preferred option to attending a day centre. One of these men emphasized the adult nature of the work situation and the value he placed on such activity in comparison to traditional day service activities.

The concept of the Third Age is not related exclusively to the years following conventional retirement. Others without the obligation or opportunity for employment and raising a family may enter this stage much earlier. For this reason, the concept of retirement has remained an ambiguous and even controversial one for people with intellectual disabilities. This situation was certainly reflected in Grampian Region where confusion existed among service providers as to whether there was an official 'retirement age' from day services and families fearful of the withdrawal of such services when their relatives attained the conventional age of retirement.

While this situation has been clarified as a result of the research – there is no official retirement age from services in the region – the issue of age-related change remained. However, a change in the pattern of service provision, as distinct from 'retirement', as an age-related break was acknowledged to be the appropriate way forward for several people over 60 years. Such an approach is consistent with the emerging view for all day service provision that it should reflect a diversity of needs and be based on accessing a range of community- and centre-based activities. We would suggest that such a model has within it a far more sensitive mechanism for adjusting to the changing needs of older people with intellectual disabilities than grouping ageing people in segregated services or retiring them from a centre-based service. Components of a varied service can be adjusted, dropped or added to as the person ages, develops or acquires new interest. What is fundamental is the availability of a flexible structure in which to pass the week, coupled with the guarantee for family carers that such provision is permanent. The use of day services for elderly people by people with intellectual disabilities appears less frequent than in the case of residential provision. Certainly the former possibility had not occurred to many service providers interviewed. One of the most impressive day services visited as part of the study was the Age Concern (Scotland) venture enjoyed by one 65-year-old woman with intellectual disabilities. Here both service users and volunteers were all over retirement age. People with a range of disabilities attended (both service users and volunteers) for a variety of leisure activities and exercise classes. The woman herself had integrated well into the group and benefited from involvement. Seven other users, some with physical or sensory disabilities, were interviewed. For them the involvement of people with intellectual disabilities was seen as not only unproblematic, but a welcome opportunity for them to contribute and share with others whom they regarded as less fortunate than themselves.

A second example of integration into a day service entailed one person with dementia and Down syndrome who spent some time at a general dementia centre. With the development of dementia services will come the opportunity to extend such specialist provision to those with intellectual disabilities.

Leisure provision was a central concern of the individuals, their families and front-line service providers. The Quality of Life Rehabilitation Questionnaire considered leisure activities in some detail. A rich menu of activities, particularly with respect to home-based entertainment, was reported. Concerns were expressed, however, about out-of-home leisure by several carers and professionals, particularly with reference to the small number of individuals with part-time or no day service. A few carers were critical of the close link between day service provision and leisure, i.e. staff making leisure provision, while the need for the carer to take the person to a leisure club or event was viewed as '… just a hindrance'.

Several barriers to leisure pursuits were reported. In both rural and urban areas, transport to activities and events was seen as a significant obstacle to community participation. For those with physical disability, wheelchair access presented difficulties. A residential keyworker reported that there should be more opportunities in a large city like Aberdeen, but in reality staff felt that leisure opportunities were restricted not only because of transport and access problems but also because of the individuals' personal acceptability and staff availability.

A small number of individuals independently accessed integrated community leisure, though this was not typical. The views of professionals, particularly in the voluntary sector, were very cautious in this respect, urging a 'thin end of the wedge' approach. This view was based in part on specific examples of failures where the behaviour of people with intellectual disabilities was regarded as unacceptable to others engaged in the activity. What did not emerge from the interviews was a positive commitment to facilitating participation in community leisure activities.

It is perhaps in the area of day activities, including education, employment and leisure, that the relation between the person and community is most manifest. Clearly specialized day services, specialized educational provision and segregated leisure activities, all identified in this study, would weaken this relation. In addition, it is in this context that opportunities for personal growth associated with the Third Age would be most evident and indeed, such development was identified for some individuals by both themselves and those associated with them. Policy decisions related to the direction and diversity of services will therefore have a pronounced impact on both community participation and the personal growth of the individuals in their later years.

HEALTH AND HEALTH CARE

Questions on ageing directed to the individuals themselves, their carers and staff naturally elicited detailed comments on health and health care. It is important to emphasize that the study was not a systematic investigation of health-related issues and we are aware in particular that information on health status from 'patients' and relatives is not, from a research standpoint, well regarded (Patrick & Erickson, 1993). Nevertheless, it would be a significant omission not to report the information our respondents considered it important to mention and offer some interpretation of this information for dealing with ageing in this older population.

Specific physical illnesses and mental health difficulties of very varying severity were reported for 27 of the 32 people in the sample. Reference was made to sensory loss, with three people reported as having cataracts and four with hearing problems, of whom three also wore glasses. Evenhuis (1995a) reports a higher prevalence of visual impairment in people with intellectual disability over the age of 60 years than in the general population, but suggests that it should be possible to reduce excess impairment by an active diagnostic and therapeutic approach from an early age onwards. Hearing loss, as indicated in Evenhuis' (1995b) sample, was only marginally greater than in the wider population. She draws attention to the importance of active screening, treatment and hygiene procedures from an early age. Three people were reported as having had a stroke or a 'heart condition' and a fourth 'periods of collapsing' from an unknown cause. A further three individuals had severe and chronic respiratory problems. Two people were reported as having ulcers, two people had hernias and two varicose veins. A number of problems affecting mobility were noted, three specifically referring to 'bad leg or foot', which included an ulcerated leg. One woman had cancer and subsequently died.

A number of neurological, psychiatric and psychological conditions were reported, affecting over 40% (n=14/32) of the sample. Six people had severe epilepsy, one person had Parkinson disease, two had a diagnosis of schizophrenia and two had 'nervous breakdowns'.

Three people were reported as having dementia. In addition to the three people noted above for whom a diagnosis of dementia was claimed, three other people, all with Down syndrome, were suspected of showing the early signs of Alzheimer dementia by keyworkers, though not their family carer. It is now acknowledged that with increasing longevity, the probability of older people with intellectual disabilities developing dementia is also greater (Janicki, 1994; Janicki et al., 1995). Attention has been drawn in particular to the high prevalence of dementia among people with Down syndrome (Dalton et al., 1993). While people with Down syndrome have a higher risk of contracting the disease, there will be more dementia sufferers without Down syndrome in the population of people with intellectual disabilities as their overall number is greater, though onset will be at an older age (Moss & Patel, 1992). Serious problems exist with the assessment and diagnosis of dementia, including Alzheimer disease, in people with intellectual disabilities (Holland, Karlinsky & Berg, 1993) and the adequacy of the diagnosis in all six individuals in the present study was, in varying degrees, suspect.

With respect to policy, it is clear that staff and agencies are being forced to think on their feet with regard to dementia and intellectual disability. There are no clear strategies with respect to day or residential provision, staff training or collaboration with specialist voluntary and statutory agencies concerned with dementia. The need for such planning is imperative. With the exception of one man, for whom a part-time day service with the mainstream voluntary organization concerned with Alzheimer dementia had been established, there was little contact with those providing services for people with intellectual disabilities and dementia.

Of the 17 women in the study, eight were past the menopause, one of whom had had a hysterectomy and one of whom was awaiting this operation. Four women reported painful or difficult periods. Three mothers noted that their daughters had irregular periods or that these had stopped. One woman had osteoporosis (in addition to Parkinson disease, mentioned above), while a second in a nursing home was suspected of having this condition or secondary cancer, leading to bone fractures.

Though the prevalence of physical and mental health conditions is high, we suspect that these estimates are on the low side. Data culled from medical records or, better still, a full medical assessment would almost certainly indicate conditions that have gone undiagnosed. This is perhaps particularly true for women as, for example, osteoporosis goes undiagnosed in a large number of the general population.

In a study which does not attempt to draw direct comparisons with the wider population of older people, it is clearly not possible to comment on how the present group's health compares to that of their peers without intellectual disability. Several studies have, however, suggested that patterns of morbidity in people with intellectual disability are broadly similar to the general ageing population (Anderson *et al.*, 1987).

For individuals in the community, the local medical centre and general practitioners were the principal providers of medical care and information, with referrals on to consultants where a significant condition was suspected. On balance, GP provision was found acceptable, but adverse comments were made to the effect that GPs did not take individuals seriously.

A specific issue that emerged in a few interviews, but which subsequent more extensive, informal exploration has suggested is of considerable importance, is that of ageing and women's health. Three mothers reported difficulties with their daughters' periods and had visited their GP, none receiving any specific treatment. Of particular concern has been the refusal of well woman clinics to accept referral of women with intellectual disabilities, on the grounds that they only deal with women who are 'sexually active'. Subsequent discussion with other service providers suggested that this refusal is more widespread. As it cannot be assumed that a woman with intellectual disabilities is sexually inactive, this is a highly discriminatory policy and one which cannot be regarded as in any way acceptable.

The adequacy of primary health care in the community received a mixed verdict, especially from family carers. The primary health care team, including the GP, is clearly under pressure to develop services in a cost-effective and efficient fashion. Steps were being taken, however, to explore the development of specialist health care teams in the community directed to adults, including older people with intellectual disabilities.

From an ecological perspective, health status and changes in it are at the heart of the ecological model with respect to both the individual and family members involved in caring. Decline in health will have an impact on all areas of life discussed above and needs to be given a more explicit position within the framing of policy on service options and individual programme planning. Strategic decisions occurring at the level of policy making by statutory agencies related to women's health care, health reviews for the over-75s and in response to dementia also need to be formulated, all 'objective' indicators of potential objective quality of life.

These will permeate through to specific service provision and become part of the wider service pattern available to individuals and their families, as well as to staff, to whom we now turn.

STAFF TRAINING FOR THOSE WORKING IN BOTH INTELLECTUAL DISABILITY SETTINGS AND IN GENERIC SERVICES FOR ELDERLY PEOPLE WHO ARE IN CONTACT WITH PEOPLE WITH INTELLECTUAL DISABILITIES

Throughout this study, the importance of staff knowledge and competence was emphasized by respondents, particularly with respect to an understanding of the needs of older people with intellectual disabilities. For some carers, this view was emphasized by saying that working with people with intellectual disabilities was a 'vocation'. However, there was an acknowledgement that in dealing with older people with intellectual disabilities, there were gaps in training and knowledge. This was the case for a wide range of service providers, including those working in day and residential services, in both statutory and voluntary sectors.

What information and training did those working in intellectual disability services indicate they needed? Principally this consisted of a fuller understanding of the ageing process as it occurred in the wider population. What is the nature of physical and psychological changes as people age? What response should be made to these with respect to the activities in which older people might engage? Staff coping with physical decline and disability in particular indicated the need for information on physical management, particularly the often untrained staff in group houses.

However, it is of some significance that it was just such untrained staff who also expressed a need for basic training with respect to intellectual disability itself. They considered their knowledge, while practically based, was limited with respect to the people with whom they worked, leaving aside the complications of ageing.

For several respondents, the issue of dementia and mental health difficulties loomed large. In another instance, day centre staff failed to read the signs of developing Alzheimer disease in one of their service users and did not attempt to deal with progressive loss of skills. At the levels of appreciating age-related change, referring the person for diagnosis and treatment and responding to these changes within the programme, staff need information on which to base their decisions to seek medical help. Moss & Patel (1992) have commented that while staff often noted changes in the mental health of older people with intellectual disabilities, they frequently failed to interpret this as pathological and did not seek advice on diagnosis and possible treatment.

It is just this kind of knowledge that those working in generic services for elderly people might be expected to have. Indeed, it was represented as a specialist area in the nursing home included in this study. From the perspective of carers and intellectual disability staff alike, lack of specialist information on intellectual disability was viewed as the principal barrier to integration into generic elderly services. The implication of this situation is to train generic staff in relevant areas of intellectual disability practice. However, it should be added that, with respect to the three women in residential settings for elderly people and a fourth woman attending a day service for general elderly people, the necessity for training was not immediately apparent nor perceived by staff. More at issue is how far the regime in these settings, deemed rightly or wrongly suitable for elderly people, is consistent with the approach to promoting personal independence in facilities for people with intellectual disabilities. However, this would seem to be primarily an issue of service philosophy rather than staff training.

The areas of training identified by staff reflect their response to ageing among their service users or residents. From a wider perspective, however, we might ask how far they have grasped the issues involved to be able to give comprehensive responses to questions regarding training needs. A broader view of what is now understood about general ageing would provoke additional questions relevant to meeting the needs of their own service users. In addition, only by defining the fundamental service objectives more clearly can the needs of staff be specified. If, for example, the primary impetus is towards integration and participation in the community, then staff need training with respect to the statutory and voluntary networks that serve elderly people and how to access them. They need fuller information on how elderly people respond to those with disability in different settings and how to facilitate transitions into both day and leisure services for elderly people. They need, therefore, not only specific information on ageing processes, but also a fuller understanding of ageing in the context of the service models to which they aspire.

This last view underlines the ecological nature of service provision for people with intellectual disabilities and its impact on their quality of life. Policy can influence specific service provision through, among other factors, staff training. This, in turn, will bear on the effectiveness with which staff meet the needs of those for whom they are responsible. Insofar as the training is directed to facilitating community participation, the relationship between the individual and the neighbourhood will be influenced.

CONCLUSION

In this chapter we have tried to capture the complexity of the situation that confronts people with intellectual disabilities as they grow older. Within an ecological framework we have identified many of the influences, some immediately in the person's experience, such as family life, and some remote, such as changes in service policy, that affect their quality of life. The data illustrate the complexities with which Goode's ecological model of quality of life attempts to deal and the necessity of adopting a comprehensive approach if we are to give a satisfactory account of quality of life in any global and holistic fashion.

It is important to emphasize the wide variability in both the characteristics of the individuals studied and in their situations. Use of qualitative methodology permits the capture of the uniqueness of the person–environment relation and in doing so offers a dynamic interpretation of the service and personal needs of the individual. While large-scale quantitative studies are essential to strategic planning of services, qualitative methodology offers a natural way in which to explore the ecological context at the centre of which the individual's quality of life is the prime concern.

REFERENCES

Anderson, D.J., Lakin, K.C., Bruinincks, R.H. and Hill, B.K. (1987) *A National Study of Residential and Support Services for Elderly Persons with Mental Retardation: Report 22*, Department of Education, University of Minneapolis, Minneapolis.

Brown, R.I. and Bayer, M.B. (1992) *Rehabilitation Questionnaire: A personal guide to the individual's quality of life – A review of the consumer's perspective*. Captus Press, Toronto.

Cantor, M. and Little, V. (1985) Aging and social care, in *Handbook of Aging and the Social Sciences*, 2nd edn, (eds R.H. Binstock and E Shanas), Van Nostrand Reinhold, New York.

Cooke, D.J. (1987) *Older Parents and their Adult Sons and Daughters with Mental Handicap: Home Living and Future Plans*. MSc thesis, Hester Adrian Research Centre, University of Manchester, Manchester.

Dalton, A.J., Seltzer, G.B., Adlin, M.S. and Wisniewski, H.M. (1993) Association between Alzheimer disease and Down syndrome: clinical observations, in *Alzheimer Disease, Down Syndrome and Their Relationship*, (eds J.M. Berg, H. Karlinsky and A.J. Holland), Oxford University Press, Oxford.

Dupont, A., Vaeth, M. and Videbech, P. (1987) Mortality, life expectancy, and causes of death of mildly mentally retarded in Denmark. *Upsala Journal of Medical Sciences*, **44**(Suppl.), 76–82.

Emerson, E. and Hatton, C. (1994) *Moving Out: The Impact of Relocation from Hospital to Community on the Quality of Life of People with Learning Disabilities*, HMSO, London.

ENABLE (1993) *Grampian Profile: A Review of Services for People with Learning Disabilities*, ENABLE, Aberdeen.

Evenhuis, H.M. (1995a) Medical aspects of ageing in a population with intellectual disability. I. Visual impairment. *Journal of Intellectual Disability Research*, **39**, 19–25.

Evenhuis, H.M. (1995b) Medical aspects of ageing in a population with intellectual disability. II. Hearing impairment. *Journal of Intellectual Disability Research*, **39**, 27–33.

Eyman, R.K., Call, T.L. and White, J.F. (1989) Mortality of elderly mentally retarded persons in California. *Journal of Applied Gerontology*, **8**, 203–15.

Eyman, R.K., Call. T. and White, J.F. (1991) Life expectancy of persons with Down syndrome. *American Journal of Mental Retardation*, **95**, 603–12.

Flynn, M.C. (1988) The social environment of adults living in their own homes, in *A Place of My Own: Independence for Adults Who are Mentally Handicapped*, (ed. M.C. Flynn), Cassell, London.

Glaser, B. and Strauss, A. (1967) *The Discovery of Grounded Theory*, Aldine, Chicago.

Goode, D.A. (1988) *Quality of Life for Person with Disabilities: A Review and Synthesis of the Literature*, Mental Retardation Institute, New York.

Grampian Regional Council & Grampian Health Board (1992) *Joint Community Care Plan: 1992–1995*, Grampian Regional Council & Grampian Health Board, Aberdeen.

Grampian Regional Council & Grampian Health Board (1993) *Joint Community Care Plan: 1993–1996*, Grampian Regional Council & Grampian Health Board, Aberdeen.

Grampian Regional Council & Grampian Health Board (1994) *Joint Community Care Plan: 1994–1997*, Grampian Regional Council & Grampian Health Board, Aberdeen.

Grant, G. (1986) Older carers, interdependence and the care of mentally handicapped adults. *Ageing and Society*, **6**, 333–51.

Hogg, J. and Moss, S.C. (1994) Characteristics of older people with intellectual disabilities in England, in *International Review of Research in Mental Retardation*, **19**, 71–96, (ed. N. Bray), Academic Press, London.

Hogg, J., Moss, S.C. and Cooke, D.J. (1988) *Ageing and Mental Handicap*, Chapman & Hall, London.

Holland, A.J., Karlinsky, H. and Berg, J.M. (1993) Alzheimer disease in persons with Down syndrome: diagnostic and management considerations, in *Alzheimer Disease, Down Syndrome and Their Relationship*, (eds J.M. Berg, H. Karlinsky and A.J. Holland), Oxford University Press, Oxford.

Janicki, M.P. (ed.) (1994) *Alzheimer Disease among Persons with Mental Retardation: Report from an International Colloquium*, New York State Office of Mental Retardation and Developmental Disabilities, Albany.

Janicki, M.P., Heller,T., Seltzer, G.B. and Hogg, J. (1995) *Practice Guidelines for the Assessment and Care Management of Alzheimer and Other Dementias among Adults with Mental Retardation*, American Association on Mental Retardation, Washington DC.

Lambe, L. and Hogg, J. (1995) *Their Face to the Wind: Service Developments for Older People with Learning Disabilities in Grampian Region*. Report of a research project commissioned by ENABLE, Grampian Healthcare (NHS) Trust, Grampian Health Board and with support from the European Union as part of the European Year of Older People and Solidarity between Generations. ENABLE, Glasgow.

Laslett, P. (1989) *A Fresh Map of Life*, Weidenfeld & Nicolson, London.

Maaskant, M.A. (1993) *Mental Handicap and Ageing*, Kavanah, Dwingeloo.

Moss, S. (1994) Quality of life and aging, in *Quality of Life for Persons with Disabilities: International Perspectives and Issues*, (ed. D.Goode), Brookline Books, Cambridge, MA.

Moss, S. and Patel, P. (1992) The prevalence of mental illness in people with intellectual disability over 50 years of age and the diagnostic importance of information from carers. *Irish Journal of Psychology*, **14**, 110–29.

Mulcahy, M. and Reynolds, A. (1984) *Census of Mental Handicap in the Republic of Ireland*, Medico-Social Research Board, Dublin.

Patrick, D.L. and Erickson, P. (1993) Assessing health-related quality of life for clinical decision-making, in *Quality of Life Assessment: Key Issues in the 1990s*, (eds R.M. Rosser and S.W. Walker), Kluwer, London.

Prosser, H. (1994) *Informal Care Networks of Older Adults with Learning Disability*. MPhil thesis, Hester Adrian Research Centre, University of Manchester, Manchester.

Reboul, H., Comte, P., Jeantet, M-C. and Rio, J. (n.d.) *Les Handicapes Mentaux Vieillissant: A la recherche de solutions adaptees, individuelles, collectives*, Centre Technique National d'Etudes et de Recherches sur les Handicaps et les Inadaptations, Vanves.

Richardson, A. and Ritchie, J. (1986) *Making the Break: Parents' Views about Adults with a Mental Handicap Leaving the Parental Home*, King's Fund, London.

Richardson, A. and Ritchie, J. (1990) *Letting Go*, Open University, Milton Keynes.

Seltzer, M.M. (1992) Aging in persons with developmental disabilities, in *Handbook of Mental Health and Aging*, 2nd edn, (eds J.E. Birren, R.B. Sloane and G.D. Cohen), Academic Press, London.

Thane, P. (1989) Old age: burden or benefit? in *The Changing Population of Britain*, (ed. H. Joshi), Blackwell, Oxford.

Wieland, H. (ed.) (1987) *Geistig behinderte Menschen im Alter: Theoretische und empirische Beitrage zu ihrer Lebenssituation in der Bundesrepublik Deutschland, in Osterreich und in der Schweiz*, Ed. Schindele, Heidelberg.

Sexual rights and sexual wrongs in the lives of people with intellectual disabilities

11

Hilary Brown

INTRODUCTION

Sexuality is an important quality issue because it tests central but often disputed civil liberties whilst also being a matter of personal protection. It is at once the site of negotiation about valued roles and lifestyles *and* an arena within which extra vulnerability must be acknowledged. Many agencies now pay lip service to the rights of people with intellectual disabilities to experience and enjoy their sexuality, but recognition of abstract rights has failed to break through the barriers of prejudice and isolation by creating real opportunities for people with intellectual disabilities to live in different kinds of partnerships and family groups or to enjoy a range of sexual relationships, contacts and activities. It is often not clear whether this is because services do not know how to achieve these things on behalf of people with intellectual disabilities or because they are ambivalent about these goals. Many services have adopted a *language* of quality which minimizes difference or difficulties, suggesting that services should court 'normality' on behalf of people with intellectual disabilities, as, for example, is advocated within the ideology of social role valorization, while failing to accept that parents, carers, staff and the general public hold more conservative views (Heyman & Huckle, 1995). This idealism may have achieved some real freedoms for individuals but it has not consistently delivered 'ordinary' options in relation to sexuality and may inadvertently have 'talked down' abuses of power, for example by reframing intimidation, exploitation or manipulation as 'individual choice'.

This chapter tackles three main issues. Firstly, a discussion of issues of sexuality and gender and why these have been left out of the quality equation. Secondly, exploration of the boundary between acceptable and abusive sexual relationships in the light of recent findings about the nature and extent of sexual abuse. Lastly, suggestion of some quality standards in the area of sexuality and personal relationships, working towards a quality framework in which the prevention of exploitation is acknowledged as a significant service competence.

In relation to quality assurance methodology, readers may want to consider whether sexuality is merely another 'worked example' which can be incorporated within the dominant paradigms of 'outcome' measurement or an issue which challenges this orthodoxy. If, as I believe, it is the latter, it may be because gender and sexuality are critical identifiers which have a pervasive and overriding role in shaping people's lives (race and social class, violence, trauma and loss may well be others) and hence cannot be compartmentalized as independent and isolated 'domains'. Felce's (1996) formulation of five domains (physical well-being, material well-being, social well-being, emotional well-being and productive well-being) would all be shaped by gender and also have a 'sexuality' dimension; also each area would be jeopardized by abuse, whether sexual, physical or financial.

Moreover, sexuality challenges traditional 'one-way' scales in that the increasing acknowledgement of sexual abuse makes it clear that measuring the absence of negatives is as important as measuring the presence of positives. Hence attention to all three components of excellence identified by Donabedian (1980) – structure, process, and outcome – is needed: focusing on outcomes as a shorthand way of reviewing service performance in this area is not enough. His formulation also identifies the importance of attending to technical input, interpersonal relationships and amenities, all of which are relevant in this context, from the details of sex education which is tailored to individual need to the sexual culture within the care service, to the facilities needed to allow individuals to make choices which reflect those which ordinary people make, such as to live in partnerships or to leave their parents' household when they reach adulthood.

Because there is no social consensus about sexual values and preferences, particularly when it comes to people with intellectual disabilities (Brown, 1994), refining outcomes is inherently problematical and leaves service agencies with a set of complex ethical dilemmas and professional judgements which the system needs to be competent to address.

WHAT DO WE ALLOW 'SEXUALITY' AND 'GENDER' TO MEAN IN THE LIVES OF PEOPLE WITH INTELLECTUAL DISABILITIES?

Sexuality is a relatively new term and tends to be used to cover a whole range of preferences, characteristics and activities. Before the term was coined, sexual behaviour was considered natural and indisputable, governed by biological and religious laws; hence, same-sex relationships and acts were framed and named as 'unnatural' as well as 'immoral' in many societies (Weeks, 1989). The emergence of a term which encapsulates sexual behaviour as a site of personal and sometimes political identity broke new ground and it is now widely used to include issues of gender, sexual attraction and orientation, sexual behaviour(s) and lifestyle, relationships and partnerships, image and projection of self through clothes and style and, as a summary term, to encapsulate how an individual presents, disguises or conceals these aspects of themselves from others. Sexuality is no longer seen as a fixed commodity but a compromise and interrelationship between personal inclination and changing social rules, rules which vary according to gender and status and which have to be negotiated and reconstructed for each generation and social group. Thus there is no 'normal' sexuality for people with intellectual disabilities. There are going to be sexualities conditioned by the particular physical and emotional cultures which characterize institutional life in hospitals and special schools or which are allowed to emerge in group homes. Sexual options and identities for many people with intellectual disabilities are constricted by the fact that many adults with intellectual disabilities do not leave their parental home and by the generally conservative attitudes of their carers (Heyman & Huckle, 1995). Furthermore, sexual feelings may be coloured by being on the receiving end of personal care into adolescence and adulthood.

Hudson & Jacot (1991, p21) suggested that there are four separate 'layers or levels of sex and gender':

1. biology;
2. gender identity;
3. object choice (i.e. choice of partners);
4. presentation of self.

People with intellectual disabilities may face special challenges in relation to each set of issues although it is arguable that, given the abnormal conditions of their lives, they meet these challenges at least as well as other people. In terms of biology, specific syndromes and aetiologies may have consequences for individuals in terms of fertility or sexual development; for example, women with spina bifida often start their periods unusually early and men with Down syndrome are usually infertile. But personal histories, social and environmental factors are likely to have an equal or greater impact in shaping the options open to most individuals. In terms of childhood development, processes of identification may be interrupted (Brown, 1991) as children with intellectual disabilities, especially those who have additional medical problems, are often separated from their familiar surroundings by prolonged stays in hospital or residential schooling. Their 'object choice' and patterns of attraction and arousal may be limited or distorted by the pervasive valuing of non-handicapped people over other potential partners (Griffiths, Quinsey & Hinsburger, 1989) and by the importance of 'staff' in their lives. Staff have a peculiarly ambiguous relationship in that they are paid to be intimate with clients and may give blurred messages about the extent and degree of their involvement (Thompson, Clare & Brown, in press). When it comes to self-image many people with intellectual disabilities do not have options for managing the way they present themselves to others on account of poverty as well as, and possibly more than, any visible disabilities they might have (Davis, Murray & Flynn, 1992; Stone, 1995). People with intellectual disabilities clearly have a struggle to overcome externally imposed barriers, to reach and then assert preferences and then to implement their choices.

Because sexuality includes all these facets, it is no longer possible to short circuit a discussion about sex in the lives of people with intellectual disabilities on the basis that they are *sexless*. The social meanings attached to their sexual behaviours and feelings, both as they are experienced by men and women with intellectual disabilities themselves and as they are responded to and reflected back by care givers, are still very much a matter of contention. Despite the clarity of social role valorization *theory*, practice has lagged behind in relation to gender and sexuality and several writers have suggested that sexuality tests the commitment to integration more than other issues (Brown, 1994; Clements, Clare & Ezelle, 1995; Giami, 1987). An implicit agenda of regulation and control of sexuality can often be seen to operate in contradiction to espoused normative values and aspirations. This tends to be expressed in terms of avoiding pregnancy and of avoiding sexual abuse/assault, the latter both on the grounds that people with intellectual disabilities need to be protected from the public and vice-versa. But the control/protection agenda often extends to the exclusion of people with intellectual disabilities from conventional gender roles.

Although services for people with intellectual disabilities have strenuously examined the values base for the work they do, neither the early formulations of normalization nor later frameworks such as O'Brien's (1986) five accomplishments made explicit the importance of gender as a key determinant of either the individual's own aspirations or the aspirations that services might have on their behalf. Services are often silent about the extent to which the values they espouse reflect, challenge or ignore the gendered assumptions which govern the way that roles at work, at home and in the wider community are shaped. While people with intellectual disabilities are excluded from mainstream gendered expectations the issue of interaction is not problematical for the community at large. Gender tends to constitute a boundary which keeps people with intellectual disabilities apart.

Moreover, gender is even more influential in structuring life experiences than sexual orientation or activity and the fact that services do not even aspire to, let alone achieve, typical gender roles and relationships fundamentally undermines attempts to establish valued social roles and relationships, as Clements, Clare & Ezelle (1995) comment:

> ... there is a high cost to be paid if a person is perceived as gender free in a gendered world. Core experiences may be denied, needs will be misunderstood and dominant but damaging value systems will be imposed ...
>
> (p426)

Chenoweth (1993) echoes this vacuum for women with intellectual disabilities who face 'double' discrimination:

> The oppression of women with disabilities goes beyond that of other women in that even female roles with some value attached which are ascribed to women in our culture ... are not readily accorded to women with disabilities. If she misses out on the wife, mother, career woman, lover, nurturer aspects of being a woman there is little left to accord her even humanness.
>
> (p26–7)

This lack of awareness leads to people living in very untypical groups and circumstances, with adults of the opposite sex who are neither family, friends nor lovers (Brown, 1994, p40). Men and women with intellectual disabilities are 'handicapped' by the lack of differentiation in their roles and by services which adopt a gender-blind approach to service design and delivery. People with intellectual disabilities who are dependent on services may interpret the absence of clear gender distinctions as a put-down when compared to the real world of their families and communities and the hierarchical structures of the services in which they live and work. Hence, people with intellectual disabilities internalize the asexual assumptions behind most service-led lifestyles. Their failure to make demands on the system for more appropriate and adult options cannot be read as satisfaction. As Felce & Perry (1995) remark:

> ... it is impossible to divorce expressions of satisfaction from their context ... satisfaction is a personal assessment, the frame of reference is personal and affected by experience and the judgement of what is possible and typical for a person in one's situation.
>
> (p56–77)

The authors argue that objective assessment or measures are necessary to guard against low or atypical expectations, but outcome measures are problematical as an alternative. Civil liberties may provide an external framework which is more sensitive to variation in values and sexual preference. Evidence suggests that people with intellectual disabilities marry less often than their non-disabled peers and have fewer children.

But should these be the benchmarks? Although the early normalization model took for granted an exclusively heterosexual model, society's values are constantly changing and in conflict. Both heterosexual and homosexual options are made available conditionally to people within our society and individuals are subject to legal sanctions and social structures which narrow their options. These include housing or service provision and benefits, the lack of communal child care facilities, the availability of information and images, all of which enforce assumptions about whom one is supposed to have sex with, live with, financially support and/or share children with. Same-sex relationships, for example, have only been decriminalized in the United Kingdom for 25 years and gay men and lesbians still struggle against prejudice and invisibility (for example, see Cambridge (1994) for a consideration of these issues as they affect men with intellectual disabilities who have sex with men). Where people with intellectual disabilities choose same-sex relationships or activities they are rarely helped to adopt an accepted identity. Hence, all people with intellectual disabilities are subject to generic prohibitions which link sexual relationships to economic independence as well as to special pressures which bar them from assuming adult roles on account of their status as disabled people (Burns, 1993).

Ambivalence can be dangerous. It leads to same-sex relationships being driven underground and devalued at a time when clear and explicit support is needed. Men with intellectual disabilities who have sex with men often lack access to basic safer sex messages or to images and language which would enable them to describe or reflect on their preference and experiences. Whether straight or gay, the challenge for people with intellectual disabilities is that there remains an assumption that they *should* be asexual and ungendered. If they resist this, by taking on ordinary roles or attributes, or develop and project an openly gay or lesbian identity, these are not responded to positively as they are seen to be inappropriate behaviours or roles *for a person with disabilities*. Clarity of purpose is usually held to be a prerequisite of quality assurance (see, for example, Berwick, 1989) but it is far from established in relation to sexual issues.

TAKING SEXUAL ABUSE INTO ACCOUNT

Despite the lack of uniform values or aspirations there are core commitments which can underpin a consistent approach to sexual issues and which emphasize the service's responsibility to assess, whether formally or informally, an individual's capacity to consent in a given situation. Definitions of sexual abuse (Brown & Turk, 1992) rest on an understanding of unequal power and its misuse: men feature predominantly as perpetrators in studies of adults with intellectual disabilities (Turk & Brown,

1993), of children (Finkelhor *et al.*, 1990) and of adults in the general population (Russell, 1986). Women feature predominantly as victims in all these groups despite an increasingly acknowledged minority of male victims (Watkins & Bentovim, 1992). The presence of sexual abuse in community services was initially denied but it's emergence can be seen positively, in that it reflects the fact that people with intellectual disabilities are beginning to speak out about their experiences and to have the confidence to discriminate between those sexual encounters which they want and those which they do not.

Any sexual behaviours, whether they involve direct contact or not, can be abusive in the absence of valid consent or in the prescence of force or intimidation. Even non-contact abuse such as voyeurism, involvement in pornography, indecent exposure, harassment, serious teasing or innuendo can be experienced as seriously abusive, especially if they take place in a threatening atmosphere. We usually think of abuse as acts done by the abuser to the person who is abused, but sometimes they involve situations where the abuser forces or persuades the abused person to do things to them. The act(s) might have happened once only or be part of an ongoing sexual relationship.

Acts may be abusive even though they are not strictly speaking illegal. Current (United Kingdom) legislation fails to take the power dynamics which exist in ongoing authority relationships into account, treating each act as a separate assault rather than as part of a long-standing pattern. In authority relationships it is very difficult for a person with an intellectual disability to challenge what they are asked to do. If you are dependent on others and if you have been encouraged throughout your life to be compliant and to be 'good', then you are not really in a position to assert yourself around sexual matters.

People with intellectual disabilities are very much at the mercy of staff even when those staff are acting in their best interests (McGill & Emerson, 1992). If workers turn the relationship around and use it to abuse, their power and control make it very difficult for people with intellectual disabilities to challenge what is being done to them.

Because capacity to consent and misuse of power are both crucial issues in determining whether a particular act, relationship or situation is abusive for the person concerned, identifying the individual's IQ is not in itself sufficient. Determining whether a given individual possesses the ability to consent or not to sexual activities or relationships is complex. There are two approaches. A *diagnostic* or *status* test makes a blanket ruling about people with a certain degree of intellectual impairment such as the legal provision contained in the United Kingdom Sexual Offences Act 1956 (Gunn, 1989) which deems *all* people with severe intellectual disabilities to be unable to give consent. The other approach involves a *functional* test which is more specific to the decision being taken and which extends to the circumstances and dynamics which surround the sexual activity or relationship (Murphy & Clare, 1995).

As a shorthand formulation there are three issues (see Brown & Turk, 1992):

1. whether the person *did* give their consent because if they did not they have been raped or assaulted like any other person;
2. whether the person *could* give their consent, that is, if they understood enough about sexual behaviour and knew what was happening;
3. a judgement has to be made as to whether the person with intellectual disabilities was under undue pressure in this particular situation, for example, due to an authority or care-giving relationship, such as might be the case if sex is initiated by a staff or family member or where force, trickery or exploitation is used. Physical force or the threat of violence or reprisals also cuts across any meaningful consent.

These need to be dealt with as discrete stages, because abuse occurs when any, not all of these conditions apply. Brown & Turk (1992) suggest that because the law specifies a distinction between people with severe intellectual impairments and those with milder degrees of disability, it would be wise for services to have a view about the capacity of individual service users who engage in sexual activities. Where people with severe intellectual disabilities have mutual relationships the service should satisfy itself of (and be prepared to defend) the reciprocity of acts or relationships. However, if people have mild learning difficulties, the service should only intervene if it has reason to believe that the person is being exploited or threatened. In fact, services often opt out, taking a *laissez-faire* stance to all service users regardless of their ability to understand risk or to protect themselves within unequal relationships.

Making judgements about other people's quality of life is a notoriously precarious business. Whether making judgements about informal matters, such as where people should live or who they mix with or what degree of activity they engage in, or making decisions of a more serious nature, such as whether to support a woman seeking an abortion, the value base from which one is operating is critical. As English law (Law Commission, 1995) struggles to come to terms with some of the contexts within which such decisions have to be made it is worth articulating the basis on which legal decisions are framed. Historically these have been twofold:

1. substitute decision making;
2. best interests.

The first acknowledges that individuals may want to live eccentric lifestyles, to make decisions which do not make sense to others but do make sense for them: the second works on the basis of what can only be termed 'enlightened paternalism'. When discussing issues of sexuality both notions are helpful. We need firstly to be mindful of the fact that individuals want different things and set parameters within which they should be empowered to make their own decisions, but sometimes, when they are not able to choose, when their actions hurt others or when they seem to others to be being exploited, there is a case for intervening in someone's best interests. Knowing when that point has been reached is not easy.

The new legislation proposed by the English Law Commission (1995) suggests that acting in someone's best interests ought to encompass the former kind of decisions, because acknowledging individuality is automatically in someone's best interests, but when it comes to sexuality and sexual decisions making, services may not be very skilled at making such judgements. The evidence is that services hang back, choosing not to do anything rather than to take explicit actions, based on explicit values or decisions. They may often avoid harm by not acting, but increasingly services are having to face up to the fact that their non-involvement in the sexual lives of the people they serve masks and sometimes causes problems. This is particularly the case when it comes to sexual abuse, sexual risk taking and abuse of others.

Fortunately, more is now known about the incidence of sexual (and other) abuses and abusing and this can be taken into account in designing quality assurance systems (see, for example, Brown, Stein & Turk, 1995; Chenoweth, 1993; Sobsey & Doe, 1991). Despite the problems of getting accurate information about such a hidden phenomenon, these and other studies have helped to identify patterns of sexual abuse involving adults with intellectual disabilities and the emerging picture is not unlike that which has been uncovered by those working in the field of child sexual abuse. The most common risks are not of 'stranger danger' in public places, but of assault or ongoing sexual abuse by a member of the person's own network. In a recent United Kingdom incidence study of reported abuse (Brown, Stein & Turk, 1995) the sexual abuse happened most often in the victim's or perpetrator's home or in their day placement.

Almost all the perpetrators were men and many had worked their way into positions of trust, either through employment or voluntary involvement in services or by establishing themselves as friends of the family. Thus they had legitimate access to vulnerable people and could often justify being alone with the person they had abused or were in a role which led them to be offering intimate care behind closed doors. However, men with intellectual disabilities formed the largest group of perpetrators reported: this may reflect their lack of sophistication in being able to keep abuse a secret, but it certainly represents a serious issue for services. Sometimes these were other people attending a day service or living in a hostel or group home or people who had used those services in the past.

Mostly these reports concerned serious sexual assaults or unconsenting sex, with almost two-thirds mentioning rape or attempted penetration, and at least half took place within ongoing abusive relationships. Just over half of those abused were women although in the two surveys undertaken the proportion of male victims reported rose from a quarter in 1989–90 to nearly a half in 1991–2. Adults of all ages and disability levels were reported as victims of sexual abuse. In a significant minority of cases the perpetrator had abused more than one person, making it very important, when allegations are made, to be sensitive to the fact that others may have been subjected to similar abuse or be at risk in the future.

WHAT DOES A SERVICE WHICH 'GETS IT RIGHT' LOOK LIKE?

It is clear that quality assurance activities need to address both positive sexual options and the protection of people with intellectual disabilities from abuse and that these are equally important and interlocking agendas.

PROTECTING RIGHTS

Despite the trend towards measurement of outcomes, sexuality may require an alternative focus. Because sexual preferences are so varied and personal, it would seem to make more sense to evaluate services in more traditional terms, using service inputs and indicators of process. Commissioners of services need to reinstate gender and sexuality as key issues in both service design and placement groupings. Sexual partnerships and choice need to be reflected in the options available. Support needs to be available to couples as well as to individuals, without the assumption that independence and autonomy are prerequisites to sexual relationships. Some single-sex services should be available for those who choose them and for those who need them. Support should also be available to people with intellectual disabilities who take on valued and ordinary roles, such as becoming carers or parents. They often do so against the odds and with a backdrop of poverty, prejudice and damaging expectations (Tymchuk, 1992; Walmsley, 1993).

A range of specialist help should be available, either through disability services which specialize in sexuality and relationship issues or through agencies which offer treatment, support and intervention to members of the general public and who are willing to develop expertise in working with people with intellectual disabilities. These arrangements all require planning and productive collaboration. Simpson (1994) found that most generic agencies were not prepared or skilled enough to offer services to people with intellectual disabilities. Moreover, fragmented service contracts tend not to build in or cost the development which would make

Table 11.1 Service inputs to support positive sexual options for people with intellectual disabilities

- Specialist one-to-one and group sex education
- Materials to support specialized education and counselling
- Facilitated women's and men's groups
- Training for sex educators
- Safer sex education for men and women, but especially for men who have sex with men
- HIV testing and counselling
- Contraceptive services for men and for women
- Sexual health and well-women and well-men clinics
- Staff training for direct support staff on personal care, sexuality and sexual rights
- Written policies and guidance for all staff
- Services for parents with intellectual disabilities

these services work. The services often fall between two stools, needing both pump-priming funding and a 'stand-by' element. Paying for service on an *ad hoc* basis may not be viable. In the United Kingdom there are several nationally recognized counselling services for people with intellectual disabilities but people living outside the capital tend not to have access to local services and while care managers may identify funding for individuals, regional planning has not been consistent. Table 11.1 sets out the range of services which should be available to support a range of positive options.

PREVENTING ABUSE

In relation to abuse, quality assurance systems must be built into individual agencies and service systems to provide an adequate level of safety to people with intellectual disabilities. There are several 'models' of protection which have been proposed in the face of the pattern of risk which has emerged (Senn, 1989). It is not realistic to suggest that any system will ensure that staff or people with intellectual disabilities will never abuse service users but it is possible to 'lower the odds' against the likelihood of abuse occurring or recurring and to expect agencies to work towards that end (ARC/NAPSAC, 1993, para 41).

Broadly there are four interlocking approaches to the issue of prevention. The services responsible can:

1. help potential 'victims' to become more assertive and able to resist sexual activities which they do not want;
2. screen out potential abusers from coming into contact with vulnerable adults;
3. stipulate and build up good practice in the area of sexuality supported by clear and unambiguous guidance to front-line staff;

4. focus on identifying abuse and acting to stop it recurring with this or any other victim. Given the propensity for abuse to be ongoing and/or to involve a series of victims, failure to report and confront abuse can be seen as a failure to prevent as well as to respond.

Compliance and communication difficulties make people with intellectual disabilities into relatively 'safe' victims and overcoming this relies on skills as well as structures. Sex education (Craft *et al.*, 1991; McCarthy & Thompson, 1993) is a prerequisite in helping individuals acquire a language to use in discussing sexual issues but is also necessary in questioning assumptions and assessing personal options. There is often confusion about how to help people acquire sexual knowledge. One major issue which needs to be resolved is for services to decide who is best placed in people's lives to teach these skills and also what are appropriate aspirations for the individual in terms of partnerships and experiences. Moreover, this must be settled within the new evolving structures with its purchaser and provider split, so that both funding and delivering agencies have to play their part in making such a service consistently available.

However, people with intellectual disabilities do find it especially difficult to get hold of accurate and unbiased information and this is best tackled through structured and explicit sex education programmes in many services. The curriculum might cover issues such as:

- naming body parts and noting which can be shown in public and which kept private;
- good and bad touch;
- appropriate sexual language;
- masturbation;
- relationships with the opposite sex;
- same-sex relationships;
- contraception and safer sex;
- parenthood;
- menstrual hygiene;
- menopause and other sexual health issues;
- assertiveness: when and how to say 'yes' and 'no';
- sexual abuse;
- appropriate behaviour in public.

There is no such thing as a standard curriculum as people vary so much. For some people the aim might be to help them understand safer sexual practices while for others a more limited goal of helping them to behave appropriately in public would be set.

Materials have been developed to cover the main points for people with both mild and severe intellectual disabilities and these often include explicit pictures. Many services have policies which say that porno-graphy should not be introduced into such programmes, because although some might argue that it is educational, there is often an under-lying inequality about the 'poses' and imagery which is not appropriate.

Staff training and support are important in enabling and legitimating sex education in day and residential services and ensuring good staff role models. Knowledge of appropriate behaviour will also enable service users to avoid putting themselves 'in the wrong' by being clear about boundaries, consent, private places and sexual acts and those who have crossed acceptable limits will be able to use it as a way of addressing and changing their attitudes and behaviours.

A dichotomy between positive or 'ordinary' sex education and educa-tion for the prevention of abuse tends to be untenable in practice as coun-sellors and educators will have to engage with the reality of service users' sexual lives and the very real possibility of disclosures of abuse in the context of their work. Thompson & McCarthy (1992) describe one service in which one-to-one counselling is offered to people thought to be engag-ing in high-risk activities. What is clear from the accounts of sex given within this setting is the pervasiveness of abusive encounters and the necessary blurring of the boundary between education for safer sex and for the prevention of sexual abuse. As the authors comment:

> Women in the project are reported as having little control; sex is some-thing the women do for men with no concept of their own sexual pleas-ure; they regularly endure sexual acts that are painful and distressing.
>
> (p8)

Meanwhile a number of men referred to the project for 'cottaging' (having sex with men in public toilets) are also reported as being the vic-tims of exploitative behaviour:

> Almost exclusively they are penetrated ... they aren't choosing ... it just happens that way without any understanding. The anal sex hurts although they are unable to do anything about it apart from 'take the pain' or 'wait till he finishes'.
>
> (p9)

What becomes clear from these first-hand accounts is the use and abuse of power in both service settings and in the sexual contacts which people with intellectual disabilities have with members of the public. In the face of this, the project advocates a more interventionist approach to protect people from high-risk or abusive sex when they are unable to take steps to protect themselves.

Even where people are able to articulate what they want, they are not always able to meet outside, and independently of, service systems. Self-advocacy groups or women's and men's groups do go some way to redressing the powerlessness of people with intellectual disabilities within their own services. For those with severe intellectual disabilities this can be achieved by the presence of independent advocates or front-line staff who are empowered to stand up for them. It would be naive to assume that people with intellectual disabilities can use generic complaints systems without help or to overstate the rhetoric of empowerment in the face of the enormous impact of threats from or promises to those on whom one depends and/or is afraid of (Lukes 1982; Wood, 1995).

Another route towards protection has been the renewed call for screening/registering of staff and volunteers who are legitimated to come into intimate contact with people with intellectual disabilities, harking back to days when caring for people with disabilities was, however unsafely, assumed to be regulated by professional registration and adherence to agreed standards. Calls for better practice in recruitment were made in relation to children's services (Warner, 1992), and these are reiterated in national guidance (ARC/NAPSAC, 1993). This would include the need to take up references, to balance good equal opportunities procedures and practice with probing interviews (Brown, 1991) and to avoid the use of short-term agency staff.

INTERLOCKING POLICIES AND GUIDANCE

Services in the United Kingdom have variously developed guidelines on sexuality concerning people with intellectual disabilities, on sexual abuse for this client group and/or on all abuse of vulnerable adults (in which procedures apply to other kinds of abuse such as financial exploitation, physical or psychological abuse or neglect and concern other groups such as older people or people with mental health problems who may also need this level of protection). This kind of guidance has been in operation since the early 1980s but has recently been redrawn in many agencies to take account of the purchaser/provider split in the United Kingdom service structures necessitating these policies to be enshrined in contracts and assured through contract compliance, inspection and regulation (Brown, 1996; Brown et al., 1996).

Good practice in relation to sexuality has focused on the development of written guidance outlining consistent approaches from direct care staff designed to reduce both the leeway staff have to act as lone agents in relation to sexual issues and the consequent stress of role ambiguity or role conflicts (Booth & Booth, 1992; Craft & Brown, 1994). Without a clear framework staff find it hard to act. Guidance also is beginning to set parameters around intimate care. People First (a prominent United Kingdom users' network) women's committee have made it clear that women with intellectual disabilities do not want to be given care by male staff, but small units find the logistics of this problematic. Policies on sexual abuse (see, for example, ARC/NAPSAC, 1993; Greenwich SS & Greenwich HA, 1992; Wiltshire CC SS, 1992) focus particularly on the importance of identifying current abuse and reporting it through official channels, so that support services can be accessed for the person who has been victimized and sanctions (or in the case of other service users who abuse, intervention) instituted against the perpetrator.

Written policies and procedures are poor predictors of service action (see, for example, Brown, Hunt & Stein, 1994; Conroy & Feinstein, 1990) but they are probably a necessary, while not sufficient, condition for coherence towards sexuality issues. Certainly they provide a useful starting point when evaluating the service culture (Mansell, 1986) in relation to sexuality and may also provide an important measure of interagency collaboration, service openness and accountability. Routes for referral and consultation should be evident in such policies, ensuring that people with intellectual disabilities are not denied assistance in their sexual lives nor confined to 'closed' systems. Without a 'money where your mouth is' commitment, direct care staff are left in a double bind in that espoused values and acceptance of risk leave them 'damned if they do' support service users in achieving their sexual aspirations, but also 'damned if they don't'.

Management in abusive regimes tends to focus on 'keeping the lid' on things (Wardhaugh & Wilding, 1993). Supporting people with disabilities around sexual issues is inevitably making visible an issue which could more easily be swept under the carpet so that mechanisms for delivering appropriate management involvement and support are critical.

> Policy is built up of fine words but the reality of what is provided for these groups denies their truth. The work is wrapped round with high-sounding terms ... but the resources and facilities made available convey to staff the low value which society puts upon their work and upon their clients. Official aspirations and standards are therefore deprived of legitimacy.
>
> (Wardhaugh & Wilding, 1993, p14)

With this in mind the functions of policy and guidelines in relation to sexual rights are:

1. to make explicit the service's commitment to uphold the sexual rights of service users, bearing in mind the often conflicting views of parents and carers. This needs to be very clearly stated to enable full advocacy on behalf of service users and to prevent individual staff imposing their own sexual attitudes and values on service users;
2. to inform staff about sexual health and local service provision;
3. to inform staff about cultural diversity in relation to sexual values and behaviours;

4. to legitimate sexuality as an area of professional concern and intervention, particularly because for any kind of sex education or counselling to be effective it has to be explicit and unambiguous;
5. to stipulate where (i.e. at what level and in which part of the service system or agency) decisions will be made and resources or expertise accessed.

In relation to sexual abuse, policy needs to fulfil the following additional functions:

1. to establish clear boundaries between the separate professional roles;
2. to develop clear and often mandatory procedures on what to do when a person with an intellectual disability discloses abuse. This prevents one individual or one part of the service from keeping abuse a 'secret' or dealing with it informally, for instance by letting an abusing member of staff resign. Such procedures aim to minimize the chance of further abuse to or by the individuals involved;
3. to suggest how to respond to the abused person after their disclosure, by accessing appropriate treatment and support services for them as they recover and assisting them throughout the process of bringing their complaint to court or to a disciplinary or other tribunal;
4. to indicate how to deal with the abuser following the victim's disclosure, including the procedure for responding to other service users who have abused or to staff members. Again, this may involve accessing appropriate services and support.

Policies aim to protect and support staff by making their responsibilities clear, for example their 'duty to report', but also setting out the limitations of their role, for example in preventing them from playing the amateur sleuth which might get in the way of an official enquiry or police investigation. In many areas policies have established a single referral point (often a multidisciplinary team) for all allegations of sexual abuse involving adults with intellectual disabilities. They may also have laid down guidance as to where and how decisions are to be taken, for example at a case conference or planning or strategy meeting, and may stipulate how long may elapse between the disclosure or complaint and the calling of such a conference. Again a range of service inputs is required to ensure that people who have been abused receive prompt support and treatment. The investigation is only one strand in a response which has to balance therapeutic and evidential requirements.

It can be seen that in relation to sexuality, evidence of good practice cannot in itself provide a guarantee against habitual abusers. Good practice therefore has to incorporate measures which acknowledge the possibility that individuals will abuse and that people with intellectual disabilities are vulnerable to sexual exploitation by virtue of their lack of

Table 11.2 Service inputs to prevent and respond to the sexual abuse of people with intellectual disabilities

- Recruitment processes which effectively screen staff and volunteers for evidence of past convictions or dismissals
- Materials which support disclosure and sensitive interviewing
- Written policies setting out how and where to report concerns or allegations
- Support for 'whistleblowers'
- Interagency agreements about roles and communication in response to alleged abuse
- Interagency collaboration to fund the development of these service options
- Services for people with intellectual disabilities who have abusive behaviours towards others
- Secure placements for people with intellectual disabilities who abuse others
- Alternative placements for people who have been victims of sexual assault or abuse
- Specialist treatment and counselling for people with intellectual disabilities who have been victims of sexual assault or abuse
- Training for professional staff responsible for investigating allegations
- Capacity to use mental health and guardianship legislation where this affords individuals needed security and protection
- Access to mainstream sex-offender programmes for sex offenders with intellectual disabilities
- Capability to monitor incidence of sexual abuse and usage of sexual health services

knowledge or power. Standard setting tends to operate on a unidimensional model with all the tension focused on whether minimum or target standards are being met but abuse (especially sexual abuse*) can occur out of this field of vision, in an otherwise competent service. Certainly it is helpful for written guidance to distinguish between:

- absolute disciplinary offences such as having any sexual contact with a client;
- reference points such as same-sex care where exceptions would need to be justified and approved;
- aspirations such as empowerment and appropriate risk taking.

Quality assurance in this field has, to some extent, to evaluate the service culture (Mansell, 1986) as well as the working structures and decision-making mechanisms (see Table 11.3). Wardhaugh & Wilding (1993) describe the 'neutralization of normal moral concerns' (p6) in abusive regimes characterized by distancing and depersonalization. Hence a service which takes this responsibility seriously is likely to be characterized by:

* Other kinds of abuse are much more likely to be systemic than sexual abuse, which does seem to be located in individual pathology.

- clear guidance for staff;
- careful assessment of capacity;
- planned interventions such as sex education and advocacy;
- individual personalized and not 'batch' decisions;
- shared and open decision making;
- good recording and individual planning;
- dignity and maturity in discussion of sexual matters (Brown, 1996).

Table 11.3 Indicators of good practice (adapted from Brown, 1996)

Generally speaking, in sensitive services:
- front-line staff will talk respectfully about sexual matters and relationships: service users' feelings will not be trivialized or their appearance made fun of
- intimate care will be offered usually by staff of the same sex
- a balance between privacy and openness will be sought in the way care is offered: for example, bathroom doors will be closed, but other staff will be around and aware of who is with a particular service user
- staff will be able to acknowledge and manage a certain amount of 'difficult' sexual behaviour such as masturbation in public areas, without taking a blaming or 'smutty' attitude
- some staff, under supervision from senior staff and/or after further training, will be able to run sex education sessions with small groups or individuals and appropriate materials will be available
- the rights of service users to have consenting sexual relationships will be respected and actively supported, whether these are heterosexual or homosexual. Sometimes this will necessitate sensitive consultation with parents, especially where people with intellectual disabilities continue to live at home into adulthood
- staff will know that service users with severe intellectual disabilities are deemed, in law, not to be able to give consent to sexual acts and will interpret this sensitively. Where uncertainties arise there should be consultation between the provider, care manager, relatives or advocates and relevant professionals in order to arrive at a shared decision
- individual and not 'blanket' decisions will be made about such issues as oral contraception and sex education
- all service users will have access to adequate health care, including attention to sexual health issues; this should include screening and access to the same range of treatments and interventions as other people of their age and gender
- staff will intervene to prevent abusive, non-consenting, exploitative or violent relationships between service users and will recognize that sex in the context of a family, caretaking or other markedly unequal relationship is an abuse of power
- staff and volunteers will be clear that they should not themselves have sex with service users because of their authority/power
- staff meetings will demonstrate that the staff team can discuss sexual issues in a professional way
- written guidance for all staff will be available reflecting these principles; individual records and care plans will show that sexual behaviour is being addressed properly
- relationships within the staff team itself will provide a good model for service users: there will not be sexual harassment or teasing between staff or lack of respect between women and men workers

WEIGHING UP THE ISSUES

Once we begin to acknowledge the importance of gender issues for service users and staff, a new and rather different agenda for quality assurance emerges. It becomes important to ask people with intellectual disabilities specifically about their aspirations in more gendered terms and to offer a wider range of activities and experiences, which enable them to both occupy and then, if they want to, to challenge the sexualized spaces which are so central to personal and community life. We need to explore ways of offering segregated space for women and men, so that they can be safe and develop a stronger sense of themselves.

Current measures tend to be gender, sexuality and abuse 'blind'. Gender is not mentioned as a defining characteristic which might weight the way items are read; for example, on several scales unemployment automatically leads to a low score for both men and women although, despite increasing trends for women to work, the role of unpaid home-maker might be a preferred option for some women with intellectual disabilities. In relation to abuse, 'measurement' raises two distinct issues. The first is its covert nature and the second is how best to evaluate its impact on and in people's lives. Would two members of staff necessarily *know* if an individual is being coerced or abused and how accurately might they assess signals of post-traumatic distress? There is encouraging evidence in the UK study reported above (Brown, Stein & Turk, 1995) that abuse awareness training does increase the likelihood that staff will recognize signals of distress and trauma and begin to name abuse as one factor in the development of emotional disturbance or challenging behaviours. This raises the issue of how to 'weight' issues of abuse in quality assurance programmes, how to balance 'positives' against the negative and oppressive impact of emotional, physical or sexual violence. High material standards do not mitigate the effects of abuse. Discrete domains identified in quality of life measures (see, for example, Keith, Schalock & Hoffman, 1986) may each need to be sensitive to abuse and its consequences. Abuse may lead to depressed scores on these measures, but its covert nature may also lead to 'false positives'. Recent reformulations (Rapley & Lobley, 1995; Schalock & Keith, 1993; Schalock, Keith & Hoffman, 1990), which have an emphasis on subjective as well as objective measures, are more likely to detect and reflect abusive situations although neither sex, gender nor abuse is directly addressed in these scales.

Approaches to quality assurance illustrated in this volume demonstrate the need for innovative bridges between quantitative and qualitative measures. Abuse is more likely to be uncovered by qualitative approaches, such as focus groups or quality circles, as these are not structured to avoid the unanticipated. Consumer satisfaction surveys are increasingly being used alongside observational data and biographical data are being used to give a longer term perspective (Walmsley, 1993). Conroy & Feinstein (1990) argue for 'both process and outcome components'.

In relation to sexual abuse one concrete measure which can be routinely monitored and learned from is the level of reporting, since underreporting is acknowledged in all client groups. Discrepancies are clear between studies which ask people with intellectual disabilities directly about abuse they have experienced and information obtained from their carers or service managers (Brown, 1994). Increased levels of reporting may be read as one indicator of service competence in recognition (without which support cannot be offered). But policies and written guidance should also be taken as evidence that the service is alert to the possibility of abuse and prepared to offer help to people who have been abused. Usage of these systems and proper record keeping should also be monitored.

Evaluating quality in this area involves consideration of undifferentiated or absent gender roles, covert phenomena such as bullying or abuse and the occasional but deliberate perversion of quality and regulatory procedures by stakeholders, whose stake is far from altruistic. A service's willingness to uphold the civil and sexual rights of individuals with intellectual disabilities should sit alongside their alertness to issues of sexual and other abuse(s) and their readiness to co-ordinate an appropriate response. Without this commitment services may achieve minimum standards and even enhance many areas of the lives of people with intellectual disabilities, but still leave them open to exploitation. Quality without safety never was, and certainly can no longer be considered, a just option.

REFERENCES

ARC/NAPSAC (1993) *It Could Never Happen Here: The Prevention and Treatment of Sexual Abuse of Adults with Learning Disabilities in Residential Settings*, ARC, Chesterfield.

Berwick, D. (1989) Continuous improvement as an ideal in health care. *New England Journal of Medicine*, **30**, 53–5.

Booth, T. and Booth, W. (1992) Practice in sexuality. *Mental Handicap*, **20**, 64–9.

Brown, H. (1991) Working with staff around sexuality and power, in *Psychotherapy and Mental Handicap*, (eds A. Waitman and S. Conboy-Hill), Sage, London.

Brown, H. (1994) Lost in the system: acknowledging the sexual abuse of adults with learning disabilities. *Care in Place*, **1**, 145–57.

Brown, H. (1996) *Towards Safer Commissioning: A Handbook on the Sexual Abuse of Adults with Learning Disabilities for Purchasers and Commissioners*, NAPSAC/Pavilion, Brighton.

Brown, H. and Turk, V. (1992) Defining sexual abuse as it affects adults with learning disabilities. *Mental Handicap*, **20, 44**–55.

Brown, H., Hunt, N. and Stein, J. (1994) 'Alarming but very necessary': working with staff groups around the sexual abuse of adults with learning disabilities. *Journal of Intellectual Disability Research*, **38**, 393–412.

Brown, H., Stein, J. and Turk, V. (1995) Report of a second two year incidence survey on the reported abuse of adults with learning disabilities, 1991 and 1992. *Mental Handicap Research*, **8**, 1–22.

Brown, H., Brammer, A., Craft A. and McKay, C. (1996) *Towards Better Safeguards: A Handbook on the Sexual Abuse of Adults with Learning for Inspectors and Registration Officers*, NAPSAC/ Pavilion, Brighton.

Burns, J. (1993) Invisible women – women who have learning disabilities. *The Psychologist: Bulletin of the British Psychological Society*, **6**, 102–5.

Cambridge, P. (1994) A practice and policy agenda for HIV and learning disability. *British Journal of Learning Disabilities*, **22**, 134–9.

Chenoweth, L. (1993) Invisible acts: violence against women with disabilities. *Australian Disability Review*, **2**, 22–7.

Clements, J., Clare, I.C.H. and Ezelle, L.A. (1995) Real men, real women, real lives? Gender issues in learning disabilities and challenging behaviour. *Disability and Society*, **10**, 425–37.

Conroy, J. and Feinstein, C. (1990) A new way of thinking about quality, in *Quality Assurance for Individuals with Developmental Disabilities*, (eds V. Bradley and H. Bersani), Brookes, New York.

Craft, A. and Brown, H. (1994) Personal relationships and sexuality: the staff role, in *Practice Issues in Sexuality and Learning Disabilities*, (ed. A. Craft), Routledge, London.

Craft, A. and members of the Nottinghamshire Sex Education Project (1991) *Living Your Life*, LDA, Cambridge.

Davis, A.M., Murray, J. and Flynn, M. (1992) *The Financial Circumstances of People with Learning Disabilities*. Paper submitted to the House of Commons Select Committee on Social Security. Hester Adrian Research Centre, Manchester.

Donabedian, A. (1980) *The Definition of Quality and Approaches to its Assessment*, Health Administration Press, Michigan.

Felce, D. (1996) Measuring quality of outcome. *Tizard Learning Disability Review*. Pavilion, Brighton, **1** (2), 38–44.

Felce, D. and Perry, J. (1995) Quality of life: its definition and measurement. *Research in Developmental Disabilities*, **16**, 51–74.

Finkelhor, D., Hotaling, G., Lewis, I.A. and Smith, C. (1990) Sexual abuse in a national survey of adult men and women: prevalence, characteristics and risk factors. *Child Abuse and Neglect*, **14**, 19–28.

Giami, A. (1987) Coping with the sexuality of the disabled: a comparison of the physically disabled and the mentally retarded. *International Journal of Rehabilitation Research*, **10**, 41–8.

Greenwich Social Services and Greenwich Health Authority (1992) *Guidelines for Staff: Recognising and Responding to the Abuse of Adults with Learning Disabilities*. Prepared in collaboration with the University of Kent's study on sexual abuse funded by the Joseph Rowntree Foundation, directed by Hilary Brown, Borough of Greenwich, London.

Griffiths, D., Quinsey, V. and Hinsburger, D. (1989) *Changing Inappropriate Sexual Behavior: A Community Based Approach for Persons with Developmental Disabilities*, Brookes, Baltimore.

Gunn, M. (1989) Can the law help? in *Thinking the Unthinkable: Papers on Sexual*

Abuse and People with Learning Disabilities, (eds H. Brown and A. Craft), FPA, London.

Heyman, B. and Huckle, S. (1995) Sexuality as a perceived hazard in the lives of adults with learning difficulties. *Disability and Society*, **10**, (2), 139–57.

Hudson, L. and Jacot, B. (1991) *The Way Men Think: Intellect, Intimacy and the Erotic Imagination*, Yale University Press, New Haven.

Keith, K., Schalock, R. and Hoffman, K. (1986) *Quality of Life: Measurement and Programmatic Implications*, Mental Retardation Service USA, Nebraska.

Law Commission (1995) *Mental Incapacity Law Commission*, No 231, HMSO, London.

Lukes, S. (1982) *Power: A Radical View*, MacMillan, Hong Kong.

Mansell, J. (1986) The nature of quality assurance, in *Evaluating Quality of Care*, (eds J. Beswick, T. Zadik and D. Felce), BILD, Kidderminster.

McCarthy, M. and Thompson, D. (1993) *Sex and the 3Rs: Rights, Responsibilities and Risks. A Sex Education Package for Working with People with Learning Disabilities*, Pavilion, Brighton.

McGill, P. and Emerson, E. (1992) Normalisation and applied behaviour analysis: values and technology in human services, in *Normalisation: A Reader for the 90s*, (eds H. Brown and H. Smith), Routledge, London.

Murphy, G. and Clare, I.C.H. (1995) Adults' capacity to make decisions affecting the person: psychologists' contribution, in *Handbook of Psychology in Legal Contexts*, (eds R. Bull and D. Carson), John Wiley, London.

O'Brien, J. (1986) A guide to personal futures planning, in *The Activities Catalogue: An Alternative Curriculum for Youth and Adults with Severe Disabilities*, (eds B. Wilcox and G.G. Bellamy), Brookes, Baltimore.

Rapley, M. and Lobley, J. (1995) Factor analysis of the Schalock and Keith (1993) Quality of Life Questionnaire: a replication. *Mental Handicap Research*, **8**, (3), 194–202.

Russell, D.E.H. (1986) *The Secret Trauma: Incest in the Lives of Girls and Women*, Basic Books, York.

Schalock, R. and Keith, K. (1993) *Quality of Life Questionnaire*, IDS Publishing, Ohio.

Schalock, R., Keith, K. and Hoffman, K (1990) *1990 Quality of Life Questionnaire Standardisation Manual*, Mental Retardation Service USA, Nebraska.

Senn, C. (1989) *Vulnerable Sexual Abuse and People with an Intellectual Handicap*, Roeher Institute, Ohio.

Simpson, D. (1994) *Sexual Abuse and People with Learning Difficulties: Developing Access to Community Service*, Family Planning Association, London.

Sobsey, D. and Doe, T. (1991) Patterns of sexual abuse and assault. *Sexuality and Disability*, **9**, 243–59.

Stone, S. (1995) The myth of bodily perfection. *Disability and Society*, **10**, (4), 413–24.

Thompson, D. and McCarthy, M. (1992) Power and confidence. *Aids Dialogue*, **18**, 8–9.

Thompson, D., Clare, I.C.H. and Brown, H. (in press) Not such an ordinary relationship: the role of women care staff in relation to men with learning disabilities who have difficult sexual behaviour. *Disability and Society*.

Turk, V. and Brown, H. (1993) The sexual abuse of adults with learning disabilities: results of a two year incidence survey. *Mental Handicap Research*, **6**, 193–216.

Tymchuk, A.J. (1992) Predicting adequacy of parenting by people with mental retardation. *Child Abuse and Neglect*, **16**, 165–73.

Walmsley, J. (1993) Contradictions in caring: reciprocity and interdependence. *Disability, Handicap and Society*, **8**, 129–43.

Warner, N. (1992) *Choosing with Care*, Department of Health/HMSO, London.

Wardhaugh, J. and Wilding, P. (1993) Towards an explanation of the corruption of care. *Critical Social Policy*, **37**, 4–31.

Watkins, B. and Bentovim, A. (1992) The sexual abuse of male children and adolescents: a review of current research. *Journal of Child Psychology and Psychiatry*, **33**, 197–248.

Weeks, J. (1989) *Sexuality*, Routledge, London.

Wiltshire County Council Social Services (1992) *Procedures and Guidance: Adults with Learning Disabilities/Sexual Abuse.* Prepared in collaboration with the University of Kent's study on sexual abuse funded by the Joseph Rowntree Foundation, directed by Hilary Brown, Wiltshire County Council, Trowbridge.

Wood, D. (1995) *Complaints Procedures in Mental Health Services: Obstacles Facing Service Users and Issues Which Commissioners Need to Address.* Tizard Centre, University of Kent, Canterbury.

Environmental design and quality of life

12

Roy V Ferguson

INTRODUCTION

Architecture is a discipline which has traditionally not been very concerned with behavioural considerations while psychology, by contrast, has tended to overlook the physical aspects of the environment (Krasner, 1980). A relatively new field of study, environmental psychology, attempts to span these two areas by regarding person–environment as an integral unit in considering the reciprocal relationships between humans and their environment (Fisher, Bell & Baum, 1984; Moore & Marans, 1995). In emphasizing that design does influence behaviour, Canter & Craik (1981) point out that the built environment should not just reflect principles of construction and aesthetics, but also should be designed with a careful view to meeting the behavioural and psychological needs of the inhabitants of the buildings. The increasing awareness of the relationship between design and behaviour has resulted in more careful attention being given to behavioural criteria in the planning of primary environments where humans spend large amounts of time. Homes, residential centres, schools and programme settings are primary environments for people with disabilities where the relationship between design and behaviour is of particular significance.

If environmental psychology is perceived from a quality of life standpoint then the issues of well-being delineated in Chapter 4 become critical. Issues of self-concept or image, choice and empowerment within and over the environment must be considered as important. These issues are central to the discussion within this chapter, for the environment can enhance or limit the individual's quality of life in each of these domains. Although persons with physical disabilities, as described in Chapter 6 have obvious concerns with changes to the built environment, the person–environment mix is no less important for individuals with other forms of disability across the lifespan. Further, environment needs to be modified in relation to all aspects of life whether in employment, home living, community contact or leisure based. The quality of life model maintains these aspects of life are interactive and therefore it is the total environment rather than selected aspects of it that must be addressed. As will be seen, shifts from institutional care to community living influence our notion of where and how we develop quality environments.

Environmental design is an important consideration for persons with disabilities as well as for those who are ageing (Brown, 1989). In fact, the environmental needs of ageing people are often remarkably similar to those of persons with disabilities. Issues such as environmental adaptation, mastery, choice, safety, comfort, convenience and accessibility are of concern to both populations.

It should be noted that the terms 'disability' and 'handicap' are often used interchangeably although a distinction can be made. Harris, Cox & Smith (1971) defined disability as the loss or reduction of functional ability while handicap is the disadvantage or restriction of activity caused by disability. One disabled friend of mine outlined this relationship quite clearly in stating, 'My body makes me disabled, but the environment makes me handicapped'.

A SHIFTING PARADIGM FOR THE CARE OF PEOPLE WITH DISABILITIES

Major changes in the philosophy of care for people with disabilities have occurred over the past years. Most pronounced was a shift away from a predominantly medical model of care towards more of a rehabilitation–educational approach (Brown & Hughson, 1993) or psychosocial rehabilitation approach (Cnaan et al., 1991). The medical model tended to treat disability as though it were an illness and the majority of care was based in institutions, designed primarily to be 'containers', which effectively removed people with disabilities from the mainstream of society. The rehabilitation–educational approach, by contrast, is predicated on the notion that people with disabilities should be integrated into the community and provided with the supports necessary for them to experience an independent, normalized life. Similarly, the psychosocial rehabilitation approach is based on the primary assumptions that individuals are motivated by a need for mastery and competence and, second, that new behaviours can be learned and that people are capable of adapting their behaviour to meet their basic needs. As the models of care shift over time, environments must be designed differently to support and reflect these changes.

DESIGN PARAMETERS

Four major parameters have been used to guide the basic design of environments for people with disabilities: cost, durability, efficiency and aesthetics. More recently, a fifth dimension has been added through the examination of behavioural factors. The psychological impact of the designed environment upon its occupants is now considered as an important part of the planning of a new building.

Consideration of the psychological factors in design for people with disabilities is a complex process, but one of vital importance. As the general awareness grows that physical and psychological functioning are not mutually exclusive entities but interdependent phenomena on a shared continuum, more effort is being applied to understanding the psychological effects of physical environments on their inhabitants and the joint effects of physical and social environments on behaviour (Cohen *et al.*, 1995). The social environment consists of interpersonal transactions while the physical environment is the setting in which these transactions occur (Wachs & Gruen, 1982). In view of this interrelationship between environment and behaviour, physical and social environments must be considered as important factors in rehabilitation programmes for people with disabilities and can be conceptualized as adaptive or therapeutic to the degree that they facilitate and support the clinical goals of the programme (Gutheil, 1992).

Consideration of the effects of the environment on behaviour is a concept or philosophy which must be carefully developed throughout the planning process in designing new buildings. In reality, the physical structures of rehabilitation environments are not often designed with a specific philosophy in mind and the use of space appropriate to the goals of the programme grows out of intuition rather than being based on concrete data (Bayes & Francklin, 1971; Nellist, 1970).

THE DESIGN PROCESS

The planning and design of a specialized environment such as a rehabilitation centre or school for people with disabilities is a long process involving many persons and input from all of the users of the new structure. Careful consideration must be given to the clinical and administrative objectives, values, priorities and philosophies of the entire organization. Only through this information can a building be designed to clearly reflect the intentions of the users.

One of the initial steps in the design process is the development of goals and objectives that relate to the specific needs of the users of the building. The aim is to achieve the greatest degree of congruence between the needs and preferences of the users and the design features of the building (Fisher, Bell & Baum, 1984). In order to achieve the best matching of form to function in the design of the building, the gap between those who design environments and those who use them must be minimized, through the use of multidisciplinary design teams sensitive to a variety of user needs. Involvement, wherever possible, of the primary users (i.e. persons with disabilities) in the design process is necessary to maximize the functionality of the new environment. Design criteria which are linked to the developmental and functional needs of persons with disabilities help to increase the congruence between the built environment and the requirements of the primary users. Establishing design criteria in this manner offsets any tendency on the part of architects to see themselves primarily as artists and ignore the functional needs and activities of the primary users of a designed environment (Gifford, 1987).

PUBLIC ATTITUDES TOWARD PERSONS WITH DISABILITIES

Before examining the relationship between architecture and disability, let us first examine some prevailing public attitudes toward people with disabilities. Such attitudes have an effect on rehabilitation and adjustment (Roeher, 1961) and much of the research suggests that these attitudes are in large part negative (Livneh, 1991; Wright, 1983). Also noted is a tendency within the public to classify people with disabilities into either inferior or superior status positions. Persons with disabilities categorized into an inferior status position are generally viewed as being less worthwhile. Conversely, the superior status position reflects the view that people with disabilities are more sensitive, kind, courageous, etc. than are ordinary people.

These stereotypic attitudes are perpetuated in part by media portrayals. Thurer (1980) argues that the portrayal of people with disabilities in art and literature is usually as sinister, evil or monstrous. Similarly, disabled people are rarely depicted as ordinary persons in comic books (Weinberg & Santana, 1978) or movies (Byrd & Elliot, 1985).

The stereotypic attitudes noted above were undoubtedly reflected in the design of environments for persons with disabilities. For example, consider the large institutional settings constructed for people with disabilities in the past. These buildings were usually large in scale, designed for efficiency rather than comfort and typically isolated from the rest of the community. They were intended to be residential facilities and yet were totally lacking in any of the design characteristics typically associated with residential dwellings inhabited by the general public. In effect, these residential institutions removed persons with disabilities from the public eye and served as monuments which contributed to the maintenance of the stereotypic attitudes noted above, in particular the negative ones. It is as Winston Churchill once said: 'We shape our buildings and then our buildings shape us'.

In contrast, thoughtful environmental design can encourage greater involvement of persons with disabilities as active participants in society. The development of small residential or home units integrated into regular communities would reduce much of the unfamiliarity with people with disabilities experienced by the general public. A more visible and active role in society would place emphasis on the wide range of things people with disabilities can do, rather than on what they cannot do, and have a pronounced effect on public attitudes toward people with disabilities. Non-institutional residential units located within the community would help to create a sense of similarity rather than difference regarding disability. Attempts to develop increased visibility within society were undoubtedly accelerated by the high-profile media coverage of athletes with disabilities in Canada such as Terry Fox and Rick Hansen. The inclusion of handicapped events with regular ones for the first time at the 1994 Commonwealth Games in Victoria (Canada) certainly indicated a move in the right direction regarding visibility for persons with disabilities. All of these recent developments will have a positive influence on public attitudes towards disability. This progress can be augmented by designing environments that integrate people with disabilities into regular communities so they continue to become a more visible element, not just at special occasions but in everyday life. This continued and regular contact is necessary in order for public attitudes towards persons with disabilities to change in a significant way.

SELF-CONCEPT AND ADAPTIVE BEHAVIOUR

Vargo (1985) points out that disability can be seen as an assault on a person's self-concept and that successful adjustment 'means not only learning how to best manage one's physical environment, but also developing a new self-concept, one that is cemented in different values regarding what it means to be worthwhile'. While managing the physical environment effectively is not the only variable in the psychological adjustment to disability, it certainly is central to the development of a positive self-concept. Shontz (1991) asserts that environmental factors are at least as important in determining psychological reactions to disabilities as are the internal states of persons who have the disabilities.

Self-concept is broadly defined as a person's perception of self which is formed through experiences/interpretations of one's environment and is greatly influenced by others (Shavelson & Bolus, 1982). A restricted physical environment negatively influences the development and maintenance of a good self-concept in a person with a disability by limiting the type and number of experiences and people who are readily available.

Again, consider the large and isolated residential institutions that were so typical in the past. These structures were designed in a manner which, because of their scale, fostered inflexible routines, depersonalization and dependency. The negative impact these institutions had on the self-concept development of their residents was tremendous.

Adaptive behaviour, defined as the ability to cope with the physical and social demands of the environment, also contributes to the development of a positive self-concept in persons with disabilities since a greater degree of adaptive behaviour means that an individual can function more independently within the community. As more adaptive behaviour is developed, greater access to the community is provided which, in turn, provides the needed experiential and social prerequisites for a strong self-concept. Also, increased access to the community will mean greater visibility which will create more familiarity with people with disabilities on the part of the general public and result in more realistic and positive attitudes towards disability.

The development of adaptive behaviours is facilitated in environments which have been modified or adapted to the particular needs of a person with a disability. To illustrate, let us consider a person whose legs are paralysed due to having polio as a child. This person, confined to a wheelchair, is able to live quite independently in the community in a unit which is designed with ramps, wide doors, bathroom hoists and modified kitchen appliances. The same person can provide their own transportation in a van that is equipped with hand controls and a hydraulic platform hoist and is able to work in an office building that has ramp access, elevators and washrooms designed for people with disabilities. Similar features in shopping centres, theatres and other public buildings extend the ability of this person to be self-sufficient. In other words, some fundamental environmental modifications can enable this person to move from a dependent role in a restrictive institutional setting to an independent and productive role in the community. The adaptive behaviours facilitated by adapted environments have an enormous effect on the self-concept of persons with disabilities.

ENVIRONMENTAL ADAPTATION, MASTERY AND CHOICE

Adaptations that have been made to the primary environment are often a good indicator of the particular coping style adopted by persons with a disability and their families. For example, if the coping style is one characterized by denial, the disability may not be accepted and dealt with realistically. Reactions such as depression, hostility, withdrawal and anger predominate and there would be little attempt to seek greater independence through environmental modifications. The view is often one that disability is a sickness from which the individual will eventually recover.

An alternative view is one where persons with a disability and their families recognize the permanent differences which exist and set out to develop environmental modifications and adjustments which promote adaptive behaviours and increased independence. The occurrence of environmental adaptations are often the earliest indicator of the development of this coping style.

Adaptive environments must be designed for persons with disabilities so that they can be more independent and achieve a sense of environmental mastery. It is important for people with disabilities, as it is for the unimpaired, to be able to exercise environmental choice. Certainly some of the choices available to people who are unimpaired and mildly impaired are closed to persons with severe disabilities. However, total environmental mastery is not even possible for people who are unimpaired. Not everyone is capable of skiing, windsurfing or mountain climbing. Environmental choices are made by people who are unimpaired on the basis of need, interest, priority, ability and situational constraint. Carver & Rodda (1978) point out that:

> Integration does not imply that every conceivable option open to all unimpaired people can be made equally available to every impaired person. It does demand, however, that there should be a sufficient range of options open to any impaired individual to enable him or her to function as a mature person and pursue a personal lifestyle as satisfying in its own way as his/her neighbour's.
>
> (p75)

The restrictiveness of an environment is not just a function of the environment, but a function of the unique needs of the person who has the disability within that environment. An environment that is unduly restrictive for one individual may be ideal for another. The quality of restrictiveness does not reside totally outside the person with a disability and exclusively in the environment. It is suggested that the concept of least restrictive environment might be replaced with the principle of most facilitative environment. The issue, then, is not necessarily to create environmental adaptations which provide every imaginable option to persons with disabilities but, more realistically, to ensure that the environment facilitates their participation in mainstream society.

Special playgrounds for children with disabilities are examples of adaptive environments designed to provide opportunities for mastery and choice. Starting with the notion that the physical environment has a rich impact on learning (Altman & Wohlwill, 1979; David & Wright, 1974) and that many of the regular playgrounds are frustrating or impossible for a child with a disability, playgrounds with 'prosthetic qualities' (Moore, 1980) began to appear. The first of these was the Adventure Playground for Handicapped Children, developed in the mid-1960s. This was a marvellous facility in the Chelsea area of London designed by Lady Allen (1968) to 'insure that the handicapped child can have rich, varied, and spontaneous experiences'. Through thoughtful design, the facility provided children with a variety of graded challenges and paced alternatives suited to a full range of abilities. The environment provided choice and the opportunity for mastery to children of all disability types. However, the playground was located behind a tall brick wall and was not made available to non-disabled children in the surrounding community. While meeting many of the developmental needs of children with disabilities admirably, it did not foster integration with other children. More recently, playgrounds such as the Playground for all Children in New York and the Boundary Park Playground in Vancouver have been designed to provide graded challenges and paced alternatives to children with disabilities, but in a setting which encourages interaction with all children. In other words, specific environmental adaptations have been made to provide opportunities for mastery and choice, but within the regular community so that the users with disabilities are not segregated.

DESIGNING FOR PEOPLE WITH DISABILITIES

There is growing awareness that the physical environment plays an important role in helping individuals compensate for various disabilities so that they can function more independently (Cohen & Day, 1993). However, too often assumptions are made by designers that people with disabilities are an homogeneous group where in actual fact, there is probably no other segment of the population that manifests such a broad diversity of individual problems and needs. In order to provide a physical environment that is safe, convenient, flexible and barrier-free, as well as one which enables choice, control and independence, the designer must be sensitive to the various needs of people with disabilities who will be inhabiting the structures (Devlin, 1992). Through the application of behavioural design criteria, physical environments can be built which assist persons with disabilities in compensating for physical and psychological difficulties.

Let us consider some examples of general behavioural design criteria which would apply to practically any programme setting for all types of disability. The opportunity for involvement in food preparation would represent a typical independence need reflected in most programme residents. Consequently, programme settings should be designed to include small-scale food preparation areas that supplement or replace (depending on the scale of the setting) the commercial kitchens which do not provide the opportunity for programme residents to be actively involved in food preparation activities. Small, non-institutional food preparation areas would be analagous to a kitchen in a home where snacks can be prepared at any time. In addition to providing increased choices and alternatives to institutionalized meal-time routines, an accessible food preparation area serves as a place where skill training can occur aimed at helping the resident move towards greater independence. In larger settings where a commercial kitchen is necessary, some of these same developmental needs can be met through the inclusion of lounge areas containing a refrigerator and microwave oven.

Another example of a general design consideration based upon a primary need of the inhabitant would be easy access to the outdoor environment. Regardless of whether the resident of a programme setting has a physical, perceptual, emotional or mental disability, there exists a need to experience the seasonal changes as well as the sights, sounds, textures and smells of the natural environment. The interactions, stimulation, choice and change afforded by being outdoors are vital to any programme resident and must be readily accessible. For some types of disability this means designing an interface between interior and exterior environments that easily accommodates wheelchairs and other wheeled forms of mobility. For others, it may mean the inclusion of a sunny courtyard or park that can be easily supervised. The main point is that the design of any programme facility must reflect this need. Too often we are witness to programme buildings for persons with disabilities which have been located in busy downtown settings that do not readily lend themselves to these considerations.

It must be recognized that people with disabilities have the same needs as others for personal independence, a choice of housing alternatives, a satisfying job, adequate income, recreational opportunities, etc. Their efforts to address these needs are often frustrated by obstacles within the physical environment. For example, a person with a moderate disability, such as loss of co-ordination, arthritis or an amputated arm, encounters difficulty in using typical design features such as stairs, water taps and door knobs. Persons in wheelchairs are restricted by narrow and/or heavy doors, stairs, small washrooms, inaccessible public transportation and elevator buttons that are placed too high.

Once it is recognized that people with disabilities have the same needs as those without, interesting and creative solutions to environmental barriers begin to emerge. In this regard I am reminded of a tremendously creative and resourceful family with whom I was involved in a rehabilitation hospital. This family had an adolescent son with a severe physical disability due to a spinal injury who was confined to a wheelchair. The boy wanted to live as typical and normal a life as possible and was encouraged in this goal by his parents and siblings. He had a number of neighbourhood friends whose company he enjoyed but he found that he was not able to play with them in the park in front of their house because his electric wheelchair would not operate over rough terrain. The parents,

ıltation with their son, designed an electric all-terrain vehicle with
ısure tyres capable of climbing curbs and negotiating all sorts of
ₒₗₐr topography. Not only did this vehicle, complete with a bucket
seat, racing harness and roll bar, enable him to navigate the park with his
friends, but it allowed him to offer rides to them.

In a similar vein, this incredible family devised an environmental
adaptation which addressed another typical, adolescent developmental
need: surfing. They rigged up a harness system on a small rubber dingy
so that their son was able to ride the waves in Hawaii and experience the
same thrill, adventure and mastery as his able-bodied counterparts. This
family was truly remarkable in their ability to find adaptations for
environmental barriers to the developmental needs of their son.

While it is not possible, within the confines of this chapter, to examine
the unique environmental needs of each type of disability, there are some
universal ones that apply to all persons across the broad range of disabilities: the need for safety, comfort, convenience/accessibility and the need
for control.

SAFETY, COMFORT, CONVENIENCE AND ACCESSIBILITY

These are important design features to incorporate in both short- and
long-term residential facilities for people with disabilities. Safety, comfort, convenience and accessibility are fundamental requirements of all
residential facilities, whether private residences, group homes or institutions. To promote safety, a facility (particularly in the case of institutional care) should permit sufficient staff surveillance to prevent
accidents or to detect them quickly when they do occur, while not creating an atmosphere lacking privacy. It has been shown that when staff
and residents in a facility are in close proximity staff may behave in
ways that encourage dependency (Harris, Lipman & Slater, 1977).
Further, design features such as handrails, safety glass and non-slip
walking surfaces should be present to prevent accidents as well as
mechanisms such as call buttons (located at appropriate heights) that
enable disabled residents to request assistance if a problem is encountered in a private area like a bathroom.

The design of environments should also promote comfort and convenience by providing orientation aids such as colour coding or universal
pictographs that facilitate way finding. While way finding aids are
absolutely essential in a larger and more complex treatment centre, they
might also be considered in the design of smaller group and individual
residential settings for residents who have visual problems or who
become easily disoriented. Hunt (1984) found that the well-being of
elderly persons moving to a new facility was related to their confidence
and ability in finding their way around the building.

Sheltered entrances, adapted toilet facilities, modified kitchen layouts and wide corridors are just a few examples of design elements that promote comfort and convenience for people with disabilities. Facilities should be designed to be warm and homelike in appearance with plenty of sensory stimulation throughout. Using bright and warm colours (as opposed to the typical institutional white, beige or pale green) (Mehrabian & Russell, 1974), considering alternatives to standard fluorescent lighting (Wandersman *et al.*, 1985), including plenty of windows (Ruys, 1970; Verderber, 1986) and utilizing less formal furniture arrangements (Holahan, 1972) will have a positive effect on the mood and behaviour of the inhabitants of the environment. It has been shown that environments designed to stimulate the auditory, visual and tactile senses increase appropriate and acceptable behaviours in institutionalized adolescents with mental disabilities (Kreger, 1971; Levy, 1974). Levy (1976) describes the physical environment as a catalytic agent in the learning process of mentally challenged persons.

Through the use of modern technology, residential environments can be designed that allow persons with disabilities to live independently. For example, persons capable only of operating a keyboard or microswitch with a single finger or by blowing into a pneumatic tube or by focusing their eyes on special sensors can activate electronic mechanisms that dial telephones, turn on lights, operate television sets, open doors and drive computerized communication systems.

Rehabilitation technology involves the use of advanced technology to enhance the lives of people with mental or physical limitations through computer applications, wheeled mobility and seating, specialized assistive devices, augmentative and alternative communication. Personal computers, in particular, are becoming a key part of adapted environments for persons with various disabilities such as head injury (Batchelor *et al.*, 1988), Alzheimer disease (Fisher, 1986), neurological problems (Batt & Lounsbury, 1990) and quadriplegia (O'Leary, Mann & Prekash, 1991). Perhaps this sort of 'high-tech' environment is what Le Corbusier had in mind when he defined a home as a 'machine for living' (Foote, 1977). At any rate, the majority of people with disabilities are able to live in their own homes or small, community-based group residences if this type of environmental support is available.

However, most persons with disabilities do not require environmental modifications as elaborate as these in order to live independently. For many it is only a matter of providing some fundamental modifications to residential structures and public buildings in order to make them accessible and functional. There are various resources that provide guidelines for the planning and design of housing for persons with disabilities. The Canadian Central Mortgage and Housing Corporation (1974), for example, has produced a manual called *Housing for the Handicapped* that provides design criteria for various types of housing alternatives ranging from single family dwellings to integrated apartment buildings. Another factual and comprehensive resource is a book by a British architect, Selwyn Goldsmith (1967), called *Designing for the Disabled*. Another useful Canadian resource on building requirements and anthropometric data for persons with disabilities, which is particularly well illustrated, is *The Section 3.7 Handbook* (Ministry of Municipal Affairs, 1984). Resources such as these and others are instrumental in the design of least restrictive environments.

CONTROL

Settings that are barrier free allow people with disabilities to move about independently and in so doing, foster a sense of personal control. This perception of control is an important factor in preventing feelings of helplessness, both real and learned. Garber & Seligman (1981) describe the ultimate consequence of loss of control as learned helplessness. If repeated efforts at establishing control in a situation result in failure, there is a tendency to stop trying which eventually becomes a response pattern generalizing to other situations. In effect, the person learns to be helpless even in situations where personal control is possible. Persons with disabilities are particularly vulnerable to the process of learned helplessness because of the many environmental barriers with which they are confronted. Until more environments are designed to be barrier free it is important to involve people with disabilities in finding solutions to aspects of the environment that function as obstacles so that learned helplessness patterns do not become established.

The design of environments for persons with disabilities should provide, whenever possible, opportunities for choice which, in turn, enhance feelings of control in the inhabitants. In a study of the effects of changes in the design of a school for people with developmental disabilities (Zimring, Weitzer & Knight, 1982) it was found that residents preferred a design alternative that gave them more control over aspects of their physical environment such as lighting and temperature and greater control of their social environment in regards to their personal interactions. Further control is provided by locating a facility in the community so that residents can choose among a variety of available services such as shopping and recreational facilities. Choice and perceived control are also facilitated through design that enhances privacy and creates a sense of personal space and territory exclusively for the individual's own use.

Personal space is defined as an invisible boundary surrounding us into which others may not trespass and regulating how closely individuals will interact (Fisher, Bell & Baum, 1984). It moves with the individual, changing in size according to the situation. Personal space has a protective function, serving as a buffer against potential emotional and physical threats such as too much stimulation, stressful over-arousal, insufficient privacy and aggression. It also serves a communication function since the distance maintained from others will indicate the level of intimacy desired in the relationship. It has been noted that people without disabilities are more comfortable interacting with people with disabilities at greater interpersonal distances (Dabbs & Stokes, 1975; Kleck *et al.*, 1968). Research has demonstrated other spatial behaviour differences. For example, Gifford & Sacilotto (1993) demonstrated that female employees of a government agency working at computer terminals in relative social isolation preferred larger interpersonal distances than did a matched group of women who worked primarily with other people. Sommer (1969) and Horowitz, Duff & Stratton (1964) found that people with schizophrenia require more space than 'normals'. Examination of the proxemics in special needs settings demonstrated that emotionally disturbed children require more personal space than undisturbed children (Fisher, 1967; Kendall *et al.*, 1976; Weinstein, 1965), as do emotionally disturbed adolescents (Newman & Pollack, 1973). Foley & Lacy (1967) suggested that because of the vulnerability of a patient with mental illness, the physical environment will have a greater impact, either positively or negatively. Interestingly, Hayduk & Mainprize (1980) found no differences in the spatial behaviour of blind and sighted individuals, although various behavioural and spatial organization differences have been described in other work.

It has been noted that individuals who use larger personal distances are perceived by others as more rejecting and aggressive (Aiello & Thompson, 1980). An effect of differences in personal space may be that certain individuals may function within interpersonal distances that lead others to attribute negative traits to them.

Territory is defined as visible, stationary and home-centred areas regulating who will interact (Sommer, 1969). Territories are places that are owned or controlled by one or more individuals. Neighbourhoods, offices, bedrooms and even particular chairs or tables are examples of territories. The work of Taylor & Strough (1978) demonstrated that defined territories increased feelings of control in subjects. Being on one's own territory or 'turf' has been shown to elicit feelings of control, security and improved performance (Barton, 1966; Holahan, 1976; Holahan & Saegert, 1973). Consequently, the design of environments for persons with disabilities should encourage individuals to personalize areas and thus create a sense of personal territory. It is important to note that most of the research on personal space and territory with people with disabilities has been done in institutional settings so that it is not certain whether the findings would generalize to home situations. However, because of the pervasiveness of these concepts, spouses and parents of people with disabilities residing in their own homes would be advised to organize the physical environment to enhance feelings of personal control.

Personal space, then, is invisible, portable and body centred and regulates how closely individuals will interact. Territory is visible, stationary and home centred and regulates who will interact. Both are key concepts in design aimed at increasing perceived environmental control for persons with disabilities.

QUALITY OF LIFE AND ENVIRONMENTS FOR PERSONS WITH DISABILITIES

The concept of quality of life usually includes considerations such as freedom of choice, personal life satisfaction, community involvement and social interaction/support. As outlined earlier, careful environmental design is an important and fundamental factor in creating choices, control, opportunities and independence for people with disabilities which, in turn, influence self-concept. Of course, all of these variables contribute to a sense of general life satisfaction. For example, Cooper & Rodman (1994) found that residents in housing co-operatives who felt the greatest degree or perceived social control over their residential environment also rated their residential quality of life the highest. Similarly, a Swedish study (Iwarsson & Isacsson, 1993) also notes the relationship between basic accessibility in domestic housing and the quality of life for persons with disabilities.

Adaptive, accessible environments for persons who are disabled mean that individuals are better able to attend visits with health care professionals in the community. Better access improves the primary health care status for persons, which has a positive influence on their quality of life. In addition to health, another domain in a comprehensive definition of quality of life is safety which includes constructs such as security, personal control, privacy, independence and autonomy. A careful environmental design process specifically directed at these dimensions contributes significantly to the comfort levels of persons within these adaptive settings. Again, designing physical environments to be sensitive to the safety needs of persons with disabilities adds to their quality of life.

Environments that are designed to be adaptive and barrier-free allow people with disabilities to be more actively involved in the community and to experience greater social interaction and support. Easy access to public buildings provides opportunities for persons with disabilities to attend theatres, sports events, concerts, plays, restaurants, libraries, museums and galleries, all of which contribute to their general quality of life. However, environments that facilitate greater participation in the community also create a spiral of change for people with disabilities. Increased community involvement means greater visibility for persons with disabilities which is necessary in the process of changing public attitudes toward them. As public attitudes change they are reflected in social policies which enable even fuller participation of people with disabilities in society and a resulting increase in their quality of life. Of course, there is still much progress to be made in this area, but the main point is that environmental adaptation is a necessary and vital first step to activate an accelerating spiral process of change in regard to quality of life for persons with disabilities.

SUMMARY

The following are the main points contained in this chapter.

- The increasing awareness of the relationship between environment and behaviour has resulted in more careful attention being paid to behavioural criteria in the design of built environments.
- The shift away from a medical model and towards a rehabilitation–educational–psychosocial model of care has influenced the type of environments being designed for persons with disabilities.
- Physical environments are an important element in rehabilitation planning and should be designed to support programme philosophies, values and objectives.
- Environmental design must be congruent with the needs and preferences of the inhabitants. The needs of people with disabilities are similar to those without but environments must be adapted in different ways for different disabilities so that these needs can be met.
- Public attitudes toward persons with disabilities tend to be stereotypic.
- Environments designed to integrate people with disabilities into regular society will facilitate the visibility and contact necessary to stimulate public attitude change towards persons with disabilities.
- Environments have a direct influence on the self-concept of people with disabilities by supporting the development of adaptive behaviours.
- Special playgrounds have been designed to provide the opportunity for challenge, mastery and choice in children with disabilities.
- Although people who have disabilities are a very heterogeneous group with respect to specific environmental needs, they have universal requirements for safety, comfort, convenience/accessibility and control.
- Through environmental adaptations and technological support, the majority of people with disabilities can live independently within the community.
- Barrier-free environments foster feelings of involvement, independence and personal control.
- The concepts of personal space and territory are key elements in design which is aimed at increasing perceived environmental control for persons with disabilities.

- Environmental adaptation is a necessary first step in activating an accelerating spiral process of change with regard to the quality of life for persons with disabilities.

REFERENCES

Aiello, J.R. and Thompson, D.E. (1980) When compensation fails: mediating effects of sex and locus of control at extended interaction distances. *Basic and Applied Social Psychology*, **1**, 65–82.

Allen, Lady, of Hurtwood (1968) *Planning for Play*, MIT Press, Cambridge.

Altman, I. and Wohlwill, J.F. (eds) (1979) *Human Behavior and Environment. Vol. 3 Children and the Environment*, Plenum Press, New York.

Barton, R. (1966) The patient's personal territory. *Hospital and Community Psychiatry*, **17**, 336.

Batchelor, J., Shores, E., Marosszeky, J., Sandanam, J. and Lovarini, M. (1988) Cognitive rehabilitation of severely closed-head-injured patients using computer-assisted and non-computerized treatment techniques. *Journal of Head Trauma Rehabilitation*, **3**, 78–85.

Batt, R.C. and Lounsbury, P.A. (1990) Case report: teaching the patient with cognitive deficits to use a computer. *American Journal of Occupational Therapy*, **44**, 364–7.

Bayes, K. and Francklin, S. (eds) (1971) *Designing for the Handicapped*, George Godwin, London.

Brown, R.I. (1989) Aging, disability and quality of life: a challenge for society. *Canadian Psychology*, **30**, 551–9.

Brown, R.I. and Hughson, E.A. (1993) *Behavioural and Social Rehabilitation and Training*, 2nd edn, Chapman & Hall, London.

Byrd, E.K. and Elliot, T.R. (1985) Feature films and disability: a descriptive study. *Rehabilitation Psychology*, **30**, 47–51.

Canter, D.V. and Craik, K.H. (1981) Environmental psychology. *Journal of Environmental Psychology*, **1**, 1–11.

Carver, V. and Rodda, M. (1978) *Disability and the Environment*, Paul Elk, London.

Central Mortgage and Housing Corporation (1974) *Housing the Handicapped*, CMHC, Ottawa.

Cnaan, R.A., Blankertz, L., Messinger, K.W. and Gardner, J.R. (1991) Psychosocial rehabilitation: toward a definition, in *The Psychological and Social Impact of Disability*, 3rd edn, (ed. R.P. Marinelli and A.E. Dell Orto), Springer, New York.

Cohen, U. and Day, K. (1993) *Contemporary Environments for People with Dementia*, Johns Hopkins University Press, Baltimore.

Cohen, U., Beer, J., Kidera, E. and Golden, W. (1995) *Mainstreaming the Handicapped: A Design Guide*, Center for Architecture and Urban Planning, University of Wisconsin, Milwaukee.

Cooper, M. and Rodman, M.C. (1994) Accessibility and quality of life in housing cooperatives. *Environment and Behavior*, **26**, 49–70.

Dabbs, J.M. and Stokes, N.A. (1975) Beauty is power: the use of space on the sidewalk. *Sociometry*, **38**, 551–7.

David, T.G. and Wright, B.D. (eds) (1974) *Learning Environments*, University of Chicago Press, Chicago.

Devlin, A.S. (1992) Psychiatric ward renovation: staff perception and patient behavior. *Environment and Behavior*, **24**, 66–84.

Fisher, J.D., Bell, P.A. and Baum, A. (1984) *Environmental Psychology*, 2nd edn, Holt, Rinehart & Winston, New York.

Fisher, R.L. (1967) Social schema of normal and disturbed school children. *Journal of Educational Psychology*, **40**, 122–5.

Fisher, S. (1986) Increasing participation with a computer in an adult day care setting. *Activities, Adaptation and Aging*, **8**, 31–44.

Foley, A. and Lacy, B. (1967) On the need for interprofessional collaboration: psychiatry and architecture. *American Journal of Psychiatry*, **123**, 1013–18.

Foote, S. (1977) *Handicapped at Home*, Quick Fox Publishers, London.

Garber, J. and Seligman, M.E.P. (eds) (1981) *Human Helplessness: Theory and Applications*, Academic Press, New York.

Gifford, R. (1987) *Environmental Psychology: Principles and Practice*, Allyn & Bacon, Boston.

Gifford, R. and Sacilotto, P.A. (1993) Social isolation and personal space: a field study. *Canadian Journal of Behavioural Science*, **25**, 165–74.

Goldsmith, S. (1967) *Designing for the Disabled*, 2nd edn, McGraw-Hill, New York.

Gutheil, I.A. (1992) Considering the physical environment: an essential component of good practice. *Social Work*, **37**, 391–6.

Harris, A.I., Cox, E. and Smith, C.R. (1971) *Handicapped and Impaired in Great Britain, Part 1*, HMSO, London.

Harris, H., Lipman, A. and Slater, R. (1977) Architectural design: the spatial location and interactions of old people. *Gerontology*, **23**, 390–400.

Hayduk, L.A. and Mainprize, S.A. (1980) Personal space of the blind. *Social Psychology Quarterly*, **43**, 216–23.

Holahan, C.J. (1972) Seating patterns and patient behavior in an experimental dayroom. *Journal of Abnormal Psychology*, **83**, 454–62.

Holahan, C.J. (1976) Environmental change in a psychiatric setting: a social systems analysis. *Human Relations*, **29**, 153–66.

Holahan, C.J. and Saegert, S. (1973) Behavioral and attitudinal effects of large-scale variation in the physical environment of psychiatric wards. *Journal of Abnormal Psychology*, **83**, 454–62.

Horowitz, M.J., Duff, D.F. and Stratton, L.O. (1964) Body buffer zone: exploration of personal space. *Archives of General Psychology*, **11**, 651–6.

Hunt, M.E. (1984) Environmental learning without being there. *Environment and Behavior*, **16**, 307–34.

Iwarsson, S. and Isacsson, A. (1993) Basic accessibility in modern housing: a key to the problems of care in the domestic setting. *Scandinavian Journal of Caring Sciences*, **7**, 155–9.

Kendall, P.C., Deardoff, P.A., Finch, A.J. and Graham, L. (1976) Proxemics, locus of control, anxiety and type of movement in emotionally disturbed and normal boys. *Journal of Abnormal Child Psychology*, **4**, 9–16.

Kleck, R.E., Buck, P.L., Geller, W.C. *et al.* (1968) Effect of stigmatizing conditions on the use of personal space. *Psychological Reports*, **23**, 111–18.

Krasner, L. (ed.) (1980) *Environmental Design and Human Behavior*, Pergamon Press, New York.

Kreger, K. (1971) Compensatory environment programming for the severely retarded behaviorally disturbed. *Mental Retardation*, **9**, 29–33.

Levy, E. (1974) *Effects of Environmental Enrichment on the Behavior of Institutionalized Mentally Retarded Adolescents*, Developmental Disabilities Office, Department of Health, Education and Welfare, Washington DC.

Levy, E. (1976) Designing environments for mentally retarded clients. *Hospital and Community Psychiatry*, **27**, 793–6.

Livneh, H. (1991) On the origins of negative attitudes toward people with disabilities, in *The Psychological and Social Impact of Disability*, 3rd edn, (eds R.P. Marinelli and A.E. Dell Orto), Springer, New York.

Mehrabian, A. and Russell, J.A. (1974) *An Approach to Environmental Psychology*, MIT Press, Cambridge.

Ministry of Municipal Affairs (1984) *The Section 3.7 Handbook*, Province of British Columbia.

Moore, G.T. (1980) *Designing Environments for Handicapped Children*, Educational Facilities Laboratories, New York.

Moore, G.T. and Marans, R.W. (eds) (1995) *Advances in Environment, Behavior and Design. Integrations, Vol. 4*, Plenum Press, New York.

Nellist, I. (1970) *Planning Buildings for Handicapped Children*, Crosby Lockwood & Son, London.

Newman, R.C. and Pollack, D. (1973) Proxemics in deviant adolescents. *Journal of Consulting and Clinical Psychology*, **40**, 148–54.

O'Leary, S., Mann, C. and Prekash, I. (1991) Access to computers for older adults: problems and solutions. *American Journal of Occupational Therapy*, **45**, 636–42.

Roeher, G.A. (1961) Significance of public attitudes in the rehabilitation of the disabled. *Rehabilitation Literature*, **22**, 66–72.

Ruys, T. (1970) Windowless offices. *Man-Environment Systems*, **1**, 49.

Shavelson, R.J. and Bolus, R. (1982) Self concept: the interplay of theory and methods. *Journal of Educational Psychology*, **74**, 3–17.

Shontz, F.C. (1991) Six principles relating disability and psychological adjustment, in *The Psychological and Social Impact of Disability*, 3rd edn, (eds R.P. Marinelli and A.E. Dell Orto), Springer, New York.

Sommer, R. (1969) *Personal Space*, Prentice-Hall, Englewood Cliffs, NJ.

Taylor, R.B. and Strough, P.R. (1978) Territorial cognition: assessing Altman's typology. *Journal of Personality and Social Psychology*, **36**, 418–23.

Thurer, S. (1980) Disability and monstrosity: a look at literary distortions of handicapping conditions. *Rehabilitation Literature*, **41**, 12–15.

Vargo, J.W. (1985) Attitudes and adjustment. *Alberta Psychology*, **14**, 5–6.

Verderber, S. (1986) Dimensions of person-window transactions in the hospital environment. *Environment and Behavior*, **18**, 450–66.

Wachs, T.D. and Gruen, G. (1982) *Early Experience and Human Development*, Plenum Press, New York.

Wandersman, A., Andrews, A., Riddle, C. and Fancett, C. (1985) Environmental psychology and prevention, in *Preventive Psychology: Theory, Research and Practice*, (eds R. Felner, S. Farber, L. Jason, and J. Moritsugu), Pergamon, New York.

Weinberg, N. and Santana, R. (1978) Comic books: champions of the disabled stereotype. *Rehabilitation Literature*, **39**, 327–31.

Weinstein, L. (1965) Social schemata of emotionally disturbed boys. *Journal of Abnormal Psychology*, **70**, 457–61.

Wright, B.A. (1983) *Physical Disability: A Psychological Approach*, 2nd edn, Harper & Row, New York.

Zimring, C., Weitzer, W. and Knight, R.C. (1982) Opportunity for control and the designed environment: the case of an institution for the developmentally disabled, in *Advances in Environmental Psychology, 4*, (eds A. Baum and J. Singer), Lawrence Erlbaum, Hillsdale, NJ.

Change and necessity: creative activity, well-being and the quality of life for persons with a disability

13

Bernie Warren

INTRODUCTION

This chapter examines some of the relationships between participation in creative activity and quality of life for persons with a disability. The emphasis of this chapter is less on the arts in general (their social construction, their role in society, etc.) and more on the potential of creative activities (e.g. painting, music, dance, drama, puppetry, storytelling, needlepoint, landscape gardening) for improving the quality of life for persons with a disability (cf Warren & Nadeau, 1988).

The chapter builds on concepts proposed by Monod (1971) to suggest that an individual's quality of life is influenced by their ability to adapt to change, not only in the person's social surroundings but also within themselves. Certain Taoist concepts (employed in both Chinese martial arts and traditional Chinese medicine) are then used to help explain the value of creative activity as a means of helping individuals adapt to change.

Finally, using examples drawn primarily from the performing arts (drama, dance and music), it is suggested that involvement in creative activities can not only help people adapt to changes but also enhance an individual's sense of well-being and may even affect how that individual is perceived by their community.

CHANCE, NECESSITY AND QUALITY OF LIFE

CHANCE AND NECESSITY

Everything existing in the universe is the fruit of chance and of necessity.
(Democritus, in Monod, 1971)

When I first read Jacques Monod's *Chance and Necessity* (almost 25 years ago) it was a ground-breaking and somewhat controversial book. Concepts first encountered in that book have stayed with me throughout my life and came to mind when I was preparing to write this chapter. It was Monod who first made me aware of the sometimes random nature of evolution, how biological organisms adapt to changing external events through a balance of chance and necessity, most often without a conscious thought. However, it was not just Monod's words but also the way in which I came across them that first made me consider their significance to this discussion of the value of the creative process to well-being.

I first encountered Monod's book when I was an undergraduate studying biochemistry. In need of a topic for a paper, I came upon his words by chance, borne of necessity. Since then I have noticed that events and experiences (books, workshops, ideas) that have had a significant effect on me have been encountered at times in my life when there has been a need for change, ranging from a relatively small impasse on a mundane problem (e.g. finding a 'hook' for this chapter) through to major life changes (e.g. my move from studying medicine to drama). These remembered 'change moments' (times when change actually occurred) are ones when not only was there a need to change, but also a receptivity to the opportunities afforded by such change. Undoubtedly there were many other potential change moments, 'missed' opportunities when I may have needed to make changes in my life but, for whatever reason, I was either unaware of the need to change or not open to the possibilities being presented to me.

DISABILITY AND THE NEED FOR CHANGE

I am not this fragile body.

(Deng, 1988)

I am not my disability, I am me.

(Swann, in Exley, 1984)

Human beings are biological organisms and in purely biological terms an organism's ability to adapt to change is essential to its survival. The majority of successful organisms thoughtlessly adapt to their surroundings not to improve their quality of life but for their very survival. Unlike other organisms, human beings can be made aware of the necessity for change and can consciously effect change in their lives. However, they must become aware of the need to change and be willing and able to do so.

In any culture it is our social performance (the way that we externalize the unspoken rules of social interaction) that enables us to remain relatively inconspicuous, thus blending in with the rest of society. The alternative is to be noticed, identified as being different which can handicap us in the eyes of our peers. The paradox that we are all different but want to be the same as everyone else is a 'myth of normality' (DeLoach & Greer, 1981). This is of particular concern to individuals coping with a disability, especially if the problem is initially visually inconspicuous (e.g. learning disability, hearing impairment) where the disability is only made visible through the individual's social interactions.

Unfortunately, one of the constants of life is that things change. In adapting to new situations, all of us can at various times produce 'impoverished performances'; performances that identify our inadequacies. Adept social actors generally learn to cope with these changes, partially because all social performances are based on a mixture of knowledge and intuition, that is, on the basis of past experiences we are able to build up a picture of what is likely to be expected of us in similar situations. However, for people who cope with a physical, intellectual or emotional disability or who have in some way been socially isolated, it is likely that they will face additional obstacles in the acquisition of what remain largely unspoken rules of social interaction. In addition, the inability to conform to prescribed social conventions may not only lead persons with a disability to become frustrated, but may also serve to additionally handicap them in the eyes of their peers. This failure and its subsequent stigmatization may exacerbate the condition by creating additional emotional problems.

As I have argued elsewhere (Warren, 1988, 1989, 1995), persons with a disability are often identified by others as being somewhat different through their social performance (by their posture, by their movement, by the way they speak). So while we all need to adapt to change it might be argued that the myth of normality means that it is even more important for persons with a disability to do so. However, they may be unaware of the need to change or their disability may create an extra challenge to their successfully adapting to change. Changes in modern society have not made the situation any easier.

TECHNOLOGICAL CHANGE AND QUALITY OF LIFE

> All around us things change their identities ... Everything is in flux. Everything flows.
>
> (Kosko, 1993)

In our current society change itself is changing the shape of our culture (the way we dress, conduct our lives, the values that we adhere to) faster than ever before. Technical innovations are rapidly transforming fantastic concepts of science fiction into reality within the space of a few short years. Change is occurring so quickly that the ability to change is rapidly becoming a necessity in modern life. The inability to adapt to change itself may create disabilities either of a behavioural kind (e.g. telling jokes that are no longer socially appropriate) or as a direct result of techno-logical illiteracy (what might be loosely termed 'computer disabled').

The prevailing wisdom seems to suggest that technological innova-tions improve our quality of life. Simply knowing how to use a computer or a labour-saving device such as a microwave or dishwasher makes our lives easier. But while these innovations can certainly improve our living conditions and in some ways make our lives easier, they may not always lead to an increased sense of well-being. They may change our lifestyle but not necessarily improve the quality of our lives.

For all people, but perhaps particularly for persons with a disability, technological change is a double-edged sword. Technological innovations have greatly improved our mobility, ability to communicate and ability to adapt to changing environmental conditions. However, these innovations have contributed to the development of other problems most of which have arisen because the ground rules of social interaction are in a con-stant state of flux. Consequently the skills needed to survive are changing rapidly.

Technological advances may save time and give the impression that they improve our lives. However, individuals frequently feel a lack of control and a sense of isolation. As Toffler (1975) points out, the speeding up of technological and social change causes severe personal and organizational dislocation. Not only are individuals out of balance with themselves, but they are out of balance with others and with their sur-roundings. From this perspective it is not surprising that although Western scientific medicine may have beaten many of the life-threatening illnesses of a few decades ago these have been replaced with other, per-haps more pernicious problems, particularly those related to stress and alienation. In many ways not only has it never been more difficult to come to terms with change, but also it has never been more necessary to step back and assess how best to adapt to these changes.

CREATIVE ACTIVITY AND QUALITY OF LIFE

THE ARTS AND CHANGE

> Each day ... we must validate our past, face our present, plan for the future.
>
> (Deng, 1988)

The arts have always had a role to play in the changing life of social com-munities. They are a cornerstone of all cultures and can be viewed as a significant indicator of the general social, physical and intellectual 'health' of any culture (Warren, 1993a; Warren & Nadeau, 1988). However, while the arts are a constant part of all cultures, they must adapt to change or, like living organisms, fade into memory, the cultural equivalent of extinction.

Changes to artistic forms occur over time as a result of both chance and necessity. The cross-fertilization of techniques among and within individual artistic disciplines such as music, dance and visual arts allows for the development of new genres, subdisciplines and even new art forms over time. This changing diversity of artistic forms allows individual artists to express themselves in an ever-widening array of media. As a result artists are better able to respond to currents within the social fabric and to both reflect and effect change.

Ultimately all of the arts provide a means by which each individual may express an inner world through symbolic means. Even the most avante-garde artistic expressions hold the mirror up to nature. While the individual participating in creative activity may not always be able to control changes, at least they are able to express their reactions to them. It is this capacity of artistic activity to enable the participant to express their response to change that has led in part to the realization that participation in creative activities is important to the general health of individuals in advanced, technological cultures.

THE ARTS AND WELL-BEING

Creative activities are rejuvenating to the mind and spirit as well as to the body.

(Miller, in Weisberg & Wilder, 1986)

Until very recently most civilized cultures (for that is how modern societies like to think of themselves) held the opinion that creativity is the responsibility of a few gifted individuals. This view was largely based on a belief that artefacts (produced as the end result of a creative process) should be used as the measure of a person's creativity because it is these artefacts which act as cultural landmarks: reminders to current and future generations of the culture of a particular epoch and geographic location. In taking this materialist view of creativity, many individuals in our technologically advanced cultures (unlike people in so-called simpler societies) were and often still are denied the opportunity to realize their creative abilities. However, it is the participation in the process, the creative activity itself, that may be of greatest value to an individual's sense of well-being and quality of life.

As Johnson (1984) points out, 'Historically, healing, community and the arts were highly integrative events with group singing, dancing and drumming at the core of the community's identity and basic to its survival'. Until very recently the notion of using the arts and other creative processes to promote and maintain good health has been extremely limited in modern industrialized societies. Thankfully, over the last three decades people have become increasingly aware of their creative potential, their need to make their mark, not because they necessarily wish to be a reminder to a future generation of a long-lost culture but because each creative mark reaffirms the self. It says 'I am here', 'I have something to express'.

Unfortunately changes in our modern society have led to the need for justification and tangible proof in almost everything we do. In the arts this has led to the 'therapy defence': the need, when questioned, to validate the use of the arts and other creative processes (particularly in professional environments) by describing all creative activity as therapy.

Elsewhere, I have suggested (Warren, 1993a) that therapy (which implies a prescribed course of treatment of a condition that produces 'ill health' with predetermined expected results for a specific diagnosed condition) and the art(s) (which at least in part suggests an exploration, one that usually finds the notion of predetermined expectation an anathema) are strange bedfellows. Happily, more and more people are becoming aware that being involved in creative activity (i.e. the *process* of creating) is every bit as important and in many cases more important than the end product. This awareness has led to an important change in how the arts are viewed when employed for, with and by persons with a disability: a move away from art(s) therapy towards 'Arts for Health' (Moss, 1987; Senior & Croall, 1993).

The Arts for Health movement reflects a move away from curing (an end product and usually something that is done to someone else) towards promoting healing and/or maintaining health, which are processes that involve some notion of self-help. Scientific and narrative research in the areas of Arts for Health and Laughter and Healing suggests that involvement in creative activity may not only motivate an individual to want to recover, but can help individuals accommodate to a specific disability or recover from a specific medical or surgical procedure (Coles, 1981; Moss, 1987; Senior & Croall, 1993). Also as I have argued elsewhere (Warren 1993b, 1994a), in certain circumstances involvement in creative activity may bring about identifiable physiological changes in the body similar to those documented in recent research on the effects of laughter in the process of healing (e.g. Cousins, 1979; Fry, 1977, 1979; Fry & Stoft, 1971; McClelland, Alexander & Marks, 1982; Saper, 1988). While some of the reports are contradictory because, as McClelland suggests (McClelland *et al.*, as quoted in Saper 1988) there are so many variables – immune factors, psychological factors, hormonal factors and illness – nevertheless there is general agreement that humour and the resulting laughter do have physiological and psychological effects on the body systems. However, in order to pursue the discussion of how creative activity may promote a sense of well-being and improve quality of life I must first make a detour to the East.

TAOISM: THE DOUBLE BALANCE AND QUALITY OF LIFE

CONNECTING THE DRAMA/THEATRE TEACHER AND THE MARTIAL ARTIST

> In the West, a fundamental split is posited between mind and body ... In the East, by contrast, the most widespread traditions assert a fundamental unity. Body and mind, spirit and matter, male and female interact in the dance which is the universe.
>
> (Payne, 1981)

My study of the martial arts began before I became interested in drama and theatre. Over the years my studies have enabled me to learn far more of significance from these experiences than mere technical expertise. Quite early on it became clear to me that despite some Western beliefs to the contrary, the martial arts (in all their infinite variations) are forms of individual expression. Anyone who has seen women demonstrate the Ju-No-Kata, the sixth Kata (fundamental or basic form) of Judo, the form of suppleness (also translated as softness or gentleness), or watched individuals participating in the solo 'exercises' of Taijiquan knows that there can be poetic expression in the execution of the prescribed movements that brings to mind classical ballet. Each in its own way is an art form and for the martial artist, like the actor or dancer, mastery of their art form requires great dedication and hours of practice.

However, beyond the external physical movements of the martial arts I discovered ways of looking at performing arts that have proved crucial to my drama/theatre teaching practice. More importantly, my continual and progressive immersion in various forms of martial arts, particularly those referred to as internal martial arts (e.g. Qigong, Taijiquan, Aikido), has had a significant effect on the development of my perspective on the value of the arts to well-being and quality of life, particularly for persons with a disability. In particular, my study of the martial arts has led me to investigate Taoist concepts of health and healing which are considerably different from orthodox Western scientific medicine.

TAOIST CONCEPTS OF HEALTH AND HEALING

> To a large extent, all systems of medicine except those based on modern Western science are almost exclusively based on a holistic concept integrating the body, the mind and the total environment.
>
> (Watts, 1961)

In orthodox Western medicine the responsibility for health promotion and maintenance has generally been assumed by a class of physician-experts and relinquished by individuals in their own regard. Patients, who expect the doctor to 'cure' them, become ever more separated from conscious participation in their own healing processes.

Taoist healers contend that no disease condition can be isolated and that exclusive focus upon disease may obscure one's vision of the patient as a whole. According to Klate (1980), the true Taoist healer cannot diagnose outside the context of the patient's holistic situation, which always includes such elements as body, mind, emotion, behaviour and the practitioner's own awareness of the patient's relationship with him (or her). Rather than a 'diagnosis', Taoist healers create a relationship.

THE ROLE OF CHI IN WELL-BEING

All things are backed by shade (Yin) and faced by light (Yang) and harmonized by the 'immaterial breath' (chi).

(Reid, 1988)

Pure energy is the root of the human body.

(Lu, 1978)

The Taoist understanding of life is based on the concepts of Chi, the five elements (Earth, Fire, Metal, Water, Air) and Yin and Yang (opposite and complementary forces such as day and night, female and male) in our ever-changing universe (Chuen, 1991). For the Taoist the universe is alive with a kind of primal power, a force they refer to as Chi. Chi (also written as Qi, Ch'i or Ki) has no direct translation in English. It is often translated simply as 'energy' but vital force, life force or creative force more accurately describe it. Taoist belief suggests that not only do all living things possess Chi but also that we all live in the midst of this vital force (Pao-p'o Tzu, in Klate, 1980). Recent developments in quantum physics have suggested that this vital force (which the physicists conceive of as a field) exists always and everywhere and is the carrier of all material phenomena (Thirring, in Capra, 1977).

While not all practitioners are Taoist, Taoist principles permeate traditional Chinese medicine. In traditional Chinese medicine, Chi is said to flow through the body and blockage of this flow is believed to be one of the major causes of illness. Taoist healers believe that the correct balance between Yin and Yang and the harmonious mixture of the five elements cause health: that the relative harmony of tendencies and forces within an individual *is* the individual's state of health. They contend that the 'opposite' is also true, that lack of balance and disharmony cause disease (Veith, 1949).

The essence of Taoist healing is to strike a double balance. Not only should the energies of the body be in balance with themselves but the body must itself be in harmony with its surroundings. The Taoist healer is not the external manipulator of the life force of another being. Rather, they are a part of the process of healing. This is the ultimate holistic perspective. Body, mind and spirit are a unity and so are patient and practitioner (Klate, 1980).

The process of identifying imbalances and re-establishing balance both physically and emotionally is one of the primary focuses of Taijiquan and of Eastern medicine (Huang, 1995). Although the methods and concepts of practitioners vary, all true Taoist healers provide a framework for engaging each patient in a dance towards wellness, utilizing the healer's knowledge of the process and their awareness of their own and the patient's role within that process. In so doing, both healer and patient are made aware that, by taking responsibility for their well-being, they can have a say in the quality of their lives.

WEI WU WEI: DO WITHOUT DOING

When you seek it, you cannot find it.

(Zen riddle in Hyams, 1982)

In a way similar to the Taoist healer, those who study internal martial arts strive to manipulate their own, other's and the universal Chi. Masters of these arts use Chi as a means of both attacking an opponent and defending against an opponent's attack. Consciously thinking through or about an action is one of the greatest impediments to progress in these and other martial arts. Overintellectualization, particularly when first learning a form (such as in Taijiquan), acts as a barrier to investing the form with flow and feeling. More importantly, it inhibits response to the subtle energies both inside and outside of the body. The result is that a living art, in which martial art and martial artist should be as one, is transformed into a mechanical act of physical choreography. The same is true of actors and dancers who try too hard or think too much about their role, resulting in all too many 'wooden' performances.

EFFORTLESS ACTION: LINKS BETWEEN THE CREATIVE AND THE MARTIAL ARTS

The mind should be nowhere in particular.

(Takuan, in Hyams, 1982)

Effortless action (a prime example of do without doing (Hoff, 1982)) is, as I have suggested elsewhere (Warren, 1994b), one of the goals of both the martial arts and creative activity. To attain this goal one must let go of conscious thought. Emptying the mind is one of the crucial elements of learning any physical activity for invariably, thinking gets in the way of doing. The martial arts, particularly the internal martial arts, teach that the mind, like water, 'must always be in the state of flowing' (Takuan, in Hyams, 1982). Just as car drivers have to learn to integrate all of the components of driving a manual-shift car so that the action of changing gear or applying the brakes is a thoughtless one, so martial artists seek to act without conscious effort so that mind, body and spirit are in perfect harmony.

Eventually, masters of martial arts reach a level of proficiency where they do not have to think about their actions: they become completely focused at a single point. To accomplish this they must step beyond technical knowledge, the physical repetition of 'steps', and seek the balance between inner knowledge and external form. They step into a meditative state in which mind, body and spirit must be perfectly balanced. This concept can be compared to stories about watching the late Glen Gould play the piano where it was said that he, the piano and the music appeared to be one.

Immersion in a creative activity provides opportunities for the participant to achieve a meditative state remarkably similar to that of the martial artist. When an individual is immersed in creative activity they can become lost in a 'creative moment' – a liminal state that brings together physical, intellectual, emotional and spiritual aspects of our being in a way that offers unique opportunities for transformation to take place.

CREATIVE MOMENTS AND THE LIMINAL STATE

> Flow with whatever may happen and let your mind be free.
>
> (Chuang-Tzu, in Hyams, 1982)

Creative activity usually pursues a cyclic pattern, one that echoes both rites of passage and the play of young children. When we engage in a creative activity, we begin with *preparation*: in this phase we get ready for the activity – how we do this often depends on the nature of the creative task. We then move to *action*: in this phase we may become lost in a creative moment in which, like children lost in play, we merge with the activity, often losing all track of time. Finally we engage in *reflection*: the third phase when we stop the activity, often pausing to reflect on it. This cycle of preparation, action and reflection is often repeated many times. While the duration of each phase may change, nevertheless when we are immersed in the activity it is as if nothing else exists.

In each creative moment an individual is able to access and engage the emotions and free the spirit. This may encourage individuals to do something because they want to and *not* just because someone else decides it is good for them. This is particularly important for individuals who are in some way disadvantaged. Often these people are confined to a state of powerlessness where they are seldom consulted in matters related to their personal aspirations or well-being. Decisions are frequently made for them in an 'omnipotent' fashion on the basis of their disability rather than their individuality. They are seldom allowed to exercise their voice, let alone develop one that is creative. However, in engaging in a creative act they express the essence of who they are as an individual and may bring physical, intellectual, emotional and spiritual aspects of themselves into balance.

From a Taoist perspective creative moments provide a way of creating a double balance: a time when the energies of the body are in balance with themselves and the body is in harmony with its surroundings. At this time, when we are 'lost to the world', it is also possible that we may become open to change. Within the balanced stillness of the creative moment, the individual focuses all their being into a 'unique creative act' and it is in that creative moment, when Chi flows freely, that they may transcend their limitations. The potential exists for changes to take place, 'in spite of ourselves'.

Providing people with a disability with access to creative activity can have a profound effect on their sense of self and on their well-being. Ultimately, creative moments are windows on each individual's explicit, personal and practical knowledge: a reflection on what that individual knows.

CREATIVE ACTIVITY AS A WAY OF KNOWING

We know more than we can say.

(Polanyi, 1962)

All creative activities make use of three general forms of knowledge:

Explicit Knowledge ... commonly held beliefs or facts;
Practical Knowledge ... The *know-how* or *skills* that are necessary for the creation of artefacts;
Personal Knowledge ... '*Unique Experience*' – that which only the individual knows; ... '*Intuition*' – what individuals know but don't know how or why they know it.

(Courtney, 1990)

Individuals involved in creative activity are able to explore and express what they know, sometimes discovering things that at a conscious level they did not know they knew. Moreover, creative activity demands that playful imagining be employed as participants exercise their knowledge in the quest for solutions to the problem at hand.

The participant in any creative activity must make choices (e.g. do I use purple or blue for the sky?). Each decision, no matter how simple it may seem, affects what is communicated both to its creator and to others. In making a creative mark the participant lost in a creative moment explores possibilities not necessarily constrained by reality and pragmatism that allow for improvization and synthesis. As Monod (1971) suggests, this is the essence of evolutionary change.

ABILITY AND CREATIVE ACTIVITY

Do not ask how intelligent I am but rather *how* I am intelligent.

(Gardner, 1984)

It is one of the great beauties of creative activity that there is no single way of doing 'it'. While there are techniques which may be learned, there are no right or wrong answers (in the way that two plus two equals four). Participants in creative activities must be allowed to fail successfully: to learn from their 'mistakes'. Only by creating new problems do we find solutions to the obstacles we face, enabling us to build on our previous knowledge.

Using what we know, each of us can create something unique and meaningful to ourselves because all human beings, irrespective of their abilities or limitations, are capable of making their own unique creative thumbprint. Each 'mark', whether it is made in sound, line, colour, form, shape or movement, is one that no one else could ever make in exactly the same way. It is this mark which states 'I exist, I have meaning' and it is a reflection of an individual as a unique human being.

A disability does not preclude successful involvement in creative activity and intellectual or physical or emotional challenges in and of themselves are not barriers to participation and expression at the participant's own level of ability. In fact, it may be argued that overly developed intellectual abilities (e.g. the ability to 'multi-task' – to consciously think about more than one activity at a time) may act as an impediment to entering the liminal state that is necessary to progress in the martial or creative arts. Moreover, artistic experience can continue throughout an individual's lifetime. Longevity, rather than being an impediment, often leads to enriched participation in the creative arts. Above all, because there are no right answers, the creation of these unique marks celebrates the diversity of the human experience.

ARTS AND THE DIVERSITY OF HUMAN EXPRESSION

There is no one way of being.

(Courtney *et al.*, 1988)

We are uniquely different people and the creative arts allow us to express this individuality. The means employed by individuals for creative expression is different for different individuals. Martha Graham's form of expression was different from Pablo Picasso's which is different from Robert Le Page's. Even when exploring the same structure, different individuals communicate differently. This is why Patrick Stewart's interpretation of 'Prospero' will be different from that of Marlon Brando or Kenneth Branagh. Moreover, the need to make a particular 'creative mark' may change with time.

While the examples given are of illustrious artists, all of the above statements are true for persons with a disability. In many cases, individuals want to express themselves in a particular medium (e.g. dance), but do not possess the technical skills to 'say' exactly what they want to. This may be the result of physical restrictions or simply of a limited experience in that medium. In order to communicate in their chosen medium they must first learn its 'language'.

THE ARTS AS LIVING LANGUAGES

The virtuoso performance is the tip of a lifetime of struggle.

(Deng, 1988)

Participants in creative activity express their emotions, thoughts and ideas by manipulating different sets of symbols (musical notes, dance steps, etc.) in an attempt to communicate to others. As such each of the arts may be considered a living language, constantly evolving but subject to certain rules that define them.

In living languages there are rules and structures that determine how individual letters combine into the words of the vocabulary and how these words are arranged in a sentence. However, while technical skills, structures and even words can be taught, the skills of communication (the way that an individual employs language in conversation) are a much more complex proposition because communication needs to be flexible to enable the individuals involved to respond immediately to any situation.

Each art form (dance, music, etc.) has its own set of grammars (its technical rules and structure) and vocabulary (forms of expression) that distinguish one art from another (e.g. a sonata from a play). These are used by individuals either directly (the dancer's body) or via an external instrument (the pianist's piano) and allow individuals to express their responses to either internal or external changes. In the arts it is possible to teach the grammars and vocabulary of a form (e.g. in learning the piano one is often taught notes, scales, arpeggios, etc.) but few will be able to speak the language fluently and fewer still will become the next Horowitz or Gould.

INDIVIDUAL EXPRESSION AND QUALITY OF LIFE

JOHN MEETS BACH: CHANGING OTHERS' PERCEPTIONS

Start from where you are.

(Way, 1967)

As suggested earlier, there is value in learning the language of an art form. An example of this concerns a young man, whom I will call John, who had been admitted at the age of 12 to a residential facility providing programmes and services to youth and their families in need of psychosocial services. He had been maltreated, neglected and was referred as being 'socially retarded' and as having a 'learning disability'. When first admitted he was lacking in even basic levels of social skills. He did not know how to eat – he would mix all his meal together – vegetables, meat, dessert – and did not know how to use cutlery. He was frequently at the receiving end of jibes made at his expense by his room mates and peers.

About a year later, he started to learn the piano as part of a creative arts programme within the facility. He still had an extremely negative self-image and a low frustration threshold. Nevertheless, it was obvious from the very beginning that although he had never had a piano lesson in his life John had a natural talent. However, it was also apparent that conventional teaching methods, similar to those in which his teacher (a classical pianist) had herself been taught, would not work with John.

The initial approach taken by his teacher did not focus on reading notes, learning scales or key signatures. Instead, it concentrated on being able to play something, no matter how short, at the end of each lesson. This approach emphasized both John's skills (he had a remarkable capacity for 'musical mimicry') and his need for instant success. As time progressed more conventional approaches to piano teaching were introduced. As John became more able to postpone his need for instant gratification, he came to realize that he had to work on pieces to be successful. Throughout this time he continued to be the recipient of various jokes and was constantly picked on by his peers. Nevertheless, John was beginning to feel better about himself because, as he put it, 'You know what's so good about piano, people can ask me questions about something I know about and they don't'.

As part of a Christmas open house, showcasing the programme's work, John played J.S. Bach's Prelude in C, a piece he had been working on for about 16 weeks. The audience at this show was very noisy. Many of the parents, siblings, teachers and residents were simply unaware of the 'etiquette' required to be a member of an audience. However, when John started to play the audience quietened to the point that you could hear a pin drop. I sat there amazed, not only at the quality of John's performance, which was excellent, but also because an audience, more used to listening to heavy metal, was silently and attentively listening to a piece of classical music.

When he had finished the audience gave John two standing ovations, but a bigger surprise was yet to come. While he was playing the other teenage participants in the show were sitting in the 'green room' watching his performance on 'live' video. Three teenagers, who were among the worst offenders for teasing John, berated the others in the room, telling them to 'shut up and listen' to John's performance. At the end of the performance they said to the others, 'When John comes in let's all clap for him'. Not only did they clap for John, but they also gave him another standing ovation.

When last heard of, John had left the institution and had been bought a piano and was working on his music. While it would be hard to argue that learning to play the piano was the panacea for all his problems, nevertheless his sense of well-being and his quality of life were changed for the better as a result of his experiences. For John, learning the language of the piano changed not only how he perceived himself but also how others perceived him. As his piano teacher put it, as a result of his performance his peers, all 'tough' kids, have discovered a new respect for John. 'For this kid, it was the greatest night of his life so far' (Ortynsky, in Warren, 1991).

INTEGRATIVE THEATRE: WORKING TOGETHER FOR CHANGE

... the starting point for performers and directors was not based on physical or mental abilities, but rather on the potential for creativity ...
(Richard, 1992)

I have been investigating factors that affect the participation of persons with a disability in drama and theatre since 1988.* During this time an array of research instruments (including audiotapes, videotapes, journals, interviews) and approaches have been used to record information and a considerable amount of data has been collected concerning factors that may make a drama/theatre experience positive for all participants irrespective of their limitations.

* I must acknowledge the generous support for this research received during this time from the McLean Foundation, the Seagram Fund, Concordia University, McGill University, the University of Windsor, the Secretary of State, Government of Canada, the Ministry of Culture, Tourism and Recreation, the Government of the Province of Ontario and the Social Science Humanities Research Council.

Some of this work, which has come to be called integrative theatre, has already been documented (Mager & Warren, 1993; Warren, 1993c; Warren & Mager, 1993; Warren & Ortynsky, 1995). Below I focus on three particular episodes which are intended to illustrate some of the ways that creative activity may influence an individual's sense of well-being or quality of life.

MERVYN AND THE SPHINX: RECOGNIZING STRENGTHS – ACCEPTING LIMITATIONS

Show us a simple riddle lift everything aside.

(Hughes, 1969)

From its inception all those who worked with 50/50 Theatre Company in Montreal were treated as equals. However, in the first production it became clear that in purely theatrical terms company members clearly did not have equal abilities. So while persons with a disability have the right to equal status within an integrative theatre company, they nevertheless require different preparation and direction. They need to be given the chance to explore and extend their unique talents starting from where they are, not from some idealized unobtainable level of parity with actors who have 20 years professional experience prior to joining a company.

As the work progressed it became clear that a performer's limitations as an actor/dancer are as interesting as their strengths. There are things that can be done by a person using a wheelchair which cannot otherwise be accomplished. That is not to suggest that performers should not be helped to improve their technique or expand their repertoire of movement, voice, etc., but it is important that all involved accept that there are some things that will never change. The ability to use these unchangeable things to one's advantage is dependent, to an extent, on the creativity of the choreographer, the director and members of the integrative theatre company and, most importantly, the person with a disability.

50/50 Theatre Company's second production was Seneca's *Oedipus*. In this production the company involved a young man with a developmental disability who used an electric wheelchair (whom I will call Mervyn). Mervyn had extremely limited verbal and motor skills, but as he had previous experience in a company of wheelchair dancers, he was desperately keen to be part of this production. He was cast as part of the chorus, but his lack of verbal skills and his restricted movements made it obvious very early on that being one of the chorus was not working. The generous decision to involve an individual with limited theatrical skills was proving to be detrimental to the production, the other company members and most importantly to Mervyn himself.

A creative solution was found by the director working in conjunction with the designer: Mervyn would become the physical embodiment of the Sphinx. A special costume was designed that was extremely light-weight and could be attached to Mervyn's wheelchair. Mervyn was given one line to be said alone in a choral section of the play and so had his moment in the sun. The decision not only changed the look of the performance for the better but also, more significantly, gave Mervyn a chance to be successful.

RACHEL AND EDNA: REFRAMING THE PROBLEM

> ... the easiest way to get rid of a Minus is to change it into a Plus.
>
> (Hoff, 1982)

All actors and dancers experience frustration in the creation of a theatri-cal performance. Persons with a disability sometimes become frustrated because they feel they cannot overcome obstacles such as accomplishing a dance step or a piece of direction at their first attempts. Working in an integrated company, persons with a disability can learn that they are not alone in their frustrations. Others, some of whom have many years of professional experience, face similar problems. Everyone can become aware that statements like 'I can't do that' frequently mean 'I think I'm incapable of doing that' or 'I'm afraid to do that'. However, with help from the director and the support of one's colleagues, these problems can be overcome.

Even when the problem is the director's, not the performer's, the knowledge contained in the members of any group is a resource for the solving of problems. One young performer with Down syndrome (I will call her Rachel) had a particularly difficult time doing an aggressive, pushing movement on stage. The director tried many different approaches to unleash greater hostility from Rachel, to no avail. Finally, Edna (the performer opposite Rachel) suggested that she could help more through her own movements. Rather than the aggressive action coming from the aggressor Rachel, Edna reacted in such a physical way as to create the illusion that she had been terrified by Rachel's attack. That solved the problem. By changing her physical response, Edna had solved two problems: those facing Rachel and those of the director. In her concern for Rachel, Edna had reacted in a way to make Rachel look good on stage. As a result Rachel got many compliments at the end of the per-formance.

SAM AND THE NINJA: DEVELOPING SELF-AWARENESS

Nothing is impossible to a willing mind.

(Hyams, 1982)

For everyone the body is an instrument of expression. Physical training exercises in voice, movement and acting can help prepare individuals not only for the theatrical stage but also for the many challenges that daily social interactions bring to us. However, many of the exercises and activities that help develop creativity, self-expression and communication are inaccessible to persons with a disability. In order for these exercises to be of benefit they have to be adapted to give persons with a disability access to the potential change moments these activities possess.

While I was working on a show with Prospero's Fools Theatre Company in Windsor, a specific event occurred which highlighted this problem. In the production *The Demon of Experiment*, persons with a disability joined with professional actors to develop an integrated theatre presentation (Warren & Ortynsky, 1995). A series of workshops preceded work on the script. A practical exercise entitled Ninja (Warren, 1993a) formed the basis for several days of exploration. When first introduced, one of the performers, a man with extremely limited theatrical experience (whom I will call Sam) and who uses a wheelchair, was unable to participate in the original form of the exercise, which requires participants to stand upright throughout.

As always with a company of mixed abilities, while I made a few contingency plans, I worked from two premises, namely that a perceived challenge does not necessarily prevent participation and that working with the person with the disability will usually produce a means of making the activity accessible to them.

Unfortunately, despite our best first efforts, a suitable means of adaptation did not present itself immediately. This proved frustrating and disappointing both to Sam and to the group. Nevertheless, over a period of two or three days Sam and I worked together (aided by the other members of the company) to find ways to adapt this exercise so that it enabled rather than disabled him.

We solved the problem of accessibility by focusing on the breathing patterns necessary to execute the original exercise successfully. Then through slight modifications (based on Qigong breathing exercises and the theatrical concepts of intention and focus), we made the changes necessary to achieve successful participation. By working on the breathing patterns, rhythms and intentions underlying the mechanical movement sequence of the exercise rather than the movement itself, it was possible to translate these qualities into movements accessible to Sam.

As can be seen from the following comments, the adapted Ninja exercise affected Sam's sense of his body image:

This exercise made me realise that acting is an entire mind/body exercise, not just isolating body parts to perform particular tasks. I was shy and withdrawn but from the Ninja exercise on, I told myself why not see what my body can do ... what does my entire body have to say? I discovered that my body is far more flexible and more capable than I gave it credit. Through this exercise I rediscovered my body.

(Warren & Ortynsky, 1995)

All his comments identify the adaptation of the Ninja exercise as a change moment: one that had influence beyond the process by which we worked on *The Demon of Experiment*. The process of adaptation also had a notable effect on me and has led to my current investigation of what approaches to physical training may have to offer the performing artist with a disability. For Sam the Ninja exercise was a turning point in his life. From that point on he left his theatrical inexperience behind. He sought as much help, advice and training as he could and became a full-time member of Prospero's Fools. Now, three years later, he has moved to a bigger city where he is happily pursuing his goal of being a professional actor.

INTEGRATIVE THEATRE AND QUALITY OF LIFE

Pounding on the piano keys may produce noise; removing them doesn't exactly further the creation of music.

(Hoff, 1982)

The individual needs of participants in integrative theatre have forced drama teachers, theatre directors and choreographers to find new and exciting ways to realize their goals so as to include persons with a disability. Integrative theatre companies are living examples of how sharing the applied knowledge of participants engaged together in a creative activity can help resolve a problem that a single individual finds insurmountable. The work of integrative theatre companies such as 50/50 Theatre Company (Montreal) and Prospero's Fools (Windsor) have documented changes in individuals due, at least in part, to their participation in integrative drama/theatre. People who have been unable to communicate or interact socially have been fully integrated within a community of learners and artists, working together for solutions to a specific dramatic problem. In addition, people who have had little or no previous experience of working with persons with a disability have had the opportunity to explore and dispel many of their preconceived notions about disability, often forming friendships with the person with a disability that extend well beyond the end of a workshop or production.

Clearly no two performers are the same. Each brings their unique qualities to their portrayal of a character. Each individual member of any drama group or theatre company brings a variety of strengths and weakness to every workshop, rehearsal and performance. However, in a good company the sum of the whole will always be stronger than that of the individual parts. The same is true of society as a whole. The problems of being accepted and finding enjoyment in integrative theatre are similar to those that face the person with a disability in many social situations.

CONCLUSION

Participation in a creative activity such as integrative theatre or playing the piano provides the chance for persons with a disability to explore problems in a supportive environment. The friendships and the experience gained from such work may enable persons with a disability to cope with change when the need arises. As I have suggested above, the ability to adapt to change is a necessary skill which affects an individual's quality of life.

REFERENCES

Capra, F. (1977) *The Tao of Physics*, Bantam Books, New York.
Chuen, Master L.K. (1991) *The Way of Energy: Mastering the Chinese Art of Internal Strength with Chi Kung Exercise*, Simon & Schuster/Fireside, New York.
Coles, P. (1981) *The Manchester Hospitals' Arts Project*, Calouste Gulbenkian, London.
Courtney, R. (1990) *Drama and Intelligence: A Cognitive Theory*, McGill/Queen's University Press, Montreal
Courtney, R., Booth, D., Emerson, T. and Kuzmich, N. (1988) *No One Way of Being: Practical Knowledge of Elementary Arts Teachers in Ontario*, Ministry of Education, Government of Ontario, Toronto.
Cousins, N. (1979) *Anatomy of an Illness*, W.W. Norton, New York.
DeLoach, C. and Greer, B. (1981) *Adjustment to Severe Physical Disability: A Metamorphosis*, McGraw-Hill, New York.
Deng, M.D. (1988) *365 Tao Daily Meditations*, Harper, San Francisco.
Exley, H. (ed.) (1984) *What It's Like to Be Me*, Exley, Watford, United Kingdom.
Fry, W.F. Jr (1977) The respiratory components of mirthful laughter. *Journal of Biological Psychology*, **19**, 39–50(b).
Fry, W.F. Jr (1979) Humour and the cardiovascular system, in *The Study of Humour*, (eds H. Mindess and J. Turek), Antioch University, Los Angeles.
Fry, W.F. Jr and Stoft, P.E. (1971) Mirth and oxygen saturation levels of peripheral blood. *Psychotherapy and Psychosomatics*, **19**, 76–84.
Gardner, H. (1983) *Frames of Mind*, Basic Books, New York.
Hoff, B. (1982) *The Tao of Pooh*, Dutton, New York.
Huang, Y-C. (1995) How to work with disabled students. *T'ai Chi*, **19**, 30–3.
Hughes, T. (1969) *Seneca's Oedipus*, Faber, London.
Hyams, J. (1982) *Zen in the Martial Arts*, Bantam Books, New York.
Johnson, D.R. (1984) The arts and communitas. *Design*, **86**, 36–9.
Klate, J.S. (1980) *The Tao of Acupuncture*, UMI, Ann Arbor, MI.

Kosko, B. (1993) *Fuzzy Thinking: The New Science of Fuzzy Logic*, Hyperion, New York.

Lu, H.C. (1978) *A Complete Translation of Nei Ching and Nan Ching (Vols. I-IV)*, The Chinese Foundation of Natural Health, Vancouver.

Mager, G.C. and Warren, B. (1993) From segregation to integration: the use of circles of friends in integrated theatre. *Journal of Practical Approaches to Developmental Handicap*, **17**, 17–25.

McClelland, D.C., Alexander, C. and Marks, E. (1982) The need for power, stress, immune function, and illness among male prisoners. *Journal of Abnormal Psychology*, **91**, 61–70.

Monod, J. (1971) *Chance and Necessity*, Alfred A. Knopf, New York.

Moss, L. (1987) *Art for Health's Sake*, Carnegie Trust, Dunfermline.

Payne, P. (1981) *Martial Arts: the Spiritual Dimension*, Crossroad, New York.

Polanyi, M. (1962) *Personal Knowledge*, Harper & Row, New York.

Reid, H. (1988) *The Way of Harmony: A Guide to Self-knowledge through the Arts of T'ai Chi Chuan, Hsing I, Pa Kua and Chi Kung*, Simon & Schuster/Fireside, New York.

Richard, R.J. (1992) *A Descriptive Analysis of Two Approaches to the Use of Drama with Persons with Disabilities*. MA thesis, Concordia University, Montreal.

Saper, B. (1988) Humour in psychiatric healing. *Psychiatric Healing*, **59**, 306–19.

Senior, P. and Croall, J. (1993) *Helping to Heal*, Calouste Gulbenkian, London.

Toffler, A. (1975) *The Eco-Spasm Report*, Bantam Books, New York.

Veith I. (1949) *Huang Ti Nei Ching Su Wen (The Yellow Emperor's Classic of Internal Medicine)*, University of California Press, Berkeley.

Warren, B. (1988) *Disability and Social Performance*, Brookline Books, Cambridge, MA.

Warren, B. (1989) The hidden stage: using drama to teach the unspoken rules of social interaction, in *Learning Difficulties and Emotional Problems*, (eds R.I. Brown and M. Chazan), Detselig, Calgary.

Warren, B. (1991a) Transforming thumbprints: thoughts on the gaps between the arts and therapy. *Journal of Creative and Expressive Arts Therapies Exchange*, **1**, 19–24.

Warren, B. (1991b) *Integration through the Theatre Arts: Relationships among Physical Humour, Disability and Social Stigma within a Theatrical Context*. Research Report, Seagram Foundation, Montreal.

Warren, B. (ed.) (1993a) *Using the Creative Arts in Therapy: A Practical Introduction*, 2nd edn, Routledge, London.

Warren, B. (1993b) *Through Chi to the Lightbulb: Creativity, Transformation and Healing*. Keynote address, AThRA Symposium, Banff School of Fine Arts.

Warren, B. (1993c) *Learning from One Another: Integrative Drama and Theatre in Education for People with Disabilities*. Paper presented at *The Relationship between Drama & Learning*, International Research Conference, Institute of Education, University of London.

Warren, B. (1994a) 'Creative Laughter: In search of the links among fools, creative activity and well-being' Colloquium, Faculty of Human and Exact Sciences, University of Algarve, Portugal.

Warren, B. (1994b) *Eastern Approaches to Creative Movement: A Practical Introduction for Artists, Educators and Other Professionals Interested in Personal Development*, University of Windsor, Windsor.

Warren, B. (ed.) (1995) *Creating a Theatre in Your Classroom*, Captus University Publications, North York.

Warren, B. and Mager, G.C. (1993) Integrative drama/theatre and education. *Drama Contact*, **17**, 13–15.

Warren, B. and Nadeau, R. (1988) Enhancing the quality of life: the role of the arts in the process of rehabilitation, in *Quality of Life for Handicapped People*, (ed. R.I. Brown), Croom Helm, London.

Warren, B. and Ortynsky, J. (1995) *The Demon of Experiment*: confronting problems of research in integrative drama/theatre, in *Drama and Theatre in Education: Contemporary Research*, (ed. J. Somers), Captus University Publications, North York, Ontario.

Watts, A. (1961) *Psychotherapy East and West*, Mentor, New York.

Way, B. (1967) *Development Through Drama*, Longmans, London.

Weisberg, N. and Wilder, R. (1986) *Creative Arts with Older Adults*, Human Sciences Press, New York.

Human spirituality in relation to quality of life 14

Aldred H Neufeldt and Patrick McGinley

INTRODUCTION

The idea of people as spiritual beings is notable by its absence from the literature on quality of life or in related literature pertaining to people with disabilities and community rehabilitation. Such neglect of spirituality might be considered somewhat surprising when one considers that the majority of the peoples in the world adopt some identifiable form of spiritual expression. Christianity, Buddhism, Islam, Hinduism and Judaism are the ones most often visible, but there are others.

Underlying reasons for silence on the topic are not hard to fathom. Some have to do with the history of scientific philosophy and the separation of science from religion in Western societies over the past several centuries. The construct of spirituality largely disappeared from educational and psychological literature somewhere around the end of the 19th century with the emergence of logical positivism as the predominant philosophy in scientific debate. Religious and spiritual concepts were seen as esoteric and unobservable. Even constructs having a 'mental' connotation were largely ignored by the behavioural and functional theorists who dominated psychological thought through the middle part of the 20th century. 'Mental' and 'emotional' constructs re-emerged in the psychological and educational literature during the 1960s and, within the past two decades, it has become acceptable to consider 'beliefs' and 'values' as useful constructs within an analytic and intervention paradigm. But there has been a studious neglect of 'spirituality' and 'religious beliefs' as important contributors to the understanding of humanity, though some research on spiritual subjects has emerged recently in relation to mental and physical health (see, for example, Gartner, Larson & Allen, 1991). Similar research in relation to disability, and in particular in relation to quality of life and disability, has yet to emerge.

Parallel arguments developed in the context of professional practice, as in research. Effective professional practice has been predicated on a stance that is non-imposing and non-judgemental. A part of professional wisdom, then, is that one avoids delving into potentially controversial areas such as religious beliefs, just as one avoids conversation about politics. The consequence, though, is that people seeking help from someone with an understanding of their spiritual beliefs usually receive at best only partial satisfaction.

The evidence of the importance of spirituality is all around us. If one travels through 'developing countries' one is often struck by the unselfconscious way religious beliefs become part of everyday discourse. Allah's name is invoked with regularity in Islamic countries. The church plays a highly visible and continuing role in most Latin American countries.

Formal religion has become less visible in high-income countries where participation in various churches (and in other formal religious groups) has dropped dramatically within the past century. Bibby (1995), a sociologist who has tracked these data in Canada, notes that weekly church attendance has dropped from about 60% in 1945 to around 20% today. But formal membership statistics do not necessarily denote loss of interest in the spiritual side of self. For example, Bibby notes that whereas the United Church of Canada only has about 700,000 formal members, over three million Canadians define themselves as its adherents. Similar data no doubt could be presented for other religious groups in many high-income countries.

Along with the established religions, there has been an emergence of 'new age' religious practices and a return to more fundamentalist forms of many of the dominant world religions. World news reports often refer to 'Islamic fundamentalists' or other similar groups as challenging state practices. Such fundamentalism is not limited to any one religion. Harvey Cox (1994), who in the 1960s predicted the imminent demise of Christianity in his book *The Secular City*, has recently written a book on the phenomenal growth of the Pentecostal movement in both low- and high-income countries.

In short, there continues to be a striving for spiritual meaning even in the most materialistic and 'logically positive' of societies. Central to this chapter is the argument that our understanding of people with disabilities, indeed all people, is incomplete unless we include some understanding of their spirituality, for two reasons. First, we suggest that full understanding of the person can be achieved only if some allowance is made for understanding spirituality, given that a large portion of the world's population clearly have spiritual beliefs. Second, much as they might assume they are free of conflict, professionals do not, in our experience, routinely monitor their own spiritual stance. Just as professionals have begun to understand that their own beliefs and values are important to both their own practices and the lives of people with whom they work, so too is the understanding of their own spirituality.

SPIRITUALITY AND PERSONHOOD

Spirituality is usually thought of in theistic terms, though it does not have to be. Examples of definitions include the following:

> Pertaining to or affecting the immaterial nature or soul of man (sic);
> Of or pertaining to God, or the soul as acted upon by the Holy Spirit.
> *(Funk & Wagnalls Dictionary*, 1986)

> The gestalt of the total process of human life and development related to the person's search for meaning and totally fulfilling relationships between oneself, other people and the encompassing universe and ontological ground of existence, whether a person understands this in terms that are theistic, atheistic, non-theistic, or any combination.
> (Canda, 1988)

These and other definitions point to an intangible, yet central dimension to the human experience. They touch on the states of awareness and human function underlying the possession of higher order values including the heroic, humanitarian, ethical, aesthetic and altruistic.

The tension between what is tangible and what is intangible to our understanding is not new, nor is 'intangibility' sufficient reason for dismissing phenomena. For example, Wilder Penfield, after a distinguished scientific career of trying to prove that the physiological brain accounts for the mind, observed that the mind seems to exist and act independently of the particular structures of the brain (Penfield, 1975). Mind and spirituality should not be considered synonymous, but they are interconnected in their intangibility and in the commonality of their human experience.

A model of the relative relationship of spirituality to various dimensions of personhood is illustrated in Figure 14.1. As a convenience, it is suggested that the definition of 'person' can be thought of as involving two main factors: our characteristics and our identity orientation. In oversimplified terms, our characteristics can be divided into those acquired and those inherited. This is consistent with the lengthy and ongoing history of research, which has amply examined the importance of both. Similarly, our source of identity is partly intrapersonal (self defined in relation to self) and partly extrapersonal (self defined in relation to others). Sample characteristics of identity are set out in each of the quadrants. We acquire skills, knowledge, insights (self–self), but we also acquire social networks (self–other) which, in turn, contribute to the definition of who we are. Similarly, we inherit biological characteristics

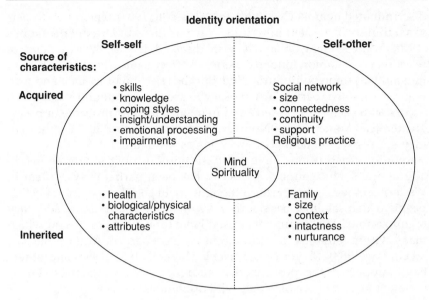

Fig. 14.1 Dimensions of personhood model.

and predispositions to various health conditions, but we also inherit our biological family and their various characteristics which, in turn, make a substantial contribution to our identity. The dotted lines dividing the quadrants denote that there is an interplay between inherited and acquired, as there is between intra- and extrapersonal loci of identity orientation. Touching all of these at the core, it is suggested, are such intangible constructs as spirituality and mind.

There is a further point. Spirituality and religious practice should not be thought of as the same. Both contribute to our identity but religious practice is observable and largely defines us in the interaction with others (self–other). We participate in Christian or Islamic or Jewish services and rites and this contributes to a sense of who we are. But this is not the same as the person's particular spiritual beliefs. The intangibility of spirituality is such that one can find deeply spiritual persons outside organized religious practice and people of little spirituality within. The strength of religious groups, though, is that they are usually composed of people seeking to strengthen their spiritual being.

RELIGIOUS PRACTICE AND PEOPLE WITH DISABILITIES

Many writers have made the point from personal observations and experience, as well as from systematic study, that people with disabilities in societies around the world routinely find themselves marginalized and discriminated against (Neufeldt & Mathieson, 1995). The insult to personal dignity is evident in writings such as those in Driedger & Gray's (1990) anthology by women who were disabled. In part, the experience of rejection is a common human experience affecting nearly all, if not all, of humanity at some point during life. But the rejection of women and men who are disabled, particularly those who are more profoundly impaired, occurs with such predictability and frequency that the probable impact is greater. Jean Vanier, Henri Nouwen and others, using religious phraseology, speak of the experience of rejection as 'wounding'.

Religious institutions have not been without their shortcomings in addressing such 'wounds'. Criticism has been particularly evident in Western societies, where critical thought about social structures affecting people with disabilities has flourished with the rise of disability advocacy organizations. The arguments raised have touched a point with which many within religious faith communities have agreed. Authors such as McGinley (1988), Meyer (1986), Webb-Mitchell (1986; 1988) and others have supported the position that churches and synagogues should become more inclusive of people with disabilities.

STUDIES OF CHURCH PARTICIPATION

Two kinds of empirical information have been gathered on the participation of people with disabilities in religious activities. Some studies have sampled groups of people with disabilities to ascertain the extent of their participation, usually in contrast to other leisure activities. Other studies have sampled congregations, with informants usually being the clergy.

An example of the first type of study is that of Scuccimara & Speece (1990) who examined the transition of mildly intellectually impaired youth from high school into community. Two years after leaving high school, church attendance was the third most frequently cited activity (63%), as contrasted with television watching (100%) and movie attendance (91%). In another study, Putnam, Pueschal & Holman (1988) found that 61% of adults with Down syndrome attended religious activities weekly, contrasting with 31% who attended clubs or other organization types of meetings. Other studies by Lavigne & Morin (1991) and Kregel *et al.* (1986) found that approximately half their samples of people with intellectual disabilities participated in religious activities. In contrast, a few studies found that religious activities ranked low in lists of frequently attended leisure activities. In Brown, Bayer & MacFarlane's (1989) study of quality of life, religious activities ranked 24th out of 28 in leisure activities. Wilhite, Reilly & Teaff (1989) also found religious activities relatively low, ranking 14th out of 21 activities.

Several observations might be made about these studies. First, they varied immensely in the age and geographic location of populations studied. Both sample age and differences in local community norms for church attendance might explain some of the differences. Second, it may well be that the data describe differences in 'beliefs' and practices of service providers rather than of the people with disabilities themselves. Third, it is noteworthy that a substantial portion of people with disabilities attend religious activities, with rates at least as high as that of population norms. It may be, though, that while attendance is relatively high, meaningful participation in activities is much lower. Kregel *et al.*'s (1986) study found that although 46% of young adults with intellectual impairments attended church services, only 14% participated in available church activities such as clubs or choirs.

In contrast, studies of congregations generally have found a disproportionately low participation rate by people with disabilities in church activities. Stubblefield (1975), in a survey of 220 clergymen in the United States from such diverse denominations as Baptist, Methodist, Church of Christ, Presbyterian, Nazarene and Catholic, found that only 9% reported any special provision for people with intellectual impairment. The implication was that very few congregations had any participants with intellectual impairments. In a more recent study of 64 congregations in one city in Canada, Stolovitsky (1992) found that people with disabilities aged 15–54 constituted less than 1% of the congregants, much less than the approximate 8% one would expect to find for this age range given available public incidence data on disability. Riordan & Vasa (1991), in a survey of 125 clergy in one mid-Western city in the United States, also found that few clergy identified individuals with disabilities in their congregations. They surmised that either clergy were unaware of disabled congregants or they did not provide opportunities for people with disabilities to participate. Barriers to inclusion, according to these and other studies, included: negative attitudes of parishioners and/or clergy, communication barriers (such as level of language and the lack of technical aids for deaf persons), architectural barriers and the lack of training of clergy (Gaventa, 1986; Stolovitsky, 1992; Wilke, 1980).

THE HISTORICAL ROLE OF FAITH COMMUNITIES

The term 'faith community' is used to refer to collections of people with a shared spiritual faith and vision who intentionally assemble on a regular or ongoing basis and who have an organizational base that can provide some assurance of continuity (Neufeldt, 1991).

While religious faith communities as represented by the people participating in churches, synagogues or mosques can be criticized for their complacency, it would be wrong to conclude that they have been more hostile environments than the surrounding society. Indeed, historically they have had a very positive role in giving dignity to disabled individuals.

Gold (1981), for example, observes that while, in general, heroes tend to be physically attractive, this has not been so for many heroes in the Jewish tradition. He gives examples from early Judaism of Moses' severe stutter, Jacob who limped following his encounter with God, Sarah who was barren for most of her life and Leah, Jacob's wife, who had 'weak eyes'. Gold notes that concern for the dignity of the diseased person is evident in sections of the Torah which deals with lepers. It was necessary to separate someone with a contagious disease, yet they were not sent away or locked up forever. They did not become non-persons; they were kept in a place on the periphery of the camp, not so far from the others, until they could rejoin the group.

Christianity has been marked from its beginnings by attention to those who were needy, weak or infirm. Among all the miracles of Jesus described in the Gospels, there is one which rehabilitation practitioners might find particularly compelling reading; a miracle which is attractively and realistically described and which is consistent with the experience of people who, after a period of blindness, are enabled to see again following surgery. The account from *Mark* (8: 22–6) follows:

> They came to Bethsaida, and some people brought Him a blind man whom they begged Him to touch. He took the blind man by the hand and led him outside the village. Then putting spittle on his eyes and laying his hands on him, He asked, 'Can you see anything?'. The man, who was beginning to see, replied, 'I can see people; they look like trees to me, but they are walking about'. Then He laid his hands upon the man's eyes again and he saw clearly; he was cured, and he could see everything plainly and distinctly. And Jesus sent him home saying, 'Do not even go into the village'.

This and other Gospel accounts of miracles are not just so many stories of magical cures demonstrating Jesus' special power over evil. They reflect a consistent attitude of Jesus towards the personal dignity of people who were blind or were impaired by leprosy, paraplegia or mental illness. The examples and sayings of Jesus provided a challenge for all Christians to take seriously the dignity of disabled people, to be caring and to include people with disabilities in the everyday life of the community. The commitment of the early Christians was such that by the fourth century of the Christian era the first formally organized means of caring for persons with various forms of disability had been established (cf. Wolfensberger, 1980).

Wolfensberger (1980) also documents how the seeds of neglect and rejection of disability were sown in the early Christian church. In this respect, the church has been vulnerable to the same human and social dynamics as other social institutions. Neufeldt & Luke (1985) describe three major cycles of neglect and enlightenment over the centuries.

Nevertheless, even during times of neglect (sometimes outright rejection), significant elements within the church continued to provide support and care for people with disabilities outside the family. Indeed, during the so-called Dark Ages, monasteries and other church institutions were the only social institutions to provide support to lepers and others with significant degrees of impairment.

Since then, many church-related organizations have emerged with a devotion to assisting 'the sick', 'the poor' and 'the disabled'. The present-day Society of St Vincent de Paul can be traced back to a priest who organized lay groups in France during the 17th century to serve the poor, foundlings and the ill. As another example, Reichgeldt (1957) gives a detailed account of the work of Canon Peter Joseph Triest (1760–1836) who founded the Sisters of Charity of Jesus and Mary and the Brothers of Charity in the early nineteenth century. The growth of the Brothers of Charity was such that by 1886 the order had 397 members, of whom 303 were Belgians, 58 were Canadians and Americans, 19 were Dutch, 13 were German and four were English. Today the Brothers of Charity work in rehabilitation, particularly with people having intellectual difficulties and mental handicaps, on five continents and 19 countries. Another church-inspired leader was William Tuke, an English Quaker who petitioned the Society of Friends in 1792 to establish a mental hospital of their own where 'a milder and more appropriate system of treatment than that usually practised might be adopted'. Other examples of participation by Christian groups and organizations up to and including the present are discussed below.

Indeed, most major human service forms in Western society, from hospitals to welfare to community housing, can be traced back to earlier versions provided by the church. Similarly, many if not most of the non-governmental agencies at work in low-income countries have their roots in the church. Provision of support to families by governments and secular non-governmental agencies is a relatively recent innovation in economically developed countries, with the vast majority of developments occurring since the beginning of the 20th century.

The Judeo-Christian religious tradition was not alone in this. Myles (1981) describes the concern for disabled persons which may be found in the early writings of Islam. According to Myles, the written revelation of Islam records specific provision for the guardianship of feeble-minded people. Islamic schools of legal interpretation discussed the rights of mentally disabled persons as early as the eighth and ninth century of the Christian era. Similarly, Ajuwon (1993) gives a number of examples where the 'heroes' of Islam were people with disabilities.

In short, it would be unfortunate to ignore the existing or potential roles of religious institutions and faith communities in the lives of disabled people. Wilson (1975) wrote: '... she (the Church) is the gathering together of the competent and the incompetent (and who is to say which is which?), in such a way as to be the sign of unity for mankind as a whole'. In an analogous way Bach (1981) described the role of the church as being opposite to the rehabilitation model. Whereas rehabilitation is generally thought of as incorporating marginalized people into ordinary society, the role of the church ... on the contrary, means this: the blind eight-year-old girl is already a member of the Body of Christ and does not have to become one. The weak members are already members of the Body of Christ. The only question is whether we act accordingly' (Bach, 1981).

In other words, problems of inclusion are a reflection of the church not living up to its mission, rather than whether people with disabilities have the privilege of joining it in the first instance. Furthermore, as Kelly & McGinley (1990) point out, people with intellectual disability are fundamentally necessary in the church as, without them, the church cannot be a complete community. Though it could be demonstrated that all of the world's major religions have not lived up to their spiritual aspirations, they also represent a potent resource when pursuing their mission along the lines expressed above.

FAITH COMMUNITIES AS SOURCES OF SUPPORT

The role of religion has not been totally ignored in studies of quality of life, as noted in some of the studies cited earlier. Generally, participation in religious activities tends to be considered in the category of how one uses one's leisure time and in relation to 'social well-being' or a similar 'subjective' category.

To the extent that spirituality as a construct overlaps with that of quality of life, inclusion in this way makes some sense. A common problem of intellectually impaired adults and others with severe levels of impairment is their impoverished social network. Family members and paid care givers tend to predominate, with other people with disabilities rarely part of their group. Participation in faith communities, then, is an indicator of one's social network, as well as an indicator of time use in a socially constructive manner.

The value of having and participating in a meaningful social network has been noted by various authors. Gottlieb (1983), for example, summarized data showing the buffering effect that social support networks had on personal health. People in supportive relationships tend to live longer, are sick less often and, when sick, recover more quickly. There also is a certain cultural validity. Most cultures encourage neighbours helping neighbours.

Though imperfect, religious faith communities have had a long history of providing support to people with disabilities, particularly in the

Christian tradition as noted above. Some of these have taken the approach of developing intentional communities outside formal church structures; others of building greater inclusiveness within existing congregational structures.

INTENTIONAL COMMUNITIES

Perhaps the best known of the intentional faith communities with an emphasis on including people with disabilities have been the L'Arche communities. L'Arche had its beginnings in 1964 when Jean Vanier chose to live with a group of intellectually impaired people in Trosly-Breuil, France (Clarke, 1974; Vanier, 1979, 1982a, b). L'Arche is the French word for 'the Ark', symbolizing Noah's Ark as a place of refuge, a community of variety and of hope (Clarke, 1974). Vanier describes the objective thus:

> Our aim is not just to have Christian assistants bound together in Christian love to 'look after' the weak and the poor. Our goal is to live in community with handicapped men and women, to create bonds with them and thus to discover their pathetic call. It is to create a community where handicapped people are fully members ... this unity in community between assistants and handicapped people is the heart and essence of L'Arche.
>
> (Vanier, 1982a)

This commitment of non-disabled assistants and people with disabilities living together with equality, pursuing a search for healing relationships, has become an inspiration around the globe. Communities now include Christians of many denominations as well as Hindus, Muslims and others (Philippe, 1982; Sadler, 1982; Vanier, 1982b). The nature of the experiences and struggles has been documented by a variety of authors (Allier, 1982; Dunne, 1986; Mosteller, 1982; Nouwen, 1986).

A community very different in form from L'Arche, though nonetheless committed to the pursuit of faith ideals, is the Botton Village Community near Danby in North Yorkshire, England. It was founded in 1955 by Carol Konig. The village houses about 300 people (200 villagers and 100 co-workers and their families) including individuals with Down syndrome, autism, brain injury, intellectual impairment, periodic depression and rage. The community does not admit people who need constant medical attention. Co-workers subscribe to the ideological motivation of Rudolf Steiner's anthroposophy, though many services and seminars are entirely optional and some villagers and co-workers attend the Church of England (Gaylord, 1974).

The Chemin d'Esperance (The Way of Hope) Community, based in Arnes, France, is a non-residential community serving adults and children with physical and intellectual impairments, with membership open to people without disabilities as well. Founded by Michel Mille in 1965, with a view to providing specialized catecheses for people with disabilities in the diocese of Arras, the movement quickly gave rise to a desire to form a basic Christian community giving priority to relationships, the welcoming of others and the sharing of daily experiences within the full meaning of Christian faith (Devestel, 1982).

Yet another approach has been that of the Fraternity of Cluizel near Lyon, France. Here men and women from different religious congregations have come together with intellectually disabled people and live together a life patterned on the discipline of religious orders. Mentally handicapped adults are asked to understand the meaning of the religious vows of chastity, poverty and obedience insofar as they can. Supported by a Christian attitude and inspiration, they may not marry and must live simply and dedicate themselves to the service of God (Devestel, 1982).

Examples of intentional communities with an emphasis on including people with disabilities also exist in North America. For example, the Hutterite Brethren, an Anabaptist Christian group that traces its emphasis on communal living back nearly 500 years, has as one of its central emphases a lifestyle reflected in joint decision making and the holding of all assets in common (cf. Hostetler, 1974; Janzen, 1990). They have a commitment to ensure that all members (including those with physical, sensory or mental impairments) have a meaningful place in their communities.

INCLUSIVENESS IN OPEN COMMUNITIES

Other faith groups have placed greater emphasis on encouraging inclusiveness of people with disabilities within existing congregational structures and programmes.

Perhaps the most concerted emphasis has been that of the Mennonites, another Anabaptist Christian group. As with the Hutterites, there has been a history of commitment to intentional sharing of resources and looking after all one's own people, though not in the communal lifestyle of the Hutterite Brethren (cf. Neufeldt, 1983). Special purpose small group residences were developed for intellectually and psychiatrically impaired members as early as the late 19th century, with residences located in the context of the towns or villages where Mennonites lived. Emphasis was and continues to be placed on encouraging participation of people with disabilities in congregational life. Within the past 20 years specific emphasis has been given to encouraging development of 'supportive care groups' within congregations with a mission to seek the full inclusion of people with severe disabilities into congregational and community life (Neufeld, 1991; Preheim-Bartel and Neufeldt, 1986).

Mennonites have not been alone. Methodists, Baptists, Lutherans, Christian Reformed, Catholics and many other denominations in North America have designated offices responsible for co-ordinating and supporting ministries related to people with disabilities. Preheim-Bartel & Neufeldt (1986) list over 30 offices of various denominations which have resource materials available for affiliated congregations.

THE INTERSECTION OF PERSONAL SUPPORT WITH SPIRITUALITY

The limits inherent in social institutions, including those of faith communities (whether intentional or open), have already been referred to. People within such communities, to a degree, experience similar influences as those outside them and succumb to similar systemic influences which lead to periodic breakdown and the need for renewal as other social institutions. Neufeldt & Breau (1991) have reflected on some of their experiences with the Mennonite and L'Arche communities, respectively. The demands of day-to-day living, the crosscurrents of social opinion and issues and differences in view and personality between individual people have been in tension with the ideals of both kinds of faith communities.

At the level of the person within a community they observe:

> ... that need for personal support and seeking personal support are two different things. It is also evident that little of what is known about personal support gives much understanding of what contributes to a successful continuing relationship, or how the mutual inter-dependence which emerges responds to the deeper beingness of man.
>
> (Neufeldt & Breau, 1991, p13)

Support is received in an unobtrusive manner in the normal circumstance, as in the support given by a parent to a child, the support of spouses to each other or of parents to schools, employers to employees and so on. Such support is noticed primarily when it is absent.

However, when one experiences a loss of some kind, then the importance of seeking out support becomes more evident. Parents who bear a child with an impairment experience loss. The loss is in the contrast between their experience and their aspiration of having a perfect child. In the same way, experience with a traumatic head injury, the discovery of cancer and so on brings with it an acute sense of change and loss. At the most basic level, such experiences expose one's 'impairment' – in the lack of knowledge one has and in the lessened capability to function. Beyond 'impairment' one may experience 'pain' – either physical or emotional. Impairments of a physiological dimension often have physical pain associated with them but the pain may be emotional as well – as when parents

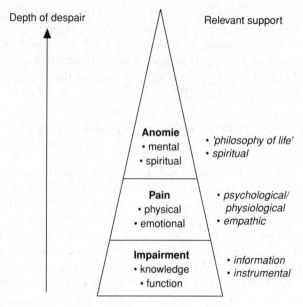

Fig. 14.2 Kinds of support in relation to felt despair.

experience the pain of watching their disabled child struggle with adversities in the world or the pain of rejection from others, the recognition of lost opportunities and so on. At times the pain is such that one may experience anomie, a sense of despair so deep that life becomes meaningless. Figure 14.2 suggests the relationship of these three levels as overlapping, but involving progressively greater experiences of despair.

Neufeldt & Breau (1991) propose that the kind of support that is valued depends on the level of despair experienced by the prospective recipient of support. Instrumental and informational supports are most easily provided by personal support networks. These help compensate for the sense of 'impairment'. At the other end of the continuum, though, the sense of anomie is likely to be beyond the capacity of most support groups to respond to. Those based in faith communities may have the capacity to provide some spiritual guidance, but the fundamental mental and spiritual dimensions of anomie are such that the person alone has to address the issue.

SPIRITUALITY IN RELATION TO QUALITY OF LIFE

We began this chapter by observing that spirituality is a topic rarely addressed in the literature on quality of life. While some quality of life studies have considered information on religious practices as part of their purview, that is not the same as considering the spiritual dimension of the person. A few authors argue that quality of life should be viewed as a 'sensitizing concept', focusing on 'broader-life defining issues by attempting to comprehend the perspective of the person with a disability (see Chapter 3). The 'broader life-defining issues' idea starts to get at the notion of spirituality, though it is not identical. Life-defining issues may indeed have a spiritual dimension, but could also represent some other important experience not affecting one's spiritual perspective. Peter (see Chapter 3) and Taylor (1994) have rightly pointed out the difficulty of trying to understand life experience from the perspective of the individual. To ascertain the spiritual perspective of the person is particularly difficult when researchers have not monitored their own stance in this regard.

A reflection on the relationship of both spirituality and religious practice to the identity of a person and the relationship of both of these to quality of life suggests that the construct of 'spirituality' lies on a different conceptual plane. 'Spirituality' implies an absolute, higher-order ideal or ethic. 'Quality of life', on the other hand, implies moral or value-based relativism. While the observable parts of religious practice lend themselves to inclusion within a quality of life framework, the interpretation of such practice presents some difficulties because of the relativism.

Brown's definition of quality of life points to the discrepancy between achieved and unmet needs and desires and the extent to which individuals increasingly control aspects of their own lives (Brown, Bayer & MacFarlane, 1989, pp57–8). Such definitions have considerable utility when examining an individual's experience over time and, in turn, provide useful insights for the provision of various community rehabilitation services. But they also have inherent limitations. Two people with roughly the same life experiences and available resources could end up concluding they have vastly different qualities of life depending on their desires and sense of control.

Differences between people do exist, of course. As such, the construct of quality of life has an elegance to it, allowing for the explanation of individual differences. But one is left wondering whether the fundamental conclusions arrived at with respect to quality of life by an individual are not based on some more fundamental ethic which lies on a plane that is orthogonal to, or surrounds, quality of life judgements.

Take as an example a person who confronts the prospect of death because of a virulent form of cancer. Prior to diagnosis, the person may well have complained considerably about their quality of life. It is commonly reported that facing the prospect of death changes one's perspective – we would say, one's spiritual perspective. The process of coming to terms with the fact that one has a life-threatening disease, the chemotherapy which saps one's life in the process of pursuing a cure, the loss of energy, all contribute to a sense of impairment, emotional and physical pain and, for many, a sense of anomie. Once the anomie has been addressed, where the person decides to accept the outcome whatever it will be, then a substantial shift in quality of life also seems to occur. Many old wants, needs and concerns are no longer relevant. The perspective has shifted. Life itself, including its frustrations, becomes much more valued. The person's 'spiritual perspective' has become the shaper of the person's quality of life.

The same may be said of other individuals who have chosen to commit themselves to a life of service in the religious-spiritual sense. For them, quality of life in the ordinary sense becomes almost irrelevant. Does quality of life make sense for a Mother Theresa who is committed to living with the poor of Calcutta? Judgements based on the values of a typical person from a high-income country might well lead to a conclusion that her quality of life was poor but the judgement from her perspective might well be that it was incredibly rich.

The mystery of this tension appears in a story told by Jean Vanier.

> A man came to see me when I was Director of the L'Arche community. He was a man with many problems: family problems, work problems and philosophical problems. ... I suppose he was normal. ... While he was sharing his sadness with me there was a knock on the door and before I could answer it, Jean Claude was in my office and laughing. Some people call Jean Claude mongoloid or Down syndrome but we just call him Jean Claude. ... He likes to come to my office and shake my hand. And that is what he did. He shook my hand and laughed. Then he shook the hand of Mr Normal and laughed and he walked out laughing. Mr Normal looked at me and said, 'Isn't it sad that there are children like that'.
>
> The great pain in all of this was that this man was totally blind. He had barriers inside of him and was unable to see that Jean Claude was happy.

(Vanier, 1991, pp94–5)

REFERENCES

Ajuwon, P. (1993) *A study on quality of Life Issues: Adults with Visual Impairment in the Nigerian Population.* PhD thesis, University of Calgary, Calgary.

Allier, H. (1982) A place of human growth, in *The Challenge of L'Arche* (ed., Jean Vanier), Darton, Longman & Todd, London.

Bach, E. (1981) *Partners in the Family of God*, World Council of Churches, Geneva.

Bibby, R. (1995) *There's Got to Be More: Connecting Churches to Canadians*, Wood Lake Books, Toronto.

Brown, R.I., Bayer, M. and MacFarlane, C. (1989) *Rehabilitation Programmes: Performance and Quality of Life of Adults with Developmental Handicaps*, Lugus, Toronto.

Canda, E. (1988) Spirituality, religious diversity, and social work practice. *Social Casework*, **69**, 238–47.

Clarke, B. (1974) *Enough Room for Joy. Jean Vanier's L'Arche: A Message for Our Time*, Darton, Longman & Todd, London.

Cox, H. (1994) *Fire from Heaven – The Rise of Pentecostal Spirituality and the Reshaping of Religion in the Twenty-First Century*, Addison Wesley, Reading, MA.

Devestel, F. (1982) *A Pastoral Approach to Mentally Handicapped Adults Living in an Institutional Setting.* Unpublished doctoral thesis, Salesian Pontifical University, Rome.

Driedger, D. and Gray, S. (1990) *Imprinting Our Image: An International Anthology by Women with Disabilities*, Gynergy Books, Charlottetown, PEI.

Dunne, J. (1986) Sense of community in L'Arche and in the writings of Jean Vanier. *Journal of Community Psychology*, **14**, 41–54.

Funk & Wagnalls *Canadian College Dictionary* (1986) Fitzhenry & Whiteside, Toronto.

Gartner, G.J., Larson D.B. and Allen, G.D. (1991) Religious commitment and mental health: a review of the empirical literature. *Journal of Psychology and Theology*, **19**, 6–25.

Gaventa, W.C. (1986) Religious ministries and services with adults with developmental disabilities, in *The Right to Grow Up: An Introduction to Adults with Developmental Disabilities*, (ed. J.A. Summers), Brookes, Baltimore.

Gaylord, R. (1974) Village Communities for the Handicapped, Polytechnic, Handicapped Persons Research Unit, Newcastle-upon-Tyne.

Gold, R.A. (1981) Judaism and persons with handicaps. *Documencap*, **15**, 9.

Gottlieb, B.H. (1983) *Social Support Strategies: Guidelines for Mental Health Practice*, Sage Publications, Beverly Hills, CA.

Hostetler, J.A. (1974) *Hutterite Society*, Johns Hopkins University Press, Baltimore.

Janzen, W. (1990) *Limits on Liberty: The Experience of Mennonite, Hutterite and Doukhobor Communities in Canada*, University of Toronto Press, Toronto.

Kelly, B. and McGinley, P. (1990) The church: the incompleat angler, in *Mental Handicap: Challenge to the Church*, (eds B. Kelly and P. McGinley), Lisieux Hall, Chorley, Lancs.

Kregel, J., Wehman, P., Seyfarth, J. and Marshall, K. (1986) Community integration of young adults with mental retardation: transition from school to adulthood. *Education and Training in Mental Retardation*, **21**, 35–42.

Lavigne, M. and Morin, J.P. (1991) *Leisure and Lifestyles of Persons with Disabilities in Canada.* Special Topic Series: The Health Activity Limitation Survey (Catalogue 82–615) Statistics Canada, Ottawa.

McGinley, P. (1988) Religion and rehabilitation: a particular challenge for Christianity, in *Quality of Life for Handicapped People*, (ed. R. I. Brown), Croom Helm, London.

Meyer, J. (1986) The religious education of persons with mental retardation. *Religious Education*, **81**, 134–9.

Mosteller, S. (1982) Living with, in *The Challenge of L'Arche*, (ed. Jean Vanier). Darton, Longman & Todd, London.

Myles, L. (1981) Some historical notes on religions, ideologies and the handicapped. *Al-Mushir (The Counsellor)*, **23**, 125–34.

Neufeld, V.H. (ed.) (1983) *If We Can Love: The Mennonite Mental Health Story*, Faith and Life Press, Newton, KS.

Neufeldt, A.H. (1991) *Supportive Care in the Congregation.* Paper presented at 'Connections and Commitment: Supporting Friends and Neighbours', a conference sponsored by the Justice Institute of British Columbia, Richmond, BC, October 3–5.

Neufeldt, A.H. and Luke, D. (1985) The history we live, in *Celebrating Differences*, (ed. A.H. Neufeldt), Faith and Life Press, Newton, KS.

Neufeldt, A.H. and Breau, Z. (1991) *Spirituality and Personal Support*. Paper presented at 'Connections and Commitment: Supporting Friends and Neighbours', a conference sponsored by the Justice Institute of British Columbia, Richmond, BC, October 3–5.

Neufeldt, A.H. and Mathieson, R. (1995) Empirical dimensions of discrimination against disabled people. *Health and Human Rights*, **1**, (2), 174–89.

Nouwen, H. (1986) *Lifesigns*, Doubleday, New York.

Penfield, W. (1975) *The Mystery of the Mind*, Princeton University Press, Princeton.

Philippe, T. (1982) Communities of the beatitudes, in *The Challenge of L'Arche*, (ed. Jean Vanier). Darton, Longman & Todd, London.

Preheim-Bartel, D.A. and Neufeldt, A.H. (1986) *Supportive Care in the Congregation*, Mennonite Central Committee, Akron, PA.

Putnam, J.W., Pueschal, S.M. and Holman, J.G. (1988) Community activities of youths and adults with Down syndrome. *British Journal of Subnormality*, **34**, 47–53.

Reichgeldt, G.J. (1957) *The Brothers of Charity 1: 1807–1880*, Brothers of Charity Central Administration, Rome.

Riordan, J. and Vasa, S.F. (1991) Accommodations for and participation of persons with disabilities in religious practice. *Education and Training in Mental Retardation*, **26**, 151–5.

Sadler, C. (1982) Rhythms of life, in *The Challenge of L'Arche*, (ed. Jean Vanier). Darton, Longman & Todd, London.

Scuccimara, D.J. and Speece, D.L. (1990) Employment outcomes and social integration of students with mild handicaps: the quality of life two years after high school. *Journal of Learning Disabilities*, **23**, 213–19.

Stolovitsky, G. (1992) *Inclusion of Adults with Disabilities in Faith Communities*. MSc thesis, University of Calgary, Calgary.

Stubblefield, H.W. (1975) The ministry and mental retardation, in *Community Services for Retarded Children: The Consumer Provider Relationship*, (ed. J.J. Dempsey), University Park Press, Baltimore.

Taylor, S. (1994) In support of research on quality of life, but against QOL, in *Quality of Life for Persons with Disabilities*, (ed. D. Goode), Brookline Books, MA.

Vanier, J. (1979) *Community and Growth*, Darton, Longman & Todd, London.

Vanier, J. (1982a) Introduction, in *The Challenge of L'Arche*. Darton, Longman & Todd, London.

Vanier, J. (1982b) A struggle for unity, in *The Challenge of L'Arche*. Darton, Longman & Todd, London.

Vanier, J. (1991) *Images of Love, Words of Hope*, Lancelot Press, Hantsport, NS.

Webb-Mitchell, B. (1986) A place for persons with disabilities of the mind and body. *Religious Education*, **81**, 522–43.

Webb-Mitchell, B. (1988) The place and power of acceptance in pastoral care with persons who are mentally retarded. *Journal of Pastoral Care*, **42**, 351–60.

Wilhite, B., Reilly, L.J. and Teaff, J.D. (1989) Recreation and leisure services and residential alternatives for persons with developmental disabilities. *Education and Training in Mental Retardation*, **24**, 333–40.

Wilke, H.H. (1980) *Creating the Caring Congregation: Guidelines for Ministering with the Handicapped*, Abingdon Press, Nashville, TN.

Wilson, D. (1975) The church, the Eucharist and the mentally handicapped. *Clergy Review*, **60**, 69–84.

Wolfensberger, W. (1980) Elemente der identität und perversionen des christlichen wohlfahrtswesens. *Diakonie*, **6**, 156–67.

Quality of life and professional education 15

Roy I Brown

INTRODUCTION

Development of quality of life models, particularly over the past decade, has opened up the prospect of advances in professional education. If it is accepted that quality of life is based on some common consensus of concepts and components, then it is pertinent to ask to what extent such principles should modify the education of personnel working within the disability field. If it is correct that quality of life models open up a new window on disabilities and enable us to perceive them from a different perspective (Brown, 1996; Taylor, 1994), then it seems reasonable to ask whether such approaches are utilized within the various service systems, to what extent staff are knowledgeable about quality of life and the degree to which this knowledge is reflected in students' initial and later professional in-service education.

ISSUES RAISED BY QUALITY OF LIFE

Other chapters in this book suggest there is little doubt that there are some commonly held views about the nature of quality of life. There has been some criticism of quality of life, in terms of the dangers it may pose in the hands of service and political systems (Wolfensberger, 1994). It has been suggested that the conceptualization of quality of life may be vague and therefore of limited scientific value (Taylor, 1994). There are those who believe that the broad conceptualization and the development of an increasingly common framework give rise to new perceptions about needs and concerns amongst persons with disabilities. The quality of life commonalities include aspects of consumers' satisfaction with their lives and well-being (material, physical, social, productive and emotional – see Chapter 4) and the notion of choice by consumers, including choice of activity, place of activity and who is involved in that activity, including the professional (Brown, 1996). The prevailing blue-prints of quality of life also take into account the fact that quality of life is holistic and involves every aspect of an individual's lifestyle. Finally, and probably most critically, most sociological, educational and psycho-logical contributors see quality of life as consumer based, unlike some approaches to quality of life in the health field (Day & Jankey, 1996; Kaplan, 1994; Parmenter, 1994), and argue that quality of life relates to perceptions held by the consumer who is receiving the service. In other words, personal perceptions (often referred to as subjective measures) are seen as a critical component of evaluation.

There are still concerns in terms of how and what to evaluate in quality of life but as Cummins (see Chapter 7) indicates, there is now a wide range of assessment devices for exploring quality of life. For those con-sumers who are more disabled and may not have verbal skills, it has been suggested (Ouellette-Kuntz & McCreary, 1996) that advocates and per-sons close to the individual consumer can express these views on the individual's behalf. However, Brown, Bayer & Brown (1992) and others have indicated that non-verbal assessment techniques need to be developed as the consumer's perceptions, in many instances, appear to differ from those of the advocate, parent or spouse. It is also recognized that quality of life is tied very closely to individual self-image and promotion of that self-image is likely to be associated with bringing about a higher quality of life from the individual's point of view. This is also likely to promote greater critical appraisal of experience (Brown, 1996), thus requiring further modification to lifestyle and therefore well-being. It is this challenging development, which occurs through applied quality of life models, which is frequently overlooked both by front-line personnel and managers.

All of the above examples provide reasons why personnel need to be aware of quality of life issues, which should be represented in the educa-tion of personnel. If quality of life-oriented services are to be provided, it is essential that practitioners are able to utilize relevant research knowledge in developing such services. While recognizing that questions of measure-ment and application remain, I believe practical experience (e.g. Brown, Bayer & Brown, 1992; Brown, Brown & Bayer 1994) demonstrates that many of the concepts, when carefully applied, work to the advantage of both consumers and their families as well as the professionals.

Quality of life models also have implications for funding, management and policy directives. It seems inappropriate to write about the education of personnel unless these additional aspects are borne in mind. But theoretical aspects of quality of life should be taught within the context of what has occurred historically in terms of intervention, with modelling of quality of life practice as a key component. For example, although there is a growing understanding that consumers should be encouraged to make choices within the context of appropriate structure, this frequently does not seem to be viewed as practical at policy level. The language of quality of life may be applied, but the changes involved in quality of life models are denied. It is the interaction, for example, between choice and structure which promotes the need for extremely effective counselling skills by front-line staff and, when choices are seen as behaviourally necessary, they require a flexibility in service delivery that is different from that which is frequently observed.

There is a very real danger in the field of disabilities that much social, psychological and educational practice becomes trapped in the latest fashion. Parents, consumers and even service providers wish to be seen at the socially acceptable cutting edge of involvement. There is a tendency to move away from previously held knowledge and experience. The rejection of medical and psychosocial models, a rigid and non-critical acceptance of normalization practices by some advocates and services and the adoption of the social construction of disability as the only explanatory model do a disservice to consumers and deny the relevance of each of these approaches. Likewise, an uncritical acceptance of quality of life models would be more than unfortunate. For example, although consumer choice is a key component of such models, it should not be seen as an isolated process but within the context of the individual's development and with their involvement. It is assumed that training practices, with their necessary structures, are available to the individual in order to promote progress. It is argued elsewhere that choice and other dimensions of quality of life require the consumer to be the primary setter of goals (Brown, Bayer & Brown, 1992) and the trainer or practitioner to give structure through counselling, intervention design and procedure, along with modifications to the environment. This suggests that, in addition to the broad base of environmental and technical innovations and behavioural, social and educational knowledge, any student of disabilities must also be a sound negotiator and have a wealth of experience in terms of psychology and social intervention.

CHALLENGES FOR THE FRONT-LINE PRACTITIONER

For ease of discussion, much of the following material relates particularly to the front-line practitioner and is consistent with the arguments of Brown, Bayer & Brown (1992) that the front-line practitioner should be seen as the most knowledgeable member of the team in terms of working with the consumer. This person is the major processor of the consumer's choices and may be a community professional or keyworker, a field practitioner, teacher, social worker or counsellor. Consistent with most counselling models, the quality of life process requires that the individual practitioner has insight into their own behaviour and, in particular, is aware of how their own philosophy of life and goals may affect the consumer. There are other general needs. The practitioner requires an understanding of quality of life terminology. However, it is not just an issue of terminology but a perceptual knowledge of issues from the consumer's perspective about needs and life experience. This affects the way the practitioner describes disability issues. It is also important that the practitioner has an understanding of the knowledge base for quality of life models, not only in historical terms but in relation to research methodology. The relevance of narrative, ethnographic and phenomenological studies and how they interface with quasi-experimental methodology is obvious.

PERSONALITY, VALUES AND CHOICE

It is obvious that certain personnel function well with particular types of consumers. If there is functional similarity between the outlook and approach of the practitioner and the needs and goals of the consumer, then a good match is more likely. But where philosophy and goals differ, then difficulties in terms of behaviour and therefore progress may well arise. For example, consider the consumer who wants to be employed in the community but shows aggressive or other antisocial behaviour in school or workshop. Personnel may reject the consumer's wishes until behaviour is modified. In so doing they are likely to promote, rather than reduce, aggressive behaviour. Acceptance of the individual's wishes is of primary importance. Within current quality of life models Brown (1996) argues that there is dignity in accepting the consumer's goals, thereby laying the groundwork for improved self-image. This does not mean that the goal will necessarily be attained, nor that there will necessarily be a direct route to the goal but, having accepted it, discussion, counselling and demonstration can take place in terms of how to achieve that particular goal. This may mean, in some instances, the subjugation of the practitioner's own philosophy and their own wishes or perceptions to those of the individual consumer. The implications for those working in the field of disability are considerable, for so many of the issues are concerned with behavioural and social adaptation and the personal views of practitioners can interfere with the development of the individual client. Views held by personnel about what is conforming behaviour, what is appropriate behaviour and what is desirable behaviour may not be held by the consumer, either because they come from a different background or because the individual conceptualizes differently as a result of their abilities and experiences.

> John, a railway worker, lost his legs in a railway accident. He stayed in hospital for many weeks, but there came a time when he was told that he had recovered physically as far as possible and should now begin to think of seeking new employment in a sedentary job. John was outraged, indicating that he had no interest in work, for he had not simply lost his legs but during his hospitalization, his wife and two children had left. John wished to deal with emotional and family issues before dealing with employment yet this was not permitted.

In this instance the rehabilitation policy as practised was at variance with the individual's choices and needs. Practices for adult rehabilitation are often employment orientated, yet there is increasing evidence that many consumers wish to deal with other personal issues first. Quality of life models argue that the consumer's view must be recognized and accepted, but this is often not the view of many government departments in terms of the policies relating to funding or consumer management. To disregard the concerns of the consumer is discriminatory and is based on a long-held view that professionals and managers know what is best for the consumer (Barnes, 1991). It must be recognized that, in the field of disability, individuals are frequently not provided with choices but rather are controlled so that (in the view of service systems) they do not make errors. They are removed from the opportunities, experiences and diversified environments enjoyed by persons without disabilities.

A further aspect, frequently unrecognized and under-researched, relates to personality profiles and attitudes of individual personnel. Again, it seems probable that such attributes are critical in determining the consumer–personnel match – an important issue at the front line. Issues around personal flexibility and values held by personnel have already been noted. As early as 1971 Grant noted that a practitioner's need to care for people could override the consumer's need to explore. Personal power issues associated with the practitioner are also relevant and need to be understood by the practitioner. It is apparent that judgement and flexibility are important attributes for personnel and the question arises of how personnel with such attributes can be selected or how skills relevant to their development can be taught. In this context the beliefs, values and attitudes of personnel seem important (Braithwaite & Scott, 1991). Such constructs not only underline the importance of studying issues such as gender and multiculturalism, but also the need for each individual to recognize their own values regarding such matters. It is not simply knowledge about issues such as sexual interests and preferences or religious or cultural practices which is important, but the development of attitudes that enable practitioners to maintain their own

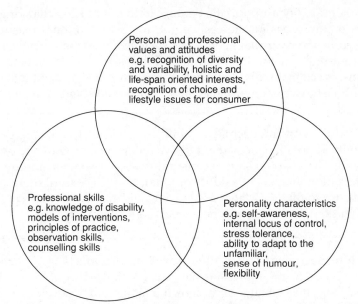

Personal and professional values and attitudes e.g. recognition of diversity and variability, holistic and life-span oriented interests, recognition of choice and lifestyle issues for consumer

Professional skills e.g. knowledge of disability, models of interventions, principles of practice, observation skills, counselling skills

Personality characteristics e.g. self-awareness, internal locus of control, stress tolerance, ability to adapt to the unfamiliar, sense of humour, flexibility

Fig. 15.1 Personal aspects of personal characteristics within professional education.

value systems while recognizing the importance of consumers' beliefs and needs. Indeed, learning how to recognize and accept the choices of others and helping them to fulfil important and socially accepted needs despite differing personal preference requires maturity, experience and judgement. It also means recognizing when one should no longer be the practitioner of choice for a particular consumer! Some of these issues are shown in Figure 15.1. They represent areas which should be explored by prospective practitioners.

THE CHOICE – MANAGEMENT GAP

The practitioner is frequently seen as a manager. They may become practically involved in various activities of the individual and arrange for others to become involved as 'need' arises, so that the individual is provided with opportunities and experience. But why should the individual necessarily succeed under such circumstances? We do not have a policy of deciding what subjects university students should study or what homes or clothes people should buy. Why, then, should we dictate the goals of people with disabilities? When so directed, the individual probably has a high chance of failure, with the result that administrators believe that the individual cannot be successful. Brown, Bayer & Brown (1992) documented the fact that many personnel not only see the individual as unable to attain certain goals, but argue that the choices made by consumers are not appropriate, because individuals keep changing their minds or the types of choices cannot, for organizational reasons, be accepted by the particular agency or management system. It is the role of the front-line practitioner, supported by appropriate management systems, to see that individual choices are recognized and put into effect. No administrative or environmental barrier should stand in the way!

An adult with intellectual disability wished to live in the community. If possible, he wanted to live on his own or with one other friend. The hospital staff accepted this was reasonable and desirable, but management said it could not take place until there was someone to fill the vacancy his move would create. The reason? The institution would lose the client's per diem allowance.

Such management policy, often based on the effects of government funding mechanisms, represents the denial of the quality of life model. In this example, it is a matter of recognizing higher order priorities, because the quality of life model maintains that the individual's wishes should predominate. At one level we can argue that this is so obvious it should not require a sophisticated and detailed model yet individuals working in service systems, generally with the best of intentions, are often unable to recognize such concepts unless they are entrenched within a model.

LEVELS OF CHOICE

It is often assumed that the right to choose is always related to major decisions. Frequently, however, choices are about minor issues which may have major consequences for the individual.

For five years Joan, who was severely multiply handicapped, had been sent on a daily basis to a training centre. At 11am she was given a glass of orange juice. A consultant espousing a quality of life model encouraged staff to introduce choices into daily living. In this instance a choice of drinks was substituted for the single glass of orange juice. The client, who had no language, was able to indicate her desire to experiment with different drinks.

Personnel often question whether it is ethical practice to meet all choices. My experience is that few people make very inappropriate or dangerous choices; this is an anxiety expressed by staff who have not worked with a 'choices' model. Traditional rehabilitation practice is replete with examples of the lack of choices. As a result individuals frequently do not make gains nor, according to their own perception, see themselves as developing (Brown, Bayer & Brown, 1992). Yet allowing the individual to work towards the selected choices often brings about considerable progress.

> Jennifer wished to learn to read. This was not thought to be possible or desirable. She was 28 years old and had failed to read when instruction had been given in the past. It was thought that social knowledge, e.g. getting around the city, would be more useful. Personnel, using a quality of life model, now argued that her choice should be honoured. Therefore, a teacher was found who was acceptable to the client. The individual made several years of reading progress over a number of months.

Individuals need to be ready to make progress and to have reached a point where they believe it is necessary to try. As they wish to succeed so changes in behaviour often occur. It is true that when individuals are encouraged to work on specific goals of their choice they may, from time to time, change their minds. Indeed, this may be a natural and adaptive process as individuals find it frustrating or impossible to modify their behaviour or learn sufficiently rapidly to satisfy their needs. Under such circumstances they may deviate from their selected goals. It is also critical to understand that progress towards goals set by the individual is likely to bring about attainment of other goals down the line. For example, there is sufficient evidence to suggest that individuals who set themselves leisure time goals or home and personal adaptation goals and attain them may then turn to employment at which they are then successful. That is, persons who have effective leisure skills are more likely to gain and maintain satisfactory employment.

The above examples, which are in no way exceptional, require changes in policy as well as changes in staff sensitivity, observation skill and flexibility. Indeed, the examples also implicitly describe consumer intra-individual variability, with the need to recognize readiness to take on challenges.

THE EDUCATION OF PERSONNEL

Given our developing knowledge in the quality of life field, it is possible to list practical skills which would be expected of professional practitioners working within a quality of life model. Some of these skills have been associated with rehabilitation and disability studies for a considerable period of time and new characteristics become relevant, particularly when personnel function in community environments. The changes result from the delineation of quality of life. The fact that the characteristics are developments rather than totally new requirements lends support to the idea that quality of life is not a totally new process but an addition to or refinement of previous experience and practice.

In quality of life models, many personnel spend much of their professional time in the client's family house or local community. Personnel may therefore be professionally isolated from colleagues. They are largely unsupervised and not part of a traditional hierarchy. Under such circumstances they need to be not only highly motivated but also able to work in isolation, using their skills to promote independence and adaptive skills. Under such circumstances personnel have additional needs. Brown, Bayer & Brown (1992) reported high levels of personnel stress. Individuals now see life from the consumer's, not the agency's, viewpoint. This necessitates observation of interaction amongst family members, along with skills to explain and mediate client needs, not all of which may be understood or supported by family members. Yet it is important that family are, wherever possible, supportive. Issues are raised about when and how to support the client, how to help them find a passage to the goal they have chosen. There is a need to counsel around challenges and difficulties and to assist parties to gain insight and modify goals or perceptions – all without abusing the client's currently held views. At times personnel will be depressed and angry with situations and still tact is required! Much of the above relates to clinical judgement and the ability to recognize one's own role. To do all this effectively means that stress counselling must be available to personnel. The need is even more apparent where there are concerns over abuse of the client. Writers such as Sobsey (1994) underscore the reality and extent of sexual abuse amongst persons with disabilities. For many, this results in the need for some trauma therapy over a considerable period of time (Nagler, 1996). This not only underlines the importance of trauma and stress counselling skills amongst practitioners, but also their own need for the resources of counselling for debriefing and grief-related concerns.

The following comments are derived from a variety of studies in the quality of life area and reflect the commentary of consumers concerning their requirements of practitioners. The work owes much to the author's practical experience reported in the quality of life study by Brown, Bayer & Brown (1992) and Brown, Bayer & MacFarlane (1989). Some of the characteristics, as previously noted, are associated with the predisposition of personnel rather than simply training expertise, but it is argued that the skilled front-line practitioner cannot simply take up this work and needs a considerable period of learning and practice through detailed education and supervision.

Experience suggests that in many practical placements students are taught in traditional and formal systems. Here it is argued that innovative programmes, where consumer choices are offered, should constitute the initial experience of students. Traditional experience is likely to teach traditional skills. Colleges and universities often find it difficult to negotiate such innovative placements, so an attempt should be made to run joint projects between flexible, exploratory services and university programmes. Alternatively, university and college programmes should develop demonstration models. In both cases, college and university personnel should be expected to demonstrate practice within a quality of life format, not simply teach in a classroom or place students initially in traditional services which model different practices.

It is expected that the rehabilitation practitioner will function within the holistic framework of a quality of life model. This means that personnel need to be comfortable working in the consumer's environment of choice. This implies that personnel are capable of supporting individuals in a variety of circumstances, whether in the home environment with other members of the family present, in employment or in the local community, dealing with social and leisure requirements. Students need to experience as well as learn. They need to have opportunities to work with consumers through a range of activities such as preparing meals, helping the person get ready for work or assisting the individual at work. This will include supporting individuals at different times of the day in leisure, recreation and community programmes, as well as a range of household tasks. The hours of involvement are set by client need, not by some inflexible management agreement. The same issues arise in relation to teaching and counselling. Here again, traditional models assume professional functions take place in professional buildings but quality of life models require changes in this formula. As seen elsewhere (Chapter 9), the issue of inclusion in education is not simply a matter of exposure to the right classroom. Within a quality of life model it means dynamic changes to a wide range of practices within school, home and community. For example, current models of teacher education do not as a general rule explore the implications of this for educational practice.

However, learning is a cyclical, not a continuous process. Individual clients who have dispensed with support from their fieldworker may later require the support to be renewed, because of stresses and strains within their environment or as a result of personal factors such as deteriorating health. Such changes require vigilance and flexibility on the part of personnel, but they also require changes in management policy. For example, it is more cost effective to supply support when needed rather than place an individual on a waiting list, which may result in greater deterioration and greater costs to the system.

Ward (1989) and others have noted that persons with disabilities often have difficulty in transferring knowledge from agency to community. Brown, Bayer & Brown (1992) suggest this is an expected phenomenon when artificial environments are employed. On the other hand, these authors recorded large improvements in learning and adaptive behaviour, along with generalization, when environments appropriate to the activity were employed. They argued this was due to improved self-image.

Considerable judgement is required of front-line personnel as they take into account the expressed needs of the consumer, but they also need sound knowledge about various aspects of rehabilitation. They require keen observation skills, should possess a sound knowledge of learning practices and have an ability to design interventions. They are the choosers of techniques, not the selectors of goals. It is important that the practitioner knows about issues of gender and recognizes that many females with a disability have a double disadvantage. The challenges set, for example, by transition (e.g. school to employment) for females with disabilities are clearly described by Wagner (1992). Practitioners need to be aware that the complexity of interacting personal attributes, including handicaps, influences self-image. Practitioners need skills to help persons with disabilities overcome controls and barriers in society (Barnes, 1991). Thus it is reasonable to expect the front-line practitioner to have a wide practical experience of the effects of different types of disabilities and how they relate to handicaps. Social and psychological aspects of disabilities tend to be general – the levels of application may differ but the principles remain the same. There is some reason to suggest it is wise to train general practitioners, rather than practitioners for specific disabilities. We are dealing with consumer choices which transcend the boundaries set by levels. The impact of society interacting with disability, which can cause further handicap, means professionals must be sensitive to the wide range of discriminations that can occur (e.g. with the bank manager, in the social welfare office, before the courts, at the shop counter). In this context a front-line practitioner has to be an educator of society as well as an enabler of the individual. Much of this can be done through appropriate modelling based on an eclectic knowledge base.

Many consumers have limitations in verbal language. It is important that cues are picked up from body or facial language, particularly where there is aggressive intent or depressive withdrawal. People move from verbal signals to non-verbal signals in many situations. Counsellors and practitioners need to have a sense of humour, to share jokes with the consumer and to be able to provide a sense of fun. Yes, interventions are seen by consumers as fun yet Brown & Goldenberg (1993) were almost alone authorities for suggesting that fun was an important consideration! Fun and enjoyment are features of motivation.

Good humour and a sense of fun influence well-being and self-image and this is clearly recognized by consumers (Brown, 1993).

Friendship is another important aspect of rehabilitation. The literature (e.g. Firth & Rapley, 1990) identifies the lack or loss of friendship as an important issue. It is likely that friendships will first grow between the front-line practitioner and the consumer. The implications of this, in terms of bonding between the two and the professional and ethical issues which can arise, are highly relevant. The practitioner needs to encourage the development of other friendships which the individual consumers have chosen. Practitioners need to be knowledgeable about social networking both in terms of their own practice and in application to consumer needs.

SKILLS AND THE CONSUMER

The following is based on skills perceived as important by consumers (see Brown, Bayer & Brown, 1992). In order to understand and recognize ways in which support can be provided, the practitioner needs good listening skills. Consumers look to a practitioner to enable them to develop or increase their motivation so they can take action. Ways of doing this involve critical skills, not only in terms of utilizing learning and cognitive theories but also from the perspective of imagery and consciousness. Counselling consumers takes time and many feel they do not receive enough time from the practitioner. Quality of life studies underscore the role of self-image and have identified choice over environment, activity and interveners as major determinants for improving self-image. Enabling people to experience success and providing opportunities for success are critical aspects of performance. The medical model has guided us towards looking at impairment and disability. The social construction of disability (Barton, Ballard & Folcher, 1991; Oliver, 1990) and quality of life models of disability point to characteristics of handicap which interact with disability and suggest key environmental factors which make it more difficult for the individual to grow and adapt. Thus, there is a pervasive political and social orientation to disabilities which argues against change. The ability to observe and unravel such environment–person interactions is a critical role of the front-line practitioner. Again, it is necessary to recognize that what individuals feel about their situation is frequently more important than the objective diagnosis.

It is what the individual feels about themselves that is often critical for human development. As Andrews (1974) noted, people respond on the basis of what they perceive, not on objective facts alone. Perception by the client may therefore be a greater determinant of behaviour and development than simply the objective diagnosis made by professionals. This does not mean that diagnosis can be overlooked or physical interventions ignored, but the front-line practitioner must recognize that perceptual processes can be utilized to assist people gain control over their lives, with a resulting increase in self-image and motivation.

Anxieties, worries and grief are all identified in quality of life studies as characteristics which the front-line practitioner be able to recognize and ameliorate. Therefore skills in counselling and emotional support in the area are critical. I am describing the 'walking counsellor' – a person who does not have a clinic but is ready to provide support and help in the individual's own community. Consumers very often confront or raise their problems when they are in situations which trigger verbal responses or other behaviour related to those difficulties. It is then that intervention can be most effective. Thus the front-line practitioner needs to be in the situation when such reactions arise.

Personal practice and behaviour, as pointed out implicitly or explicitly, are critical (Chambers, Wedel & Rodwell, 1992; Schalock, 1995). Honesty and straightforwardness, ethical and professional practice skills are more than relevant, but so are other characteristics (Brown, 1993). For example, many consumers feel that the voice skills of practitioners are poor and complain that practitioners often sound boring or uninterested in what they are doing. Such 'monotonous behaviour' is perceived by the client as a negative which leads to reinforcement of the client's poor image and decreases motivation. Front-line practitioners should use gender-appropriate and culture-sensitive language, along with appropriate body language to suit the occasion.

THE FAMILY AND THE PRACTITIONER

Quite frequently family members also have difficulties in allowing a person to develop and grow. They, too, have concerns over care and protection. These are issues where counselling is required. Help and support can be provided so that the individual is enabled to grow, while ensuring that any necessary protection or support is in place. Many traditional practitioners and families still supply only care and support to consumers and in so doing reduce opportunities for the client to take action. It should be recognized that in order to develop and grow the person with the disability also needs to share and give and do things for others (Lichty & hnson, 1992). This should be enabled within the rehabilitation process.

ality of life studies have stressed the need to develop self-image.
arents and other family members also cite the need to encourage
behaviour and the need to deal with emotional challenges.
s have not been dealt with effectively in most traditional
programmes. Indeed, the very nature of traditional pro-
decrease the opportunities to resolve these aspects of
of attitudes which support conformity, protection and

group treatment. Frequently, family members are concerned about autonomy over such issues as residence, employment, expressions of leisure interests, sexual preference, partnerships and marriage.

Front-line workers should be able to mediate between different members of the family. Where there are disparities between client and family perceptions of events (Brown, Bayer & Brown, 1992) the family is likely to be less supportive and helpful. It is the role of a front-line practitioner to clarify and reduce such discrepancies. Thus, the front-line practitioner is a translator and mediator, bringing about integration of feelings and enhancing the opportunities for effective rehabilitation. Skills in conflict resolution and stress management come into play.

MANAGEMENT AND EVALUATION

However, the above views alone ignore the needs of the family. Quality of life models stress the importance of environmental context. The relations between the various individuals are complementary. The practitioner, while recognizing the central focus of their role with the person who is disabled, also needs to take into account the effects of stress, loss and grief within the family and the impact these have on the client. Involvement may therefore include counselling the family to provide a more supportive framework for the individual. The practitioner may need to judge the degree to which they can personally do this and the extent to which other counselling supports are required.

As the individual grows and develops, specialized skills and resources will have to be tapped. Matching of clients to more advanced generic services, including colleges, universities and institutes, which not only provide academic programmes but opportunities for other rewarding activities such as drama, music and visual arts, will be required.

CONCLUSION

It is important to recognize that the process of rehabilitation, in the field of developmental or acquired disabilities, is predetermined to some degree by the previous experiences and personality of the individual. I have argued for the relevance of social constructs of disability along with basic changes in social attitudes towards disability. Quality of life models, which have received growing attention in the field of disabilities over recent years, are set within the context of a wide human network. In this context the application of quality of life models to the needs of children becomes relevant. Indeed, the emotional and social development of young children with or without disabilities leaves so much to be desired in Western culture. This in itself argues for the holistic education of personnel, not just in the education and health fields but throughout the administrative, political and economic system. In the same way as the work ethic of society and, more recently, economic rationalism have affected our communities, so now a more liberal and social message involving individualized values and choices needs to be portrayed. There are many who will argue that choices need to be related to society as a whole yet it is readily apparent, in examining the development of children and persons with disabilities, particularly in early learning stages and during times of stress and difficulty, that choices are frequently related to more concrete and personal constructs. It is only later that more altruistic choices may be developed.

However, there are challenges within the model. How do individuals make choices when they have not had an opportunity to experience a wide range of possibilities? The answer seems to lie in the openness of the individual's environment to opportunities for exploration. This needs to be developed in the context of effective and personal counselling by the individual who is chosen as a professional partner by the client. This can give rise to major problems for organizations and individual personnel. They are not used to being selected or rejected. They frequently function within a model which simply delivers a professional service to the individual. In a quality of life model, the selection should ideally be made by the consumer. This means the consumer must have the opportunity to get to know a number of potential front-line personnel, in order to make choices about whom they feel can work with them most effectively. There has been little exploration of this issue, though Fewster & Curtis (1989) indicate the importance of such an approach. Extensive research is now required to observe personal attitudes and values of personnel and the reasons for choices by consumers. Thumlert (1995) has argued persuasively for the exploration of these dynamic attributes within the context of a quality of life model. Indeed, our Western model of intervention and education, whether in generic or specialized systems, often assumes that exposure or teaching is sufficient. Consumers do not feel included when systems are designed and applied on their behalf. They respond when their actions and understanding are interwoven into the overall plan. Quality of life models deal with personal views, information and emotional content. They direct us to other attributes such as assertion and self-image. It then ~comes important to develop a more flexible, entrepreneurial system ~re these issues can be at the forefront of decision making. Today, emphasis is placed on the use of generic services. However, ~ this is important and generic personnel require education ~eeds of persons with disabilities, the front-line worker who is ~nd enabler of the individual with a disability is critical. ~essional education may be seen as a decisive component ~ork of quality of life constructs.

REFERENCES

Andrews, F.M. (1974) Social indicators of perceived life quality. *Social Indicators Research*, **1**, 279–99.

Barnes, C. (1991) *Disabled People in Britain and Discrimination: A Case for Anti-Discrimination Legislation*, Hurst, London and University of Calgary, Calgary.

Barton, L., Ballard, K. and Folcher, G. (1991) *Disability and the Necessity for a Socio-Political Perspective*, Monograph 51, University of New Hampshire, Durham.

Braithwaite, V.A. and Scott, W.A. (1991) Values, in *Measures of Personality and Social Psychological Attitudes*, (eds J.P. Robinson, P.R. Shauver and L. Wrightman), Academic Press, New York.

Brown, P.M. and Goldenberg, S. (1993) Change in self image: the impact of individualised intervention involving consumer choice. *Australia and New Zealand Journal of Developmental Disabilities*, **18**, 209–18.

Brown, R.I. (1993) Some challenges to counselling in the field of disabilities, in *Rehabilitation Counselling: Approaches in the Field of Disability*, (eds S. Robertson and R. Brown), Chapman & Hall, London.

Brown, R.I. (1996) People with developmental disabilities: applying quality of life to assessment and intervention, in *Quality of Life in Health Promotion and Rehabilitation: Conceptual Approaches, Issues and Applications*, (eds R. Renwick, I. Brown and M. Nagler), Sage, Thousand Oaks, CA.

Brown, R.I., Bayer, M. and MacFarlane, C. (1989) *Rehabilitation Programmes*, Lugus, Toronto.

Brown, R.I., Bayer, M.B. and Brown, P.M. (1992) *Empowerment and Developmental Handicaps: Choices and Quality of Life*, Chapman & Hall, London.

Brown, R.I., Brown, P.M. and Bayer, M.B. (1994) A quality of life model: new challenges arising from a six year study, in *Quality of Life for Persons with Disabilities: International Perspectives and Issues*, (ed. D. Goode), Brookline Books, Cambridge, MA.

Chambers, D.E., Wedel, K.R. and Rodwell, M.K. (1992) *Evaluating Social Programs*, Simon & Schuster, Massachusetts.

Day, H. and Jankey, S. (1996) Lessons from the literature: toward a holistic model of quality of life, in *Quality of Life in Health Promotion and Rehabilitation: Conceptual Approaches, Issues, and Applications*, (eds R. Renwick, I. Brown and M. Nagler), Sage, Thousand Oaks, CA.

Fewster, G. and Curtis, J. (1989) Creating options: designing a radical children's mental health program, in *Learning Difficulties and Emotional Problems*, (eds R. Brown and M. Chazan), Detselig, Calgary.

Firth, H. and Rapley, M. (1990) *From Acquaintance to Friendship: Issues for People with Learning Disabilities*, British Institute of Mental Handicap, Kidderminster.

Grant, W.B. (1971) *Some Management Problems of Providing Work for the Mentally Disordered with Particular Reference to Mental Handicap*. Unpublished MSc thesis, University of Manchester.

Kaplan, R.M. (1994) Using quality of life information to set priorities in health policy. *Social Indicators Research*, **33**, 121–63.

Lichty, J. and Johnson, P. (1992) Client intervention: one team's experience, in *Empowerment and Developmental Handicaps: Choices and Quality of Life*, (eds R.I. Brown, M.B. Bayer and P.M. Brown), York University, York.

Nagler, M. (1996) Qualify of life of people with disabilities who have experienced sexual abuse, in *Quality of Life in Health Promotion and Rehabilitation*, (eds R. Renwick, I. Brown and M. Nagler), Sage, Beverly Hills.

Oliver, M. (1990) *The Politics of Disablement*, Macmillan, London.

Oullette-Kuntz, H. and McCreary, B. (1996) Quality of life assessment for persons with severe development disabilities, in *Quality of Life in Health Promotion and Rehabilitation: Conceptual Approaches, Issues, and Applications*, (eds R. Renwick, I. Brown and M. Nagler), Sage, Thousand Oaks, CA.

Parmenter, T.R. (1994) Quality of life as a concept and measurable entity, in *Improving the Quality of Life*, (eds D.M. Romney, R.I. Brown and P.S. Fry), Kluwer, Boston.

Schalock, R.L. (1995) *Outcome-Based Evaluation*, Plenum, New York.

Sobsey, D. (1994) *Violence and Abuse in the Lives of People with Disabilities: The End of Silent Acceptance?* Brooks, Baltimore.

Taylor, S.J. (1994) In support of research on quality of life, but against QOL, in *Quality of Life for Persons with Disabilities: International Perspectives and Issues*, (ed. D. Goode), Brookline Books, Cambridge, MA.

Thumlert, I. (1995) *Attitudes, Values, and Beliefs of Personnel Serving Persons with Disabilities: A Research to Practice Challenge.* Unpublished PhD thesis, University of Victoria, Canada.

Wagner, H. (1992) *Being Female – a Secondary Disability? Gender Differences in the Transition Experience of Young People with Disabilities.* Special Education, Special Interest Group of the American Educational Research Association, Annual Meeting.

Ward, J. (1989) Obtaining generalization outcome in developmentally disabled persons: a review of the current methodologies, in *Learning Difficulties and Emotional Problems*, (eds R. Brown and M. Chazan), Detselig, Calgary.

Wolfensberger, W. (1994) Let's hang up 'quality of life' as a hopeless term, in *Quality of Life for Persons with Disabilities: International Perspectives and Issues*, (ed. D. Goode), Brookline Books, Cambridge, MA.

The concept of quality of life in 21st century disability programmes

16

Robert L Schalock

INTRODUCTION

The Spanish philosopher Ortega V. Gasset once stated that 'Human life is a constant preoccupation with the future'. In this chapter, I would like to suggest that we think about the nature and characteristics of 21st century programmes for persons with developmental disabilities.

Today, programmes for persons with developmental disabilities are undergoing significant changes related to both service delivery philosophy and services. Four major changes include:

1. a transformed vision of what constitutes the life possibilities for people with developmental disabilities. This vision includes an emphasis on strengths and capabilities, importance of normalized and typical environments, provision of age-appropriate services, development of individualized support systems, enhanced adaptive functioning and role status and increased empowerment (Luckasson *et al.*, 1992);
2. an interfacing of the concept of quality of life with quality enhancement, quality assurance, quality management and outcome-based evaluation (Albin, 1992; Schalock, 1994 a,b);
3. a focus on major life activity areas and functional limitations which become a 'disability' only as the person interacts with environmental demands (Institute of Medicine, 1991). Thus, the focus of (re)habilitation is to reduce a person's functional limitations and thereby reduce the associated 'disability';
4. a supports paradigm that is currently reflected in supported living and employment programmes (Bradley, Ashbaugh & Blaney, 1994) and person-centred planning (Smull & Danehey, 1994).

Not only are these major changes having significant impacts on service delivery philosophy and practices, but they are also providing the foundation for 21st century disability policy and programmes. The purpose of this chapter is to assist our thinking of what those 21st century programmes might look like and what action will be required to get us there. The chapter is divided into two sections: the suggested characteristics of 21st century disability programmes and four action steps required to get there.

CHARACTERISTICS OF THE 21ST CENTURY DEVELOPMENTAL DISABILITY SYSTEM

My feeling is that four characteristics will drive 21st century developmental disability (DD) programmes. They include:

1. a changing conception of disability;
2. a focus on quality of life;
3. services based on supports;
4. the critical importance of valued, person-referenced outcomes.

THE CHANGING CONCEPTION OF DISABILITY

We are beginning to rethink the relationship among terms such as pathology, impairment, functional limitations and disability (Institute of

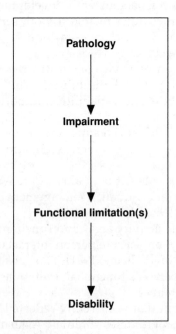

Fig. 16.1 The disabling process.

Medicine, 1991). This relationship is summarized in Figure 16.1. In this four-stage conceptualization of the disabling process, the 'pathology' is associated with an abnormality at the cellular or tissue level, such as tuberous sclerosis. The pathology then produces an 'impairment' at the organ or organ system, such as brain dysfunction. The brain dysfunction then produces a 'functional limitation' at the organism level, such as low intelligence. The functional limitation becomes a 'disability' only when it impacts or interferes with the person's social role.

This four-stage conceptualization of the disabling process has a number of implications for the field of developmental disabilities. Among the more important (Schalock, 1995a) are:

- disability is neither fixed nor dichotomized. Rather it is fluid, continuous, changing and an evolving set of characteristics depending upon the characteristics of and supports available within a person's environment;
- one lessens functional limitations (and hence a person's disability) by providing interventions or services and supports that focus on adaptive behaviours and role status.

The changing conception of disabilities also necessitates a number of significant changes in one's thinking and service provision. First, one cannot overlook the significant roles that environments and supports play in the manifestation of a disabling condition. Second, categories based on only one aspect of the person (for example, level of disability based primarily on intelligence level) are not sufficiently descriptive or predictive to characterize or fully describe persons with developmental disabilities. Third, the new emphasis on functioning requires a greater clarity in describing behaviour as suggested in the 1992 definition of mental retardation (Luckasson et al., 1992). And fourth, the focus of (re)habilitation programmes is to reduce the person's functional limitations and thereby reduce the 'disability'.

A FOCUS ON QUALITY OF LIFE

The current emphasis on the quality of life of persons with developmental disabilities is part of the larger social-cultural quality revolution (Schalock, 1995b). This book on quality of life for people with disabilities underscores the significant role that the concept of quality of life plays in current public policy, (re)habilitation programmes and research.

To me, quality of life can be defined quite simply: it is a person's desired conditions of living related primarily to home and community living, school or work and health and wellness. This concept is shown in Figure 16.2 that depicts the relationship between a person's perceived quality of life and their experiences with the three basic life domains of home and

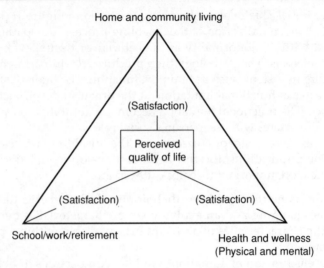

Fig. 16.2 Quality of life model (reproduced with permission from Schalock, 1995a).

community living, school or work and health and wellness. The model not only reflects my efforts over the last ten years to conceptualize, measure and apply the quality of life concept to persons with developmental disabilities, but also provides the basis later in the chapter for interfacing support intensities with person-referenced quality of life outcomes (see Fig. 16.5).

SERVICES BASED ON SUPPORTS

The concept of supports is integrally related to current service provision for persons with developmental disabilities as reflected in the popularity of supported living and employment programmes throughout the world. Supports can be defined (Schalock, 1995c) as resources and strategies that:

- enhance the functioning of individuals with or without disabilities;
- enable persons to access resources, information and relationships inherent within integrated school, work and community environments;
- result in an individual's enhanced independence/interdependence, productivity, community integration and satisfaction.

There are currently a number of ways to conceptualize the source of supports, along with their functions, intensities and desired outcomes (Bradley, Ashbaugh & Blaney, 1994; Kiernan, Schalock & Sailor, 1993; Luckasson *et al.*, 1992; Schalock, 1995c). A heuristic supports model is presented in Figure 16.3. As shown in Figure 16.3, support resources include the individual, other people, technology and/or services. Exemplary support functions include those eight listed, but they should

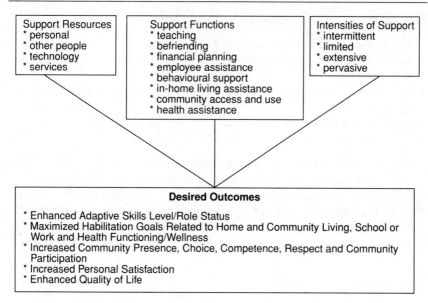

Support Resources	Support Functions	Intensities of Support
* personal	* teaching	* intermittent
* other people	* befriending	* limited
* technology	* financial planning	* extensive
* services	* employee assistance	* pervasive
	* behavioural support	
	* in-home living assistance	
	* community access and use	
	* health assistance	

Desired Outcomes

* Enhanced Adaptive Skills Level/Role Status
* Maximized Habilitation Goals Related to Home and Community Living, School or Work and Health Functioning/Wellness
* Increased Community Presence, Choice, Competence, Respect and Community Participation
* Increased Personal Satisfaction
* Enhanced Quality of Life

Fig. 16.3 Supports – outcome model.

not be considered exhaustive. The four intensities of support – intermittent, limited, extensive and pervasive – are explained in Table 16.1 (Luckasson *et al.*, 1992).

Table 16.1 Definition and examples of intensities of supports

Intermittent
Supports on an episodic 'as needed basis'. Characterized by episodic nature, person not always needing the support(s), or short-term supports needed during lifespan transitions (e.g. job loss or an acute medical crisis). Intermittent supports may be high or low intensity when provided.

Limited
An intensity of supports occurring on some dimensions on a regular basis for a short period of time of an intermittent nature. May require fewer staff members and less cost than more intense levels of support (e.g. time-limited employment training or transitional supports provided during the school to adult period).

Extensive
Supports characterized by ongoing, regular involvement (e.g. daily) in at least some environments (such as work or home) and not time-limited (e.g. long-term support and long-term home living support).

Pervasive
Supports characterized by their constancy and high intensity. Supports are provided in several environments and are potentially life sustaining in nature. Pervasive supports typically are more intensive and involve more staff members than do extensive or limited supports.

Desired outcomes from a supports model include:

- enhanced adaptive skills level and role status;
- maximized habilitation goals related to home and community living, school or work and health and wellness;
- increased community presence, choice, competence, respect and participation;
- increased personal satisfaction;
- enhanced quality of life.

Although the concept of needed supports is by no means new, what is new is the belief that the judicious application of appropriate supports can improve the functional capabilities of individuals with developmental disabilities. Hopefully, the supports outcome model presented in Figure 16.3 will facilitate the work needed in operationalizing and implementing a supports model for (re)habilitation services in the 21st century.

PERSON-REFERENCED OUTCOMES

The fourth characteristic of 21st century developmental disability services will undoubtedly stress the importance of valued, person-referenced outcomes. Throughout public law, human services and self-advocate groups, there is an increased emphasis on accountability and specific goals for persons with developmental disabilities. Figure 16.4 summarizes a simple

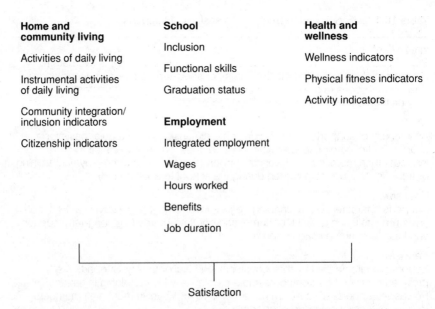

Fig. 16.4 Quality of life areas and valued person-referenced outcomes.

way to relate valued, person-referenced outcomes to the concept of quality of life and personal satisfaction.

In selecting valued, person-referenced outcomes, one needs to consider the following five criteria (Schalock, 1995a):

1. valued by the person in that the outcome reflects an enhanced skill level or role status in the community;
2. multidimensional in that outcomes need to be evaluated across a number of domains such as home and community living, school or work and health and wellness;
3. objective and measurable so that programme evaluation studies can be done. However, this criterion should not minimize the critical importance of the subjective nature of quality of life;
4. connected logically to the programme. Only when this criterion is met can meaningful programme evaluation be done;
5. evaluated longitudinally. This criterion is important since the immediate effects of (re)habilitation programmes or interventions are not always the same as those noted over time. Indeed, some intervention effects that appear to be effective in the short run do not show sustained effects and conversely, some that produce little or no effect immediately after intervention show significant effects sometime later. Additionally, an individual's role status changes slowly.

Thus, four characteristics of 21st century DD programmes – a changing conception of disability, a focus on quality of life, services based on the support needs of persons and valued, person-referenced outcomes – will both guide the delivery of services for persons with developmental disabilities and serve as the basis for the evaluation of those services. If this is true, then how might we bring about those changes in the service system so that our mission and goals are aligned with our services and desired outcomes? This requires a number of action steps, four of which are discussed in the next section. Each of these action steps represents a significant challenge to current thinking and practice.

ACTION STEPS TO GET US TO THE 21ST CENTURY

In a very few years, we will be into the 21st century. This reality, plus the current window of opportunity provided by the entrepreneurial spirit discussed shortly, is most exciting and challenging. This section of the chapter briefly discusses four action steps that are both realistic and potentially productive as we bring the current system into alignment with those four characteristics of the 21st century just discussed. These four action steps are:

1. begin with the end in mind;
2. operationalize supports;

3. restructure the service delivery system;
4. capitalize on the entrepreneurial spirit.

BEGIN WITH THE END IN MIND

Yogi Berra once said that 'The problem with not knowing where you are going is that you might end up somewhere else'. Steven Clovey, in his most successful book (Clovey, 1989) describing the seven habits of highly effective people, made the same point by stressing the need to begin with a clear notion of where you are going. As discussed earlier, there is no doubt in my mind that we are heading very fast into a quality of life-referenced outcome paradigm based on a supports model.

There is considerable evidence that one gets what one pays for and if outcomes are desired, they will be achieved. For example, as part of an ongoing project by the Institute for Community Inclusion in Boston, we have surveyed over 700 facilities regarding their day and employment programmes over a ten-year period (McGaughey *et al.*, 1994; Schalock, McGaughey & Kiernan, 1989). In our last survey (McGaughey *et al.*, 1994), among other data-based questions we asked two questions regarding the movement of persons into integrated work environments and factors that had contributed to the movement. The first question was, 'What factors contributed to your agency's expansion of integrated employment?'; the second, 'What incentives have been helpful in expanding integrated employment?'. Across facilities, the factors that contributed the most to the agency's expansion into integrated employment included:

- a philosophy that emphasizes integrated employment;
- state/federal funding policies;
- family requests.

Similarly, the incentives that were specified as the most helpful in expanding into integrated employment included:

- funding tied to a commitment to expand integrated employment;
- higher rates of funding provided for integrated employment;
- additional training and technical assistance for integrated employment;
- social security work incentives.

The implications of these results are clear: funding streams and advocacy play a critical role in obtaining desired person-referenced outcomes. Thus, the first action step requires that we are clear in establishing those programme models and funding streams that have the highest probability of producing the person-referenced outcomes that consumers, policymakers, funding agencies and (re)habilitation programmes are demanding.

Table 16.2 Variables to consider in developing measurable indicators of support intensities

Variable	Examples
Time	Duration of support Frequency of support Period of individual's life during which supports are needed Predictable schedule vs as needed
Location	Number of environments in which support is required Home vs out-of-home Isolated vs in the community
Resources	Number of people required to implement supports Specialities of personnel Costs
Intrusiveness	Consistency with principle of normalization Desirability of the support Purpose of the support

OPERATIONALIZE SUPPORTS

As we continue to move towards a supports model, two major tasks face us. First, we need to define support intensities better and second, we need to develop appropriate support standards that will be required increasingly for funding, licensure/accreditation and programme evaluation efforts.

Support intensities

Table 16.1 summarized four intensities of support that vary from intermittent to pervasive. Since support intensities vary across people, situations and life stages, one of the major challenges facing the developmentally disabled community over the next five years is to develop better quantitative measures of each of the four proposed support intensities. Four variables that need consideration in developing objective and measurable indicators of the intensity of support are summarized in Table 16.2.

In efforts to operationalize supports, it is very important to distinguish between support intensities, such as intermittent, limited, extensive and pervasive, and disability levels, such as mild, moderate, severe and profound. They are not the same and should not be equated for either convenience or administrative purposes. Supports are different from levels of disability in at least six ways (Schalock *et al.*, 1994):

1. The intensities of needed supports are based upon a person's strengths and limitations in the four dimensions of intellectual functioning and adaptive skills, psychological/emotional, physical and health and environment.

Table 16.3 Proposed support standards

1. Supports occur in regular, integrated environments.
2. Support activities are performed primarily by individuals normally working, living, educating or recreating within that environment.
3. Support activities are individualized and person referenced.
4. Supports are co-ordinated through someone such as a supports manager.
5. Outcomes from the use of supports are evaluated against quality indicators and person-referenced outcomes.
6. The use of supports can fluctuate during different stages of life.
7. Supports should not be withdrawn unless the service provider continues to monitor the person's current and future intensities of needed supports.

2. Support assessment involves many disciplines working as a team and analysing a variety of assessment findings.
3. Levels of needed supports are founded upon the strengths and limitations of the person and their environment, not simply upon an individual's intellectual limitations.
4. Levels of needed support are viewed as potentially changing and thus requiring reassessment, not as static descriptions of intellectual traits.
5. With an individual's support profile at any given time, there is likely to be a varied array of needed supports and intensities, making a global summary label meaningless.
6. Support predictions are simply not ability predictions.

Support standards

As the support model continues to direct developmental disability services in the 21st century, there will be an increasing need (and demand) for the development of support standards. An initial list of seven support standards is summarized in Table 16.3. As currently envisioned, these standards are consistent with both the four major changes in the current developmental disability service delivery system and the four projected 21st century characteristics.

RESTRUCTURE SERVICE DELIVERY SYSTEM

The concepts of supports, quality of life and valued, person-referenced outcomes are already resulting in significant changes to and restructuring of the developmental disability service delivery system. What might the restructuring look like in the 21st century, based on these three aspects? A simple answer is shown in Figure 16.5. This matrix is not meant to be exhaustive, but it does depict clearly the relationship between the different intensities of support reflective of the supports model (Fig. 16.3) and the desired person-referenced outcomes related to home and community living, school or work and health and wellness (Fig. 16.4).

Intensity of support	Quality of life area		
	Home and community living	**Employment**	**Health and wellness**
Intermittent	Banking/financial affairs Counselling/crisis management Transitioning Legal affairs	Advocating Job counselling Transitioning Trouble shooting	Medical appointments Wellness counselling Nutrition awareness

Limited	Community living training
	In-home assistance
	Shopping
	Transportation
	Behavioural support
		Job training
		Job accommodation
		Transportation
			Nutrition training and
			  assistance
			Medical alert devices
			Recreation and leisure
			Training and
			  opportunities
			Safety training

Extensive	Homemaker services Overnight Assistance/supervision Personal care assistance	Long-term assistance/support Transportation Supervision Prosthetics Job accommodation	Nutrition provided Meals on wheels Home health
Pervasive	24-hour care 24-hour supervision Respite care	High intensity Supervision Prosthetics Job accommodation	Nutrition provided Health care availability Health care assistance Attendant care

Outcomes →	Activities of daily living
	Instrumental activities of
	  daily living
	Community integration
	  indicators
	Citizenship indicators
		Wages
		Hours worked
		Benefits
		Level of integration
		Job duration
			Wellness indicators
			Physical fitness
			  indicators
			Activity indicators

Fig. 16.5 Service array based on intensity of support and quality of life outcomes.

The impact on the service delivery system of operationalizing and implementing such a service array is potentially revolutionary. It will require not only person-centred planning, but also unbundling services so that the service system makes effective use of community resources, is flexible and responsive and offers real choices with effective competition (Smull & Danehey, 1994). As stated so well by Gettings (1994, p169):

> The key to crossing this threshold and entering the new era is to restructure existing methods of organizing, delivering, and financing services so that the consumer becomes the hub, rather then the hubcap, of the service delivery process.

CAPITALIZE ON THE ENTREPRENEURIAL SPIRIT

One of the most popular books today is Osborne & Gaebler's (1993) *Reinventing Government: How the Entrepreneurial Spirit is Transforming the Public Sector*. In this text, the authors discuss the paradigm shift in government that is providing that previously mentioned 'window of opportunity'. Common threads that reflect this paradigm shift include:

- promoting competition between service providers;
- empowering citizens by pushing control out of the bureaucracy into the community;
- embracing participatory management;
- measuring outcomes;
- being driven by goals, not rules and regulations;
- redefining clients as customers and offering them choices;
- putting energy into making money, not just spending it;
- preferring market to bureaucratic mechanisms;
- galvanizing all sectors (public, private, voluntary) into action to solve problems.

If we are to capitalize on this entrepreneurial spirit, we need first to understand it and second to be part of it. Recently (Hisrich, 1990) a hybrid form of entrepreneur, referred to as an 'intrapreneur', has been described as one who exists in current organizations and is essential to systems change. Current work in this area has taken a person-environment approach that includes the climate for entrepreneurship and the characteristics of intrapreneurs. Lets look briefly at each.

Climate for entrepreneurship

The climate for entrepreneurship generally includes such things as: support for new ideas, experimentation is encouraged, available resources, multidiscipline work teams and task groups, and the reinforcement of intrapreneurship. From all indications, the current *zeitgeist* ('mood of the time') supports this climate.

Characteristics of entrepreneurs

Common characteristics include: understanding the environment, being visionary and flexible, creating management and service options, encouraging work teams, encouraging open discussion, building a coalition of supports and persisting. Thus, we each need to ask the question, 'Am I an intrapreneur, and can I use my intrapreneurial capabilities to help bring about those four changes to the 21st century developmental disability service delivery system discussed above?'

SUMMARY

In 1929 John Dewey suggested that 'Every great advance in science issued from a new audacity of the imagination'. Today, we are embarking on a great advance in how we view persons with developmental disabilities and how our service delivery systems need to change to reflect concepts such as vision, empowerment, equity, capability, supports and valued, person-referenced outcomes.

The challenges are both apparent and real. Apart from those characteristics of 21st century developmental disability programmes discussed in this chapter, the real challenge to future developmental disability programmes is to believe that the quality of life of persons with developmental disabilities can be enhanced. Once we believe that, we have the capability to make those changes in both programme philosophy and services that will truly revolutionize developmental disability services. Key action steps in that process include:

BEGIN WITH THE END IN MIND

- Establish programme models and funding streams that have a high probability of producing valued, person-referenced outcomes.
- Establish agreed quality of life areas such as: rights and dignity, individual control, community membership, relationships, personal growth and accomplishment and personal well-being.

OPERATIONALIZE THE SUPPORTS MODEL

- Develop quantitative measures of support levels.
- Develop support standards.

RESTRUCTURE THE SERVICE DELIVERY SYSTEM

- Implement a service delivery system built upon a matrix of major life activity areas and support intensities.
- Change the current system from a downstream, deficit model to an upstream, growth and development model.
- Base funding mechanisms on the support needs of the person.
- Measure valued, person-referenced outcomes.

CAPITALIZE ON THE ENTREPRENEURIAL SPIRIT

- Recognize the 'three Cs' of the 21st century: customer first, competition and change.
- Be intrapreneurs.

REFERENCES

Albin, J.M. (1992) *Quality Improvement in Employment and Other Human Services: Managing for Quality through Change*, Brookes, Baltimore.

Bradley, V.J., Ashbaugh, J.W. and Blaney, B.C. (1994) *Creating Individual Supports for People with Developmental Disabilities: A Mandate for Change at Many Levels*, Brookes, Baltimore.

Clovey, S.R. (1989) *The Seven Habits of Highly Effective People: Restoring the Character Ethics*, Simon & Schuster, New York.

Dewey, J. (1929) *The American City*, Macmillan, New York.

Gettings, R.M. (1994) The link between public financing and systemic change, in *Creating Individual Supports for People with Developmental Disabilities: A Mandate for Change at Many Levels*, (eds V.J. Bradley, J.W. Ashbaugh and B.C. Blaney), Brookes, Baltimore.

Hisrich, R.D. (1990) Entrepreneurship/intrapreneurship. *American Psychologist*, **45**, 209–22.

Institute of Medicine (1991) *Disability in America: Toward a National Agenda for Prevention*, National Academy Press, Washington DC.

Kiernan, W.E., Schalock, R.L. and Sailor, W. (1993) *Enhancing the Use of Natural Supports for People with Severe Disabilities*, Institute for Community Inclusion, Children's Hospital, Boston.

Luckasson, R., Coulter, D.L., Polloway, E.A. *et al.* (1992) *Mental Retardation: Definition, Classification and Systems of Supports*, American Association on Mental Retardation, Washington DC.

McGaughey, M.J., Kiernan, W.E., McNally, L.C., Gilmore, D.S. and Keith, G.R. (1994) *Beyond the Workshop: National Perspectives on Integrated Employment*, Institute for Community Inclusion, Children's Hospital, Boston.

Osborne, D. and Gaebler, T. (1993) *Reinventing Government: How the Entrepreneurial Spirit is Transforming the Public Sector*, Penguin Books, New York.

Schalock, R.L. (1994a) Promoting quality through quality enhancement techniques and outcome based evaluation. *Journal on Developmental Disabilities*, **3**, 1–16.

Schalock, R.L. (1994b) Quality of life, quality enhancement, and quality assurance: implications for programme planning and evaluation in the field of mental retardation and developmental disabilities. *Evaluation and Programme Planning*, **17**, 121–31.

Schalock, R.L. (1995a) *Outcome Based Evaluation*, Plenum, New York.

Schalock, R.L. (ed.) (1995b) *Quality of Life: Its Conceptualization, Measurement and Use*, American Association on Mental Retardation, Washington DC.

Schalock, R.L. (1995c) The assessment of natural supports in community rehabilitation services, in *Rehabilitation Services in the Community*, (eds O.C. Karan and S. Greenspan), Andover Medical, New York.

Schalock, R.L., McGaughey, M.J. and Kiernan, W.E. (1989) Placement into non-sheltered employment: findings from national employment surveys. *American Journal on Mental Retardation*, **94**, 80–7.

Schalock, R.L., Stark, J.A., Snell, M.E. *et al.* (1994) The changing conception of mental retardation: implications for the field. *Mental Retardation*, **32**, 181–93.

Smull, M.E. and Danehey, A.J. (1994) Increasing quality while reducing costs: the challenge of the 1990s, in *Creating Individual Supports for People with Developmental Disabilities: A Mandate for Change at Many Levels*, (eds V.J. Bradley, J.W. Ashbaugh and B.C. Blaney), Brookes, Baltimore.

Author Index

Subject Index